Problems of Normal and Genetically Abnormal Retinas

ACADEMIC PRESS INC. (LONDON) LTD.
24/28 Oval Road
London NW1

United States Edition Published by
ACADEMIC PRESS INC.
111 Fifth Avenue
New York, New York 10003

British Library Cataloguing in Publication Data
Problems of normal and genetically abnormal retinas.
1. Retina—Diseases—Congresses
I. Clayton, R.M.
617.7'3   RE551

ISBN 0-12-176180-0

Printed in Great Britain

CONTRIBUTORS

AGUIRRE, G. *School of Veterinary Medicine, University of Pennsylvania, Philadelphia, Pennsylvania 19104, USA.*

ANDERSON, R.E. *Cullen Eye Institute, Baylor College of Medicine, Houston, Texas 77030, USA.*

ARDEN, G.B. *Dept of Visual Science, Institute of Ophthalmology, Judd Street, London, UK.*

ARRUTI, G. *INSERM U. 118, CNRS ERA 842, Unité de Recherches Gérontologiques, Paris, France. (On leave from Montevideo Faculdad de Medicina, Uruguay.)*

BARNETT, K.C. *Comparative Ophthalmology Unit, Animal Health Trust Small Animals Centre, Lanwades Park, Kennett, Newmarket, Suffolk OB8 7PN, UK.*

BARRITUALT, D. *INSERM U. 86, Laboratoire d'Opthalmologie de l'Hotel Dieu, 75001 Paris, France; University of Paris XII, UER Sciences, 94100 Créteil, France.*

BEALE, R. *Nuffield Laboratory of Ophthalmology, Walton Street, Oxford OX2 6AW, UK.*

BERMAN, E.R. *Eye Biochemistry Unit, Dept. of Ophthalmology, Hadassah University Hospital, Jerusalem, Israel.*

BIRD, A.C. *Dept. of Clinical Ophthalmology, Moorfields Eye Hospital, London, UK.*

BUYUKMIOHI, N. *School of Veterinary Medicine, University of Pennsylvania, Philadelphia, Pennsylvania 19104, USA.*

CHADER, G.J. *Laboratory of Vision Research, National Eye Institute, National Institutes of Health, Bethesda, Maryland 20205, USA.*

CHAN, I.P.R. *Dept. of Visual Science, Institute of Ophthalmology, University of London, UK.*

CHASE, D.G. *Jules Stein Eye Institute, UCLA School of Medicine, Los Angeles, California 90024, USA: Developmental Neurology Laboratory and the Cell Biology Research Laboratory, Veterans Administration Medical Centre, Sepulveda, California 91343, USA.*

CLAYTON, R.M. *Dept. of Genetics, University of Edinburgh, West Mains Road, Edinburgh EH9 3JN, UK.*

CONVERSE, C.A. *Dept. of Pharmacy, University of Strathclyde, Glasgow G1 1XW, UK.*

COURTOIS, Y. *INSERM U.118 — CNRS ERA 842 — Unité de Recherches Gérontologiques, Paris, France.*

CRISANTI-COMBES, P.   *CNRS ER 231 and INSERM U178, Hôpital Brous-sais, 96 rue Didot, 75674 Paris, Cedex 14, France.*

CUTHBERT, J.   *Dept. of Genetics, University of Edinburgh, West Mains Road, Edinburgh EH9 3JN, UK.*

DAEMEN, F.J.M.   *Dept. of Biochemistry, University of Nij-megen, PO Box 9101, 6500 HB Nijmegen, The Netherlands.*

EGUCHI, G.   *Institute of Molecular Biology, Faculty of Science, Nagoya University, Nagoya 464, Japan.*

FARBER, D.B.   *Jules Stein Eye Institute, UCLA School of Medicine, Los Angeles, California 90024, USA: Develop-mental Neurology Laboratory and the Cell Biology Research Laboratory, Veterans Administration Medical Centre, Sepulveda, California 91343, USA.*

GIRARD, A.   *CNRS ER 231 and INSERM U178, Hôpital Broussais, 96 rue Didot, 75674 Paris, Cedex 14, France.*

GIUSTO, N.M.   *Cullen Eye Institute, Baylor College of Medicine, Houston, Texas 77030, USA.*

GORRIN, G.   *Dept. of Anatomy, University of California, San Francisco, School of Medicine, San Francisco, CA 94143, USA.*

DE GRIP, W.J.   *Dept. of Biochemistry, University of Nijmegen, P.O. Box 9101, 6500 HB Nijmegen, The Netherlands.*

HAYWOOD, J.   *Dept. of Biochemistry, University of Edinburgh, Edinburgh EH8 9XD, UK.*

HOLLYFIELD, J.G.   *Cullen Eye Institute, Baylor College of Medicine, Houston, Texas 77006, USA.*

HUSSAIN, A.A.   *Dept. of Visual Science, Institute of Ophthal-mology, University of London, UK.*

IKEDA, H.   *Vision Research Unit, The Rayne Institute, St. Thomas' Hospital, London SE1 7EH, UK.*

JACOBSON, S.G.   *Vision Research Unit, The Rayne Institute, St. Thomas' Hospital, London SE1 7EH, UK*

JANSEN, P.A.A.   *Dept. of Biochemistry, University of Nij-megen, PO Box 9101, 6500 HB Nijmegen, The Netherlands.*

KAITZ, M.   *Vision Research Laboratory, Dept. of Ophthalmology, Hadassah University Hospital, Jerusalem, Israel.*

KOH, S.-W.M.   *Laboratory of Vision Research, National Eye Institute, National Institutes of Health, Bethseda, MD 20205, USA.*

LAVAIL, M.M.   *Dept. of Anatomy, University of California, San Francisco, School of Medicine, San Francisco, CA 94143, USA.*

LEE, W.   *The University Depts. of Pathology and Ophthalmology, The University of Glasgow, Glasgow G11 6NT, UK.*

LOLLEY, R.N.   *Developmental Neurology laboratory, Veterans Administration Medical Centre, Sepulveda, California 91343: Dept. of Anatomy, UCLA School of Medicine, Los Angeles, California 90024, USA.*

MacINNES, D.G. *MRC Brain Metabolism Unit, Dept. of Pharmacology, University of Edinburgh, 1 George Square, Edinburgh EH8 9JZ, UK.*

McDEVITT, D.S. *Dept. of Animal Biology, University of Pennsylvania, School of Veterinary Medicine, Philadelphia, Pennsylvania 19104, USA.*

MARGRY, R.C.J.F. *Dept. of Biochemistry, University of Nijmegen, P.O. Box 9101, 6500 HB Nijmegen, The Netherlands.*

MARSHALL, J. *Dept. of Visual Science, Institute of Ophthalmology, University of London, London, UK.*

MASTERSON, E. *Laboratory of Vision Research, National Eye Institute, National Institutes of Health, Bethesda, MD 20205, USA.*

MAURICE, D. *INSERM U. 86, Laboratoire d'Opthalmologie de l'Hotel Dieu, 75001 Paris, France.*

MOSCONA, A.A. *Laboratory for Developmental Biology, Cummings Life Science Centre, University of Chicago, Chicago, Illinois 60637, USA.*

MOSKAL, J.R. *National Heart, Lung, and Blood Institute, National Institutes of Health, Bethesda, Maryland 20205, USA.*

NEUHOFF, V. *Nuffield Laboratory of Ophthalmology, Walton, Street, Oxford OX2 6AW, UK.*

NIRENBERG, M. *National Heart, Lung and Blood Institute, National Institutes of Health, Bethesda, Maryland 20205, USA.*

O'BRIEN, P. *National Eye Institute, National Institutes of Health, Bethesda, Maryland 20205, USA.*

OKADA, T.S. *Dept. of Biophysics, Faculty of Science, University of Kyoto, Kyoto 606, Japan.*

OSBORNE, N.N. *Nuffield Laboratory of Ophthalmology, Walton Street, Oxford OX2 6AW, UK.*

PESSAC, B. *CNRS ER 231 and INSERM U.178, Hôpital Broussais, 96 rue Didot, 75674 Paris, Cedex 14, France.*

PINTO, L.H. *Dept. of Anatomy, University of California, San Francisco, School of Medicine, San Francisco, CA 94143, USA.*

PLOUET, J. *INSERM U. 118, CNRS ERA 842, Unité de Recherches Gérontologiques Paris, France.*

POLLOCK, B.J. *Dept. of Genetics, University of Edinburgh, West Mains Road, Edinburgh EH9 3JN, UK.*

DE POMERAI, D.I. *Dept. of Zoology, University of Nottingham, Nottingham NG7 2RD, UK.*

RANDALL, C.J. *Ministry of Agriculture, Veterinary Laboratory, Eskgrove, Lasswade, Midlothian, UK.*

RAPP, L.M. *Cullen Eye Institute, Baylor College of Medicine, Houston, Texas 77030, USA.*

READING, H.W.   *MRC Brain Metabolism Unit, Dept. of Pharmacology, University of Edinburgh, Edinburgh EH8 9JZ, UK.*

ROMEY, G.   *Centre de Biochimie, CNRS, Université de Nice, Parc Valrose, 06034 Nice, France.*

SANYAL, S.   *Dept. of Anatomy, Erasmus University, Medical Faculty, Postbox 1738, 3000 DR Rotterdam, The Netherlands.*

SCHNEIDER, M.D.   *National Heart, Lung and Blood Institute, National Institutes of Health, Bethesda, Maryland 20205, USA.*

SEGAL, N.   *Eye Biochemistry Unit, Dept. of Ophthalmology, Hadassah University Hospital, Jerusalem, Israel.*

SHEARDOWN, M.J.   *Vision Research Unit, The Rayne Institute, St. Thomas' Hospital, London SE1 7EH, UK.*

SHINDE, S.L.   *Institute of Molecular Biology, Faculty of Science, Nagoya University, Nagoya 464, Japan.*

THOMPSON, P.   *INSERM U. 86, Laboratoire d'Opthalmologie de l'Hotel Dieu, 75001 Paris, France.*

TRISLER, G.D.   *National Heart, Lung and Blood Institute, National Institutes of Health, Bethesda, Maryland 20205, USA.*

VOADEN, M.J.   *Dept. of Visual Science, Institute of Ophthalmology, University of London, UK.*

WIEGAND, R.D.   *Cullen Eye Institute, Baylor College of Medicine, Houston, Texas 77030, USA.*

WILSON, M.A.   *Dept. of Genetics, University of Edinburgh, West Mains Road, Edinburgh EH9 3JN, UK.*

WIRZ, K.   *Abteilung Augenheilkunde der Medizinischen Fakultat, 5100 Aachen, Goethestrasse 27/29, W. Germany.*

WOLF, E.D.   *Dept. of Comparative Ophthalmology, College of Veterinary Medicine, University of Florida, Gainesville, Florida, USA.*

YASUMURA, D.   *Dept. of Anatomy, University of California, San Francisco, School of Medicine, San Francisco, CA 94143, USA.*

PREFACE

This book represents an attempt to cover the biological,
structural and functional aspects of inherited degenerative
conditions of vertebrate retina, by discussing modern concepts of normal retinal developmental processes and some
of the control mechanisms which may go awry and so be involved in cellular degeneration. The volume represents the
contributions and discussions of an International Workshop on
this topic, held in Edinburgh during September 1981.

In planning the workshop with this book in mind, the
Editors have endeavoured to present an overall presentation
which would be of interest to experienced and new workers in
the field, as well as the scientists and clinicians interested
in these problems.

The original concept arose out of our combined interest in
the problem of primary pigmentary degeneration of the retina,
with special reference to human retinitis pigmentosa. No
recent, up-to-date books covering wider aspects of this
problem exist, and no International meetings addressed to
the topic have been held for a number of years so that the
time is opportune for an update. Retinitis pigmentosa, in
the UK accounts for more than 10% of the adult registered
sufferers from blindness. The causes of this condition are
unknown so that specific treatment is unavailable. In the
last decade, very significant progress has been made in
understanding the cellular and biochemical heterogeneity of
the normal retina and the molecular mechanisms involved in the
visual process. Several animal models with inherited retinal
degeneration have been described, and their study has further
revealed mechanisms involved in abnormal retinal function.
Much of the research is being carried out by workers in widely
separated disciplines so the need was felt for an integrated
interdisciplinary meeting. The workshop achieved this
objective and provided a basis for discussion of the animal
models of retinal dystrophy and their relevance to retinitis
pigmentosa in man as well as an opportunity to outline stra-
tegies for future research.

It is difficult to point to specific research programmes

which offer the greatest promise, but the significant recent
advances would appear to be those concerned with biological
study of developing retinal tissues, tissue culture methodo-
logy, the inter-relationships between the neural retina and
the pigment epithelium and analysis of genetic background
and histories.   Until more is known about the stages of
normal retinal development and differentiation of the different neuronal layers and the different biomolecular events
associated with this development, progress on unravelling
the aetiology of inherited retinal degeneration will be
slow.   In the field of molecular biology, the discovery of
abnormalities in cyclic nucleotide metabolism associated
with the condition in experimental animals may prove to
offer some means of interfering with the relentless progress
of the lesion.

The Workshop was organized by the Editors of this book,
together with Dr C. Beevers, Mr D. Curr and Professor C.I.
Phillips.

CONTENTS

SECTION 1: CELLULAR AND MOLECULAR BIOLOGY OF THE RETINA

SECTION 3: ANIMAL MODELS AND HUMAN DISEASE

Part 1

ACKNOWLEDGEMENTS

Our special gratitude goes to Dr Alan Laties of the University
of Pennsylvania, Philadelphia, USA. Without his active support and encouragement, this meeting would not have taken
place and this book would not exist.
  We are also grateful for financial support which made the
workshop possible, from the following:

  The Retinitis Pigmentosa Foundation (USA)
  The Wellcome Trust
  The International Society for Developmental Biology
  The Humane Research Trust

  Astra Clinical Research Unit
  Bank of Scotland
  B.P. Trading Co. Ltd.
  City of Edinburgh Lions Club
  Corstorphine Round Table
  Dema Glass Ltd.
  Dunfermline Ladies Circle
  International Enzymes
  Marks and Spencers (Edinburgh)
  Safeway Stores (Edinburgh)
  Scottish Life Assurance
  Sigma (London) Chemical Co.
  Syntex Research Centre (Syntex Pharmaceuticals Ltd.)
  Uniscience

We are also indebted to numerous individuals who helped,
and to many individual members of the Edinburgh branch of
the British Retinitis Pigmentosa Society. We are grateful
to Ms M. Alexander, Genetics Department, University of
Edinburgh and Ms H.C. Tyler of Academic Press, London, for
their help with the preparation of this book.

CELLULAR AND MOLECULAR BIOLOGY OF THE RETINA: INTRODUCTION

R.M. CLAYTON

Institute of Animal Genetics, West Mains Road, Edinburgh, EH9 3JN, UK

Clinicians, pathologists, electrophysiologists, neuropharmacologists, and biochemists who are interested in the retina are all accustomed to the differentiated structure and its properties and functions, and to the changes in these characteristics associated with the various genetic dysplasias and degenerations known and studied in humans, and in animal models.

The developmental biologist, interested in molecular and cell biology, and using the retina as a model system, will have much to learn from these specialists in the retina but also much to offer them, since many conditions of concern to the clinician will have developmental antecedents, and it is by a study of the parameters of differentiation and of developmental potential that we may be able to understand better some of the postnatal consequences of early lesions. Even if we are considering a heritable degeneration detectable only relatively late in life, the locus of the first changes, and pattern of the spread of damage across the retina suggest some process superimposed on a pre-existing cellular heterogeneity, or a cellular gradient. The papers in this section deal with several different aspects of developmental cell research, into properties which are probably found in the retinas of all vertebrates.

PERMANENT CELL LINES DERIVED FROM
QUAIL AND MOUSE RETINAS

BERNARD PESSAC*, PATRICIA CRISANTI-COMBES*, GEORGES ROMEY**
AND ARLETTE GIRARD*

*CNRS ER 231 and INSERM U178, Hôpital Broussais, 96 rue Didot,
75674 Paris Cedex 14, France

**Centre de Biochimie, CNRS, Université de Nice, Parc Valrose,
06034 Nice, France

INTRODUCTION

The aim of the work presented here is to develop permanent
cell lines from the neural retina. The main advantage of
established cell lines which originate from single cell clones
is that they represent a homogenous material which is obtain-
able in unlimited amounts. Cell lines with neuronal or glial
properties which were established from the peripheral and
central nervous system had provided information on the
properties of neurones and glial cells as well as on their
lineage.
  The neural retina is an evagination of the central nervous
system; its structure and physiology have been well
documented (Dowling, 1975). It is made up of a limited
number of cell types: Müller (astroglial) cells, photoreceptors,
and four main classes of neurones: horizontal, bipolar,
amacrine, and ganglion cells which can be further subdivided
into several groups. Most of the cell lines derived from
the nervous system have either been obtained from spontaneous
tumors, or from tumors resulting from the injection of a
chemical carcinogen. An alternative approach, which had not
been previously investigated with the neural tissues, is the
infection of cells with an oncogenic virus.
  We had observed that infection of the quail neural crest
or mouse cerebellum cells by, respectively, the oncogenic
viruses Rous sarcoma virus (RSV) and simian virus 40 (SV-40)
leads to permanent cell lines which have retained differen-

tiated properties (Pessac *et al.*, manuscript in prep.;
Pessac *et al.*, 1978). It was therefore decided to transform
quail embryo neuroretinal (NR) cells with RSV, and mouse
retina with SV-40. Permanently established cultures have
been obtained in both systems and some of their properties
are described.

QUAIL CELL LINE

In the first system, primary cultures from 7 day quail embryo
NR cells were infected with a conditional mutant of RSV which
transforms cells at the permissive temperature ($36^{\circ}C$), but not
at the non permissive temperature ($41^{\circ}C$). The cultures were
nonetheless kept at $39^{\circ}C$ as this is the upper limit compatible
with the maintenance of quail NR cells. The establishment
of a permanent culture proceeded through a multiple step
process. During the initial stage, RSV-induced cellular
proliferation was very active. Two neuronal markers were
detected in these cultures: a large number, (up to 50%), of
the morphologically transformed, round cells (Fig. 1), bound
tetanus toxin (as seen by the indirect immunofluorescence
assay), thus indicating the neuronal nature of these cells

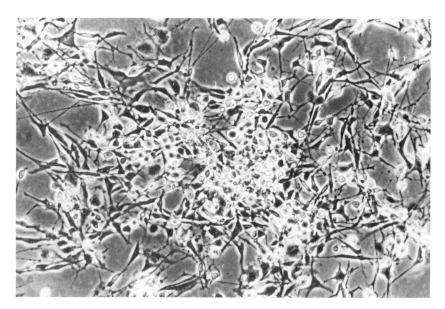

Fig. 1 *Phase micrograph of the quail neuroretina cell line
(× 125). Note the clusters of round transformed cells.*

(Mirsky *et al.*, 1978; Pettman *et al.*, 1979) (Fig. 2). Also
the specific activity of the enzyme glutamic acid decarboxylase (GAD) responsible for the synthesis of the neurotransmitter gamma-aminobutyric acid (GABA) was markedly stimulated
(Crisanti-Combes *et al.* 1982). The cultures were passaged
several times over a period of 3 to 4 months; then, for 2 to 3
months, the cell population did not increase; after this
"crisis", cell multiplication resumed. At that time, GAD
specific activity was still high (about 10 nmoles CO_2/mg of
protein/h); the electrophysiological studies showed that a
minority of cells responded to electrical stimulation with
a weak partial response or a "delayed rectification".

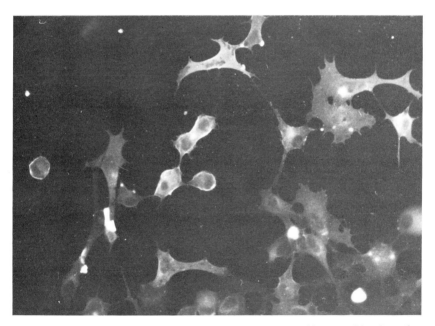

Fig. 2 *Visualization of tetanus toxin binding cells by the
double immunofluorescence technique. About 30% of the cells
are stained on their surface.*

After 18 months, two major changes occurred in these cultures. For one thing, the GAD activity disappeared, and
for another, about 10% of the electrode impaled cells were
able to produce action potentials upon electrical stimulation.
These action potentials were completely blocked in 5 min by
the presence of 10^{-7} M tetrodotoxin. The cultures have,
to date, been passaged 20 times since the first recording of
these action potentials and their electrophysiological
properties have not changed. These action potential positive

cells are either single, or associated with other cells in
clumps. They do not have a distinct morphology. In
addition to the cells which can generate action potentials,
other cells still display the weak signs of excitability
recorded earlier (Pessac *et al.*, manuscript submitted).
    These permanently established quail NR cultures raise many
questions:

1) Which *"in vivo"* cell type is the counterpart of the cells
which are able to produce action potentials? Since amacrine
and ganglion cells are probably the only ones which depolarize
"in vivo", the action potential positive neurones could be
either cell type. It is however possible that cells that
do not generate action potentials *"in vivo"* can do so *"in
vitro"* after transformation by RSV.
2) How many different cell types (photoreceptors, neurones,
astroglial) are the cultures made of? Since 30 to 50% of
the cells specifically bind tetanus toxin to their plasma
membranes, it is reasonable to assume that this is the lower
limit for an estimation of the number of neurones present in
the cultures. However, as we found no marker for quail
Müller cells in culture, we do not know if the tetanus toxin
negative cells are astroglial.
3) The coexistence of an apparently constant proportion of
cells with different properties over a long period of time
is somewhat surprising, and could be accounted for by two
hypotheses. One could envisage that the different cell
populations might have an identical cell cycle time. On the
other hand, it is possible that the cultures might be composed of uni- or pluri-potential, precursor cells, which eventually mature into differentiated neurones.

These questions might be answered if we succeed in obtaining
populations developed from single cell clones. Cloning of
these cells is rendered difficult by the fact that they permanently replicate the RSV, which is partially lytic. A few
clones have, nevertheless, been developed recently and we are
currently studying some of their properties.

MOUSE CELL LINE

The other cultures we have permanently established *"in vitro"*
are retina cells taken from embryonic or post-natal mice
and transformed by SV-40 (Pessac *et al.*, 1976). Many permanent cell lines have been obtained from these cultures
in this way, but we shall restrict ourselves to a description

of the one which has been most extensively studied. This
culture was started from retinas of one day old mice and
infected 24 h later with SV-40. Foci of transformed cells
appeared 4 weeks later and multiplied actively. Cloning
was done at the third subculture and has been repeated 3
times; the properties described are therefore those of a
single cell clone (R-ClB, manuscript in preparation).

The cells of this clone appear to be astroglial, since
all cells in monolayer cultures are specifically stained
with a reference antiglial fibrillary acidic protein serum
(Bignami et al., 1980). Secondly, they apparently have a GAD
specific activity (10 nmoles CO_2/mg of protein/h) which is
similar to that of the adult mouse retina. This result seems
somewhat surprising, as it would mean that Müller cells can
synthetize GABA. Thirdly, in collaboration with Maurice P.
Dubois (INRA, Laboratoire de Neuroendocrinologie Sexuelle),
we have detected an immunoreactivity to many neuropeptides.
Of the peptides which have been assayed by indirect immunofluorescence: i.e. alpha- and beta-MSH, alpha- and beta-
endorphin, somatostatin, methionine- and leucine-enkephalin,
TRH and Substance P, only the last one was not detected. A
large majority (about 80%) of the cells are immunoreactive
for each of these peptides. Thus most peptides, if not all,
are probably present in every cell. Although appropriate
controls have indicated that the immunoreactivity was
specific for each of these peptides, experiments are underway (with P. Emson, Medical Research Council, Cambridge) to
identify these peptides with biochemical techniques. Since
reactive peptides are detected in cells kept in serum-free
medium, they would appear to be synthesized by the ClB cells.
We do not yet know if these peptides are present in the
Müller cells of the post natal mouse "in vivo", and the
physiological significance of peptides in these presumptive
Müller cells in culture therefore still needs to be determined.

These results show that permanent cell lines from retina
acquire, and/or keep, differentiated properties after transformation with an oncogenic virus. They could be useful
tools to study the properties of various neuroretina cell
types at the cellular and molecular levels.

ACKNOWLEDGEMENTS

This work was supported by grants from the Centre National
de la Recherche Scientifique, the Institut National de la
Santé et de la Recherche Médicale (ATP No 81-79-113), the

Délégation Générale à la Recherche Scientifique et Technique
(No 78-7-2777) and the Fondation pour la Recherche Médicale
Francaise.

REFERENCES

Bignami, A., Dahl, D. and Rueger, D.C. (1980). Glial fibrillary acidic protein (GFA) in normal neural cells and in
  pathological conditions. *Adv. Cell. Neurobiol.* 1, 285—310.
Crisanti—Combes, P., Lorinet, A.M., Girard, A., Pessac, B.,
  Wassef, M. and Calothy, G. (1982). Expression of neuronal
  markers in chick and quail embryo neuroretina cultures
  infected with Rous sarcoma virus. *Cell Different.*, 11,
  45—54.
Dowling, J.E. (1975). The vertebrate retina. In "The Ner-
  vous System" (Ed. D.B. Tower), Vol. 1, pp. 91—100. Raven
  Press, New York.
Mirsky, R., Wendon, L.M.B., Blacks, P., Stolkin, C. and Bray,
  D. (1978). Tetanus toxin: a cell surface marker for
  neurons in culture. *Brain Res*. 148, 251—259.
Pessac, B., Alliot, F., Girard, A., Crisanti-Combes, P.,
  Guerinot, F., Privat, A. and Drian, M.J. (1-78). Pro-
  perties of mouse cerebellum cells transformed by SV-40.
  Neurosci. Lett. (suppl. 1), S39 (abstract).
Pessac, B., Calothy, G. and Alliot, F. (1976). Transforma-
  tion de cellules retiniennes de Souris par le virus
  simien 40. *Compt. Rend. Acad. Sci. (Paris)*, 283, 87—90.
Pettman, B., Louis, J.C. and Sensenbrenner, M. (1979).
  Morphological and biochemical maturation of neurones cul-
  tured in the absence of glial cells. *Nature* 281, 378—380.

THE CHARACTERIZATION OF CELL CULTURES
OF NEONATAL RETINA

RICHARD BEALE, VOLKER NEUHOFF* and NEVILLE N. OSBORNE

*Nuffield Laboratory of Ophthalmology,
Walton Street, Oxford OX2 6AW, UK*

INTRODUCTION

We are studying the biochemistry and development of the
individual cell types of the retina. Dissociation of the
retina affords opportunities to purify the various cell
types by physical or immunological techniques. Subsequent
culture of the cells allows both a stringent test of their
viability and study of their development in a simplified
environment. However, some means must be found to identify
the dissociated cells. To this end we have characterized
rat retinal cell cultures using a number of immunofluorescence
and autoradiographic techniques.

METHODS AND RESULTS

Tetanus Toxin

It is generally accepted that tetanus toxin binds specifically
to neurones in central and peripheral nervous systems
(Dimpfel *et al.*, 1975; Mirsky *et al.*, 1978). An indirect
immunofluorescence assay for tetanus toxin binding revealed
preferential binding of the toxin to the surfaces of large
spheroid cells with long processes (Fig. 1). In frozen
sections of formaldehyde-fixed rat retina, a similar assay
revealed intense binding to the inner plexiform layer; the
outer plexiform and inner nuclear layers were also labelled
while the outer nuclear layer was essentially unlabelled
(Fig. 2a). A similar labelling pattern was obtained after
autoradiography of frozen sections incubated with ^{125}I-
tetanus toxin. These results suggest that tetanus toxin
binds much more intensely to the cell bodies and processes

*Max-Planck-Institut für Experimentelle Medizin, Forschungs-
stelle Neurochemie, 3400 Göttingen (FRG).

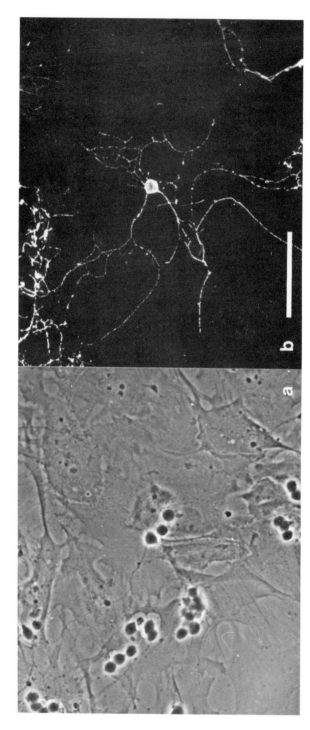

Fig. 1 Tetanus toxin indirect immunofluorescence on rat retinal cell cultures 6d in vitro: (a) phase contrast and (b) epifluorescence images of same field. Scale bar = 50 µm.

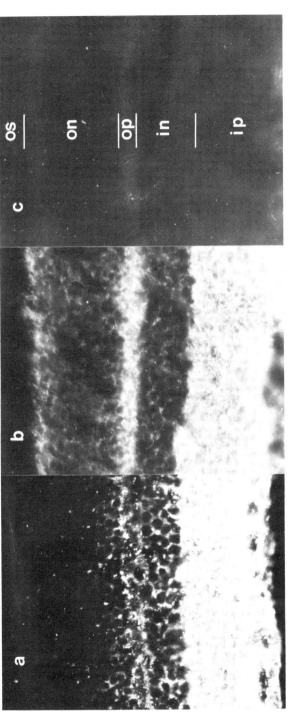

Fig. 2 Indirect immunofluorescence on frozen sections of adult rat retina: (a) tetanus toxin; (b) monoclonal antibody A4; (c) monoclonal antibody Ran-2 (control for A4; tetanus toxin had a similar appearance). os: outer segments; on: outer nuclear layer; op: outer plexiform layer; in: inner nuclear layer; ip: inner plexiform layer. Scale bars (dividing lines in c) = 20 μm.

of retinal neurones than to photoreceptor perikarya.

A4

A4 is a monoclonal antibody which binds to the surfaces of
central but not peripheral neurones (Cohen and Selvendran,
1981). Indirect immunofluorescence studies with A4 showed
the antibody to associate with the surfaces of virtually
all spheroid cells in cultures of rat retina. On frozen
sections of retina the antibody labelled all layers except
the area corresponding to photoreceptor outer segments: in
particular clear ring fluorescence was evident around cell
bodies of both inner and outer nuclear layers (Fig. 2b).
Thus A4 appears to bind to the surfaces of photoreceptors as
well as retinal neurones.

   In summary, the A4 and tetanus toxin immunofluorescence
studies indicate that the surfaces of photoreceptor cell
bodies share an antigen (defined by A4) with central neurones,
but seem to lack gangliosides GD1b, GT1b and GQ1, thought
to be the tetanus toxin "receptors" (Van Heyningen and
Mellanby, 1971; Holmgren *et al.*, 1980; Rodgers and Snyder,
1981).

Autoradiography of D-aspartate Uptake

When retinal cell cultures were incubated with micromolar
concentrations of [^{3}H]-D-aspartate and then processed for
autoradiography, moderately high concentrations of silver
grains appeared above the majority of small spheroidal
cells: the class of cells corresponding to those unlabelled
by tetanus toxin immunofluorescence (Fig. 3a). A minority
of larger multipolar cells also accumulated radioactivity,
while flattened cells were only lightly labelled.
   Autoradiograms of intact rat retinas incubated with
[^{3}H]-D-aspartate showed that the majority of photoreceptor
cells and a minority of inner nuclear layer cells had accumulated radio-activity. These results are similar to those already
described to occur for the uptake of aspartate by human and rat
retinas (Lam and Hollyfield, 1980; Voaden *et al.*, 1980). D-
aspartate therefore appears to be preferentially taken up by
photoreceptors and neurones situated in the inner nuclear layer
in intact retinas. The similar labelling of small spheroid
cells in retinal cultures, and the fact that tetanus toxin
appears not to bind to these cells, supports the opinion
that these cells are immature photoreceptors. It is interesting to note that they appear to retain this differentiated
property after dissociation in spite of their lack of
morphological differentiation.

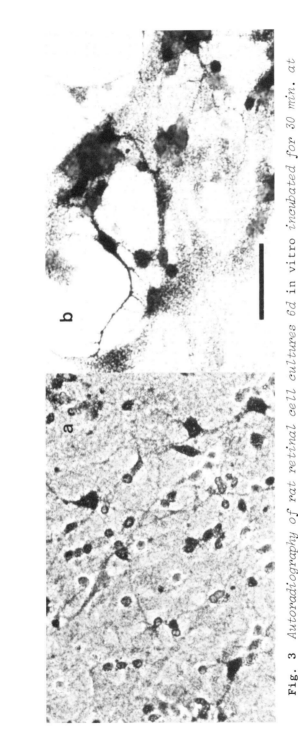

Fig. 3 *Autoradiography of rat retinal cell cultures 6d in vitro incubated for 30 min. at room temperature with: (a) 0.4 μM ³H–D–aspartate; (b) 1 μM ³H–glycine. (a) shows a phase contrast and (b) a bright field image of autoradiograms stained through the emulsion with methylene blue. Scale bar = 50 μm.*

Autoradiography of GABA and Glycine Uptake

In mammalian retinas only a sub-class of amacrine cells
accumulates exogenous [^{3}H]-glycine, whereas [^{3}H]-GABA
appears to be taken up by Müller cells as well as amacrine
cells (Neal and Iversen, 1972; Ehinger, 1977; Lam and
Hollyfield, 1980; Kong *et al.*, 1980; Pourcho, 1980). Rat
retinal cell cultures processed for autoradiography following incubation in micromolar concentrations of [^{3}H]-glycine
and [^{3}H]-GABA revealed sub-classes of the larger spheroidal
cells bearing long processes to be heavily labelled (Fig.
3b and 4a). Autoradiography combined with immunofluorescence
studies on the same preparations showed that tetanus toxin
binds to these cells which suggests that they are neurones
(Fig. 4b). Flattened cells were only slightly labelled
by radioactivity following exposure to [^{3}H]-glycine or
[^{3}H]-GABA.

GFAP and Ran-2

Glial fibrillary acidic protein (GFAP) has been localized to
astrocytes by immunohistochemistry (Bignami *et al.*, 1972).
In the retina, strong binding of anti-GFAP serum to similar
fibrils in Müller cells has only been reported after injury
to the eye (Bignami and Dahl, 1979). In retinal cell cultures
anti-GFAP associated to a varying extent with the majority
of flattened cells. Some showed strong binding similar to
the reported studies on cultured astrocytes (e.g. Raff
et al., 1979), but the majority were labelled only marginally
more than controls. The former cells are likely to have
been retinal astrocytes and the latter Müller cells. In
agreement with a previous report (Bartlett, *et al.*, 1981)
the majority of flattened cells were surface-labelled with
monoclonal antibody Ran-2. A minority of flattened cells
were unlabelled by Ran-2 or anti-GFAP. These cells are
likely to have been endothelial cells, pigment epithelial
cells or fibroblasts (Fig. 5).

DISCUSSION

In cell cultures prepared from rat retinas 3 basic classes
of cells may be recognized:

1)   Glial cells (Müller cells and astrocytes) are flattened
to the substrate. Their surfaces bind monoclonal antibody
Ran-2, and they are lightly labelled with radioactivity
following incubation with micromolar concentrations of

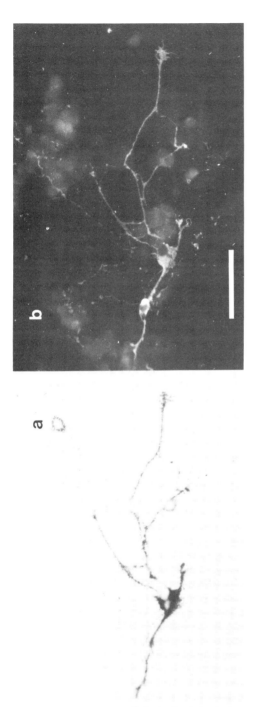

Fig. 4 *Combined autoradiography and tetanus toxin immunofluorescence of rat retinal cell culture 6d in vitro: (a) bright field and (b) epifluorescence images of same field. Dim, diffuse non-specific fluorescence also appears in (b). Note that the bright tetanus toxin-specific fluorescence duplicates the image of the large cell heavily labelled in (a), but not that of the more lightly labelled cell in the top right corner of the same picture. Scale bar = 50 μm.*

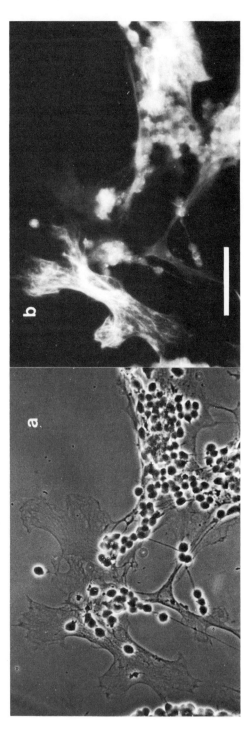

Fig. 5 Indirect immunofluorescence of anti-GFAP serum on rat retinal cell culture 4d in vitro: (a) phase contrast and (b) epifluorescence images of the same field. Note that diffuse labelling of spheroid cells also occurs in controls. Scale bar = 50 μm.

[^{3}H]-glycine; [^{3}H]-GABA or [^{3}H]-D-aspartate.

2) Immature photoreceptors are spheroid and lack long processes. They accumulate [^{3}H]-D-aspartate and their surfaces bind neither tetanus toxin nor Ran-2.

3) Retinal neurones are bipolar or multipolar spheroid cells and are the only cell type in our cultures to which tetanus toxin binds. Subclasses of multipolar spheroidal cells show intense labelling after autoradiography of cultures incubated in micromolar concentrations of [^{3}H]-GABA, [^{3}H]-glycine, or [^{3}H]-D-aspartate. These cells have similar sizes and shapes to those of amacrine neurons in intact retinas. Other "tetanus-positive" cells are similar in appearance to bipolar, horizontal and ganglion neurons, but we have as yet found no more certain way to identify these cell types.

Our ability to identify cultured cells by surface chemistry and physiology encourages us to believe that these and other cell-type-specific properties are retained *in vitro* where they may be more easily investigated. These identification methods will also enable us to monitor our efforts to produce populations of cells enriched in certain cell types. Such cell populations of defined specificity should then allow detailed study of the chemistry, physiology and pharmacology of specific retinal cell-types.

ACKNOWLEDGEMENTS

We are grateful to Erika Abney, Jim Cohen, Lawrence Eng and Martin Raff for gifts of antisera, to R.O. Thomson and Prof. E. Habermann for gifts of native and ^{125}I-labelled tetanus toxin respectively, and to Kathy Andersen for typing the manuscript. We are also indebted to Stifftung Volkswagenwerk for financial support.

REFERENCES

Bartlett, P.F., Noble, M.D., Pruss, R.M., Raff, M.C., Rattray, S. and Williams, C.A. (1981). Rat neural antigen-2 (Ran-2): a cell surface antigen on astrocytes, ependymal cells, Müller cells and lepto-meninges defined by a monoclonal antibody. *Brain Res.* **204**, 339-351.

Bignami, A. and Dahl, D. (1979). Radial glia of Muller in the rat retina and their response to injury: immuno-fluorescence study with antibodies to the glial fibrillary (GFA) protein. *Exp. Eye Res.* **28**, 63-69.

Bignami, A., Eng, L.F., Dahl, D. and Uyeda, C.T. (1972).

Localization of the glial fibrillary acidic protein in astrocytes by immunofluorescence. *Brain Res*. **43**, 429-435.

Cohen, J. and Selvendran, S.Y. (1981). A neuronal cell-surface antigen is found in the CNS but not in peripheral neurones. *Nature, Lond*. **291**, 421-423.

Dimpfel, W., Neale, J.H. and Habermann, E. (1975). ^{125}I-labelled tetanus toxin as a neuronal marker in tissue cultures derived from embryonic CNS, *Naunyn-Schmiedeberg's Arch. exp. Path. Pharmak*. **290**, 329-333.

Ehinger, B. (1977). Glial and neuronal uptake of GABA, glutamic acid, glutamine, and glutathione in the rabbit retina. *Exp. Eye Res*. **25**, 221-234.

Holmgren, J., Elwing, H., Fredman, P., Strannegard, O., and Svennerholm, I. (1980). Gangliosides as receptors for bacterial toxins and sendai virus. In "Structure and Function of Gangliosides" (Eds. L. Svennerholm, P. Mandel, H. Dreyfus and P.F. Urban), pp. 453-470. Plenum Press, New York.

Kong, Y.C., Fung, S.C. and Lam, D.M.K. (1980). Post-natal development of glycinergic neurons in the rabbit retina. *J. Comp. Neurol*. **193**, 1127-1135.

Lam, D.M.K. and Hollyfield, J.C. (1980). Localization of putative amino acid neurotransmitters in the human retina. *Exp. Eye Res*. **31**, 729-732.

Mirsky, R., Wendon, L.M.B., Black, P., Stolkin, C. and Bray, D. (1978). Tetanus toxin: a cell surface marker for neurones in culture. *Brain Res*. **148**, 251-259.

Neal, M.J. and Iversen, L.L. (1972). Autoradiographic localization of ^{3}H-GABA in rat retina. *Nature New Biol*. **235**, 217-218.

Pourcho, R.G. (1980). Uptake of ^{3}H-glycine and ^{3}H-GABA by amacrine cells in the cat retina. *Brain Res*. **198**, 333-346.

Raff, M.C., Fields, K.L., Hakomori, S.-I., Mirsky, R., Pruss, R.M. and Winter, J. (1979). Cell-type-specific markers for distinguishing and studying neurons and the major classes of glial cells in culture. *Brain Res*. **174**, 283-308.

Rogers, T.B. and Snyder, S.H. (1981). High affinity binding of tetanus toxin to mammalian brain membranes. *J. Biol. Chem*. **256**, 2402-2407.

Van Heyningen, W.E. and Mellanby, J. (1971). Tetanus toxin. In "Microbial Toxins". (Eds S. Kadis, T.C. Montie, and S.J. Ajl) Vol. 2A, pp. 69-108. Academic Press, New York.

Voaden, M.J., Morjaria, B. and Oraedu, A.C. (1980). The localization and metabolism of glutamate aspartate and GABA in the rat retina. *Neurochem*. **1**, 151-165.

THE RETINA AND IRIS IN REGENERATION
OF THE EYE LENS

DAVID S. MCDEVITT

*Department of Animal Biology, University of Pennsylvania,
School of Veterinary Medicine, Philadelphia,
Pennsylvania 19104, USA*

INTRODUCTION

The ability to regenerate the lens of the eye in adult vertebrates is restricted to a group of urodele amphibians (Stone,
1967; Berardi and McDevitt, 1982). Complete removal of the
lens in these animals is followed by formation of a new lens
at the dorsal pupillary margin. The classical idea that the
source of this regenerated lens is the dorsal iris epithelial
cells now has strong experimental support (for reviews, see
Yamada, 1977; Reyer, 1977). Notwithstanding the long history
and intrinsic interest of this system, little is known concerning the causal factors of lens regeneration, or the biochemical composition of the regenerated lens. I would now
like to report the progress which our laboratory has made
in analysis of the structural proteins, the crystallins, of
the regenerating and the regenerated lens, as well as to
identify some of the paradoxes and dilemmas inherent in this
phenomenon and their relation to iris and retinal tissues.

METHODS AND MATERIALS

Adult *Notophthalmus viridescens*, the common spotted newt of
the eastern United States, were collected in the field
(Mountain Lake Biological Station of the University of Virginia, Giles Co., Virginia; Wayne Co., Pennsylvania) or
obtained commercially (Bill Lee Newt Farm, Oak Ridge,
Tennessee). The animals were lentectomized via a naso-
temporal incision of the cornea, as described by McDevitt
and Brahma (1982*a*), and maintained in aquaria for periods of
up to six months. The regenerated lens completes its histo-

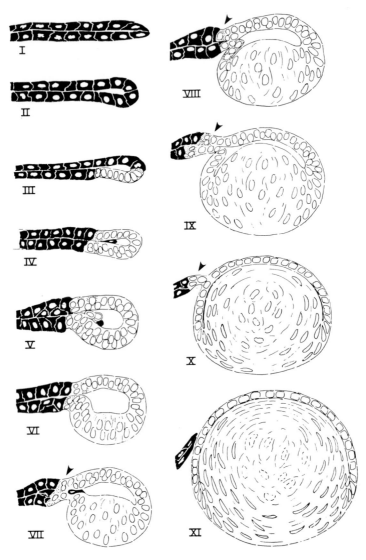

Fig. 1 *Diagrams showing morphological stages of Wolffian lens regeneration (from the dorsal iris) in adult* Notophthalamus viridescens, *the Eastern Spotted newt. Sections are through the mid-dorsal pupillary margin of the iris, oriented perpendicular to the main body axis. Cornea above, retina below, dorsal to the left. The pigmented iris cells are indicated by black cytoplasm; depigmented regenerate cells by white cytoplasm. Incomplete depigmentation is shown with dots. Arrows indicate stalk of the regenerate noted in the Discussion.*

genesis within 30 to 35 days at room temperature, but requires five to six months to attain the size of the former adult "normal" lens. Lens regenerates were staged (Fig. 1) according to Yamada (1967). The crystallins of the normal and 5 to 6 month regenerated lenses were separated by Sephadex G-200 Superfine (Pharmacia) chromatography, according to McDevitt and Brahma (1981; 1982*b*). Immunofluorescence was performed on median sections through the regenerating lens rudiment (McDevitt and Brahma, 1982*a*), using antibodies made specific for the α, β and γ crystallin classes as derived from G-200 chromatography of adult normal lenses. Peptide mapping was performed on tryptic digests of γ crystallin fractions using the method of McDevitt and Croft (1977).

RESULTS AND DISCUSSION

Indirect immunofluorescence analyses (summarized in Table 1) revealed that β crystallins appeared in the thickening layer of the lens regenerate at Stage V (Fig. 1) and in the external layer at Stage VIII. The γ crystallins appeared, albeit erratically, in a few cells of the internal layer at Stage V, and could not be detected in the epithelium. The α crystallins were first detectable at Stage VII in a few cells of the developing fibre region, and in the external layer/presumptive lens epithelium at Stage VIII (beginning of secondary fibre information). An example of the results and specificity obtained (here, for β crystallins) can be seen in Fig. 2. These results differ from those obtained in an immunofluorescence study of normal *embryonic* lens development in *N. viridescens* (McDevitt and Brahma, 1981), e.g., no α crystallins could be detected in the lens epithelium through metamorphosis, and β crystallins appeared prior to γ crystallins. Thus the ontogeny and localization of the crystallins differ in development and regeneration, even though the end result of both processes, the lens, appears to be at least superficially similar in each.

    Gel-filtration chromatography of total normal adult and regenerated crystallins resulted in four major fractions, identified in the bovine (Bloemendal, 1977) as α; βHigh Molecular Weight; βLow Molecular Weight; and γ crystallins (Figs 3 and 4). The first (putative α crystallin) peak obtained in both, however, contained both α and β crystallins,

---

Iris stroma cells and amoeboid cells are not shown (from Yamada, 1967, with permission of the author and Academic Press).

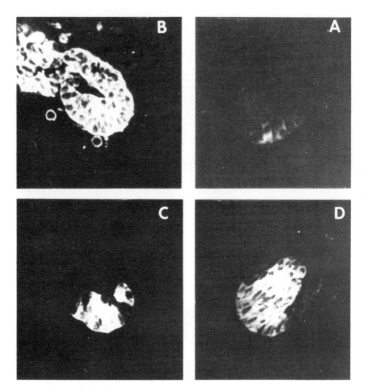

Fig. 2 *Darkfield photomicrographs of sections through the regenerating lens of* N. viridescens *treated with antibody to* N. viridescens *total β crystallins. Orientation: cornea of lentectomized eye to the top, retina to the bottom, dorsal iris laterally. Refer also to the illustrations in Fig. 1.*
  A *Stage V (immunofluorescence). β crystallins appear for the first time in a few cells of the vesicle internal layer.*
  B *Tungsten illumination, as an identical histological reference for* C *Stage VII. β crystallins at this stage of regenerate morphogenesis exhibit a characteristic "patchy" distribution, with negative cells sharply delimited by positive cell areas in the internal layer.* D *Stage VIII (immunofluorescence); some cells of the external layer are now weakly positive for β crystallins.*

as seen in immunoelectrophoresis and S.D.S. electrophoresis (data not shown). Analysis of Figs 3 and 4 reveals that the β crystallins (peaks B and C) of the regenerated lens elute as more heterogenous and polydisperse than those of the normal lens, with the β_H fraction much reduced. γ crystallins also

TABLE 1

[1] Detection of Crystallins in the Regenerating Lens of N. _viridescens_ by Immunofluorescence

STAGE		Anti-α E	Anti-α F	Anti-β E	Anti-β F	Anti-γ E	Anti-γ F
V		-	-	-	+	-	+
VI		-	-	-	+	-	+
VII		-	+	-	+	-	+
VIII		+	+	+	+	-	+
IX		+	+	+	+	-	+
X		+	+	+	+	-	+
XI		+	+	+	+	-	+

E = Epithelium (includes external layer of early lens regenerate; stalk <u>always</u> negative)
F = Fibers (includes internal layer of early lens regenerate)
+ = Positive immunofluorescence for designated crystallin (No distinction made for intensity of immunofluorescence or % of total area positive)
- = Negative; no immunofluorescence observed

(From McDevitt and Brahma, 1982a; with permission of Academic Press)

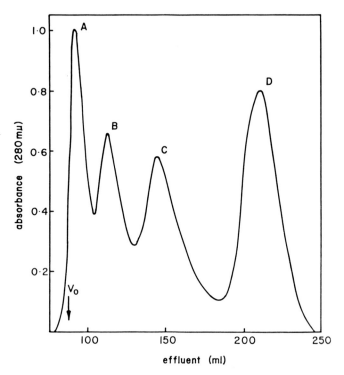

Fig. 3 *Representative gel-filtration chromatography of adult*
N. viridescens *total soluble lens proteins on Sephadex G-200*
Superfine. 74 mg of protein was added to a 2.6 cm × 48.5 cm
column, and eluted with 0.05 M tris-Cl buffer, pH 7.2, with
0.1 M KCl, 5mM β mercaptoethanol and 1mM EDTA. Fractions were
collected as 1.9 ml aliquots. Vo = Void Volume, determined
using Blue Detran 2000; bovine thyroglobulin (M.W. 6.7 × 10⁵)
also eluted before peak A.

comprise a much larger percentage (52% vs. 37%) of the elution
profile of the regenerated lens crystallins. In addition,
peptide mapping of the total γ crystallins (peak D) derived
from regenerated lenses (Fig. 5) demonstrates the presence of
"embryonic/fetal" γ crystallin subfractions analogous to
bovine γIII and γIV (Slingsby and Croft, 1973) not seen in the
adult lenses. Twenty peptides were common to each γ crystallin
sample, but 3 peptides could be found only in the regenerated
lens γ crystallins and 4 peptides only in those γ crystallins of
the normal adult lens. These results suggest the mature regenerated lens as exhibiting "embryonic" features (i.e., increased amounts of γ crystallins and decreased amounts of
$β_H$ crystallins (Asselbergs *et al.*, 1979), yet indicate that
the genome in terminally-differentiated iris tissue is still

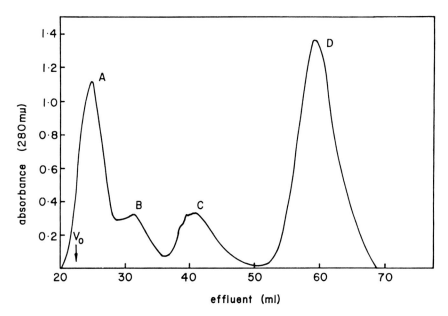

Fig. 4 *Sephadex G-200 Superfine chromatography of total soluble lens proteins derived from six-month regenerated* N. viridescens *lenses. 23 mg of protein was added to a 1.6 cm × 35 cm column, and eluted with 0.05M tris-Cl buffer, pH 7.2, with 0.1 KCl, 5mM β mercaptoethanol and 1mM EDTA. Fractions were collected as 0.5ml aliquots. Vo = Void Volume, determined using Blue Dextran 2000 and thyroglobulin.*

capable of producing proteins, specific for another ocular tissue, that never would have been synthesized by it in the normal course of events.

   I would like to continue with a discussion of only two of many intriguing aspects of lens regeneration. A major difference between normal lens development and lens regeneration is that in the latter, the lens rudiment does not separate early from surrounding tissue, but remains connected to the iris epithelium and continues to receive cells from it (Reyer, 1971), until Stage XI. This is accomplished via a recognizable "stalk", itself depigmented from Stage VII on. The boundary between the stalk and the lens regenerate is histologically imprecise and difficult to determine at most Stages (Fig. 1 - arrows). Even when depigmented (as is the lens regenerate), this structure never exhibits a positive immunofluorescence reaction with any crystallin antibody (c.f. Fig. 2D; and McDevitt and Brahma, 1982a). Moreover, without

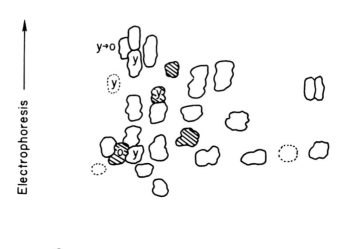

Fig. 5 *Peptide maps of tryptic digests of* N. viridescens
*adult normal and regenerated γ crystallins (Figs 3 and 4, D)
oxidized with performic acid. Low-voltage electrophoresis
was performed with pH 3.6 pyridine-acetate buffer; chromatography was performed at 90° to the electrophoresis direction
in the solvent BAWP (butan-1-ol-acetic acid-water-pyridine
15:3: 12:10, v/v). Cross hatched circles, peptides present
only in normal γ crystallins; broken circles, peptides present
only in regenerated γ crystallins; solid circles, peptides
common to both. (From McDevitt and Brahma, 1982b; with the
permission of Academic Press).*

exception, the external layer/lens epithelium adjoining the
stalk is the last area (until Stage VIII) to acquire an immunofluorescence reaction for crystallins. In a mature (Stage
IX to X) regenerate, the positive immunofluorescence reaction
for α or β crystallins in the lens epithelium, with the
negative, histologically-indistinguishable adjacent stalk
cells, permits discrimination of the boundaries between the
two. The hitherto neglected role of the stalk of the lens
regenerate in determination of the timing of the acquisition
of "lensness", i.e., expression of crystallins, bears further
investigation.

It has been well-documented for several decades that lens
regeneration *in situ* from the dorsal iris is dependent upon
a stimulus coming from the neural retina, that is, if the
neural retina is removed, lens regeneration is delayed until
the neural retina has itself regenerated (for reviews, see

Reyer, 1977; Yamada, 1977). Despite much research, such a
"factor(s)" — in the classical sense — has not been idenfitied
or characterized. Iris epithelial cells in cell culture, however, can be found to transform into lens cells without the
presence of retina (Eguchi *et al.*, 1974; Yamada, 1977); the
effect of neural retina thus appears to be permissive rather
than instructive, and its presence is not an absolute condition for transformation of iris epithelial cells into lens
cells. Yamada and Beauchamp (1978) have suggested that the
neural retinal "factor" involved in lens regeneration acts
indirectly, to preferentially shorten the cell cycle time in
the dorsal iris epithelial cells *in vivo* as compared to
ventral iris (which cannot regenerate a lens *in vivo*). This
would permit the dorsal iris epithelial cells to go through
the requisite number of cell cycles (6 to 7) for conversion
into lens cells, before mitosis ceases once again in the iris
epithelium. They point to *in vitro* observations (Yamada
and McDevitt, 1974; Eguchi *et al.*, 1974) that both dorsal and
ventral iris epithelial cells have similar cell cycle times
and similar abilities to convert into lens cells. This interesting hypothesis does not, however, address itself to the
paradox of dorsal iris competence vs. ventral iris incom-
petence to regenerate a lens *in situ*. It must also be presumed that any neural retinal "factor" must be available to
both sectors of iris tissue.

This intriguing phenomenon of regeneration of the eye
lens, with important implications for practical application,
recommends itself as a fertile subject for vision research.
It remains for the new techniques of molecular biology,
concomitant with new insights into long-recognized problems,
to elucidate the mechanism(s) that permits transformation of
iris tissue, in the presence of neural retina, into lens.

ACKNOWLEDGEMENTS

Samir K. Brahma, Laurie Croft, Sharon DiRienzo and Tuneo
Yamada provided invaluable collaboration on much of the work
discussed. This research was supported by the National Eye
Institue, N.I.H. (EY-02534).

REFERENCES

Asselbergs, F.A.M., Koopmans, M., van Venrooij, W.J. and
    Bloemendal, H. (1979). β crystallin synthesis in
    oocytes. *Exp. Eye Res.* **28**, 475–482.
Berardi, C.A. and McDevitt, D.S. (1982). Lens regeneration

from the dorsal iris in *Eurycea bislineata*, the two-lined
salamander. *Experientia* **38**, 851-852.

Bloemendal, H. (1977). The vertebrate eye lens. *Science* **197**,
127–138.

Eguchi, G., Abe, S. and Watanabe, K. (1974). Differentiation
of lenslike structure from newt iris epithelial cells *in
vitro*. *Proc. Natl. Acad. Sci. U.S.A.* **71**, 5052–5056.

McDevitt, D.S. and Brahma, S.K. (1981). Ontogeny and
localization of the α, β and γ crystallins in newt eye
lens development. *Dev. Biol.* **84**, 449-454.

McDevitt, D.S. and Brahma, S.K. (1982a). α, β and γ crystallins in the regenerating lens of *Notophthalmus viridescens*.
Exp. Eye Res. **34**, 587-594.

McDevitt, D.S. and Brahma, S.K. (1982b). Ontogeny and localization of the crystallins in eye lens development and
regeneration. In "Cell Biology of the Eye" (Ed D.S.
McDevitt), Academic Press, New York, pp. 143-191.

McDevitt, D.S. and Croft, L.R. (1977). On the existence of
γ crystallin in the bird lens. *Exp. Eye Res.* **25**,
473–481.

Reyer, R.W. (1971). DNA synthesis and the incorporation of
labelled iris cells into the lens during lens regeneration
in adult newts. *Devel. Biol.* **24**, 535–558.

Reyer, R.W. (1977). The amphibian eye, development and regeneration. In "Handbook of Sensory Physiology" *VII/5*;
Visual System in Vertebrates, (Ed. F. Crescitelli) pp.
309-390, Springer, Berlin.

Slingsby, C. and Croft, L.R. (1973). Developmental changes
in the low molecular weight proteins of the bovine lens.
Exp. Eye Res. **17**, 369–376.

Stone, L.S. (1967). An investigation recording all sala-
manders which can and cannot regenerate a lens from the
dorsal iris. *J. Exp. Zool.* **164**, 87–104.

Yamada, T. (1967). Cellular and subcellular events in
Wolffian lens regeneration. *Curr. Top. Devel. Biol.* **2**,
247–283.

Yamada, T. (1977). Control mechanisms in cell type conversion in newt lens regeneration. "Monographs in Developmental Biology" (Ed. A. Wolsky) Vol. 13, Karger, Basel.

Yamada, T. and Beauchamp, J.J. (1978). The cell cycle of
cultured iris epithelial cells: its possible role in cell-
type conversion. *Devel. Biol.* **66**, 275–278.

Yamada, T. and McDevitt, D.S. (1974). Direct evidence for
transformation of differentiated iris epithelial cells
into lens cells. *Devel. Biol.* **38**, 104–118.

MOLECULAR OVERLAPS AND INTERCONVERSIONS BETWEEN RETINA AND OTHER TISSUES: A BRIEF OUTLINE

R.M. CLAYTON

Institute of Animal Genetics, University of Edinburgh, West Mains Road, Edinburgh EH9 3JN, UK

The genetics of RP in man and the description of RP-like conditions in animals both lead to the conclusion that there must be a variety of distinct mechanisms, all of which can lead to breakdown and degeneration in the photoreceptor-pigment epithelium region of the retina, and this, in principle, could be due to a defect in the pigment epithelium, in the photoreceptors, in both, or be extrinsic to both. An important aim of RP research must ultimately be the elucidation of the primary defect, both for the development of possible therapies and for the detection of heterozygotes or individuals at risk, yet retina biopsies cannot be regarded as a serious possibility. However, recent information on the nature of tissue differentiation in general and on interconversions of ocular tissues in particular are not only of interest in themselves but hold out some hope that the molecular lesions may be sought for in more accessible tissues.

Interconversions of different tissues of the eye were first shown to be possible by experimental manipulations of the amphibian eye *in situ*, when it was found that lens can be regenerated from iris, and that neural retina and pigment epithelium could regenerate each other and that the iris could also be regenerated (reviewed, Stone, 1959; Reyer 1977; and see McDevitt, this volume). Retinal structures have also been obtained *in vivo* from extraocular sources (reviewed Clayton, 1982*a*).

A significant development in this field was made by Eguchi and Okada (1973) and Okada *et al.* (1975), who showed that pigment epithelium and neural retina of the chick could both redifferentiate in cell culture conditions, to give rise to lens cells expressing lens crystallins. Neural retina could also give rise to pigment cells. This phenomenon, which

they termed transdifferentiation, has been found in all
vertebrate species so far examined, including the human foetus
(reviews Eguchi, 1979; Okada, 1980; Eguchi and Itoh, 1981;
Clayton 1979).

A wide range of tissues have been found to have this property of transdifferentiation to lens, including cornea, iris,
neural retina, pigmented retina, and embryo adenohypophysis
(reviewed Clayton, 1978; 1982*a,b*). Furthermore, other interconversions are possible in appropriate *in vitro* conditions,
including the formation of neuronal cells from retinal pigment
epithelium (Tsunematsu and Coulombre, 1981) as well as the
formation of pigment epithelium from neural retina (Okada
et al., 1975) and the formation of pigmented cells and neurone-
like cells from lens epithelim (Patek and Clayton, 1982;
Clayton and Patek, 1982), while both pigment epithelium and
neural retina, including photoreceptors, have been obtained
from iris (Hoperskaya and Zviadadze, 1981).

The use of techniques of great sensitivity and high re-
solution has shown in recent years that many substances once
thought of as tissue specific may be detected, at low levels,
in several other tissues which may be developmentally and
functionally distinct from the tissue which is the major
source of the gene product in question (reviewed Clayton 1982*a*,
b). There is some evidence suggesting that interconversions
may be associated with the expression, in the starting tissue,
of gene products at low levels, which normally are found at
high levels in the tissue to which the interconversion takes
place (Clayton *et al.*, 1979). Lens proteins (crystallins)
or crystallin mRNA have been detected at low levels in iris,
neural retina, pigmented retina and embryo adenohypophysis;
and some other tissues which may give rise to non-lenticular
lens cells (reviewed Clayton 1982*a,b*). During transdifferentiation of chick neural retina, retinal pigment epithelium, or
embryo eye cup to lens cells, it can be shown that crystallin
mRNA and crystallin proteins increase steadily, (Thomson
et al., 1978, 1981; Clayton *et al.*, 1979; Yasuda *et al.*, 1981)
and the cells eventually obtained have characteristic lens
ultrastructure (reviews, Eguchi 1979; Eguchi and Itoh, 1981;
Okada, 1980; Clayton, 1978, 1982*a,b*).

δ crystallin has also been detected in chick and quail
embryonic mid-brain, (Barabanov, 1982), which has not yet
been shown to be capable of transdifferentiation to lens,
but which is the region of the brain from which light sensitive cells are obtained during development. (Salvini-Plawen
and Mayr, 1977). δ crystallin has also been found in single
cells derived from chick embryo limb (Kodama and Eguchi,
1982), following the type of manipulation which is most
commonly used to obtain transdifferentiation *in vitro*. The

authors suggest a neural crest origin for these cells.   Just
as crystallin mRNAs have been detected in retina, so lens
cells have also been found to express, at low levels, mRNA
species which are abundant in pigment epithelium and in
neural retina (Jackson *et al*., 1978).   This may be related
to the production of the pigmented and neurone-like cells from
lens epithelium in culture, referred to above, but the biochemical nature of these cells remains to be investigated.
There are numerous other examples both direct and indirect, of
molecular species characteristic of retina which may also be
detected in other tissues, including iris, lens, choroid, uvea
and cornea, and in some cases, extraocular tissues such as
brain, skin, kidney or liver, (see for example Clayton *et al*.,
1968; Mikhailov and Barabanov, 1975; Benezra, 1976; Brinkman
et al., 1978, from which papers further references may be
obtained).   Some of these retina antigens have been shown
to differ in their spectrum of cross reactivities, ontogeny
and quantitiative level of expression.   Molecular species
important in photoreceptor cells may be detected elsewhere.
Figure 1 shows immunofluorescent localization, possibly of cell
membrane components in the Xenopus retina, using a total lens
antiserum.   Antibodies to bovine rhodopsin (generally considered to be characteristic of and confined to the photoreceptors) were found to react with retina extract and also
with determinants in cornea, choroid, and sclera, (Brinkman
et al., 1979); while Deguchi (1981) found a rhodopsin-like
photosensitivity in chick pineal.   There is also cross reactivity between species for certain retina antigens (Brinkman *et al*., 1980), holding out hope that human tissues may

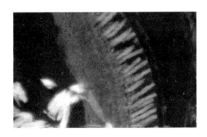 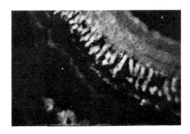

A   B

*Fig. 1 Immunofluorescence of Xenopus tadpole retina with
antiserum to total chick lens (1A) or to total Xenopus lens
(1B) shows species cross reactive material tending to
localize in retina cell membranes (Clayton and Campbell,
unpubl.).   The maximum localization is on the lens, fragments
of which are fluorescing brightly.   In the retina the maximum
localization is on the photoreceptors.*

be examined by heterologous reagents. Belehadrek *et al.*
(1979) used antisera to guinea pig retina to detect antigens
on human retinoblastoma cells, thus pointing both to species
cross reactivity and to the retention of retina antigens
on cultured malignant cell lines. Long term cultures of rat
lens cells lost crystallin expression, but acquired an antigen characteristic of normal retina (Hamada *et al.*, 1979).

We have begun to examine the possibility that mutants
affecting retinal integrity may affect the course of transdifferentiation. The *rdd* chick mutant, (Wilson *et al.*, this
volume), shows programmed cell death of a subset of neural
retina cells in culture, affecting subsequent transdifferentiation events but not those occurring earlier (Kondoh *et al.*,
1980*a*). The Hy-1 chick, which has effects both on lens and
retina cells, and on crystallin gene expression in both lens
and transdifferentiating neural retina, (reviewed Clayton,
1982*a*) also shows a change in the proportion of neuroepithelial
and neuronal cells differentiating in cultures of early
embryos (Kondoh *et al.*, 1980*b*). The *beg* mutant shows accelerated transdifferentiation of neural andpigment epithelium
to lens (Pollock *et al.*, this volume and in prep). The time
required for transdifferentiation is governed by the level
of crystallin mRNA, the number of retina cells expressing
crystallin mRNA and their capacity for cell-cell contacts
(Thomson *et al.*, 1981; Clayton 1982). The defect in *beg* may
therefore affect one of these parameters.

Retinal cells may be obtained from other tissues, molecular
species important in retina may be detected elsewhere, and
the process of transdifferentiation itself may be an indicator
of genetic lesions. The wider potential for RP research of
transdifferentiation phenomena remains to be explored.

REFERENCES

Barabanov, V.M. (1982). Extra-lenticular localisation of
    δ-crystallin in *coturnix japonica, TES. Doklady Akademii
    Nauk S.S.S.R.* **262**, 1491-1494.
Belehradek, J. Jr., Block-Michel, E., Faure, J-P., Campinchi,
    R. and Thonier, R. (1979). Expression of organ-specific
    antigen(s) in long-term cultured human retinoblastoma
    cells. In "Immunology and Immunopathology of the Eye"
    (Eds A.M. Silverstein and G.R. O'Connor), pp. 197-201.
    Masson, New York.
Benezra, D. (1976). Experimental specific memory reaction
    to cornea, lens and retina antigens. *Arch. Ophthalmol.* **94**,
    661-664.
Braverman, M. Cohen, C. and Katoh, A. (1969). Cytotoxicity
    of lens antisera to dissociated chick neural retina cells
    in tissue culture. *J. Emb. exp. Morph.* **21**, 391-406.

Brinkman, C.J.J., Oerlemans-van Zutphen, M.P.J. and Broekhuyse, R.M. (1978). Demonstration of common antigenicity
in corneal epithelium and other tissues in the bovine eye.
Exp. Eye Res. **27**, 81-86.

Brinkman, C.J.J., Oerlemans-van Zutphen, M.P.J. and Broekhuyse, R.M. (1979). Ocular antigens X. Bovine rohdopsin
and α-crystallin: a study of their immunogenicity in the
rabbit and antigenic relationships with various ocular
tissues. *Exp. Eye Res*. **29**, 609-617.

Brinkman, C.J.J., Tolhuizen, R.F.J. and Broekhuyse, R.M. (1980).
Ocular antigenz XI. Common antigenic determinants in the
soluble retinal fractions of man, monkey, pig and calf.
Exp. Eye Res. **30**, 391-400.

Clayton, R.M. (1978). Divergence and Convergence in lens
cell differentiation: Regulation of the formation and
specific content of lens fibre cells. In "Stem Cells and
Tissue Homeostasis" (Eds B.I. Lord, C.S. Potten and R.J.
Cole), pp. 115-138. Cambridge University Press, Cambridge.

Clayton, R.M. (1982*a*). Cellular and molecular aspects of
differentiation and transdifferentiation of ocular tissues
in vitro. In "Differentiation *in Vitro*" British Society
for Cell Biology Symposium 4. (Eds M.M. Yeoman and D.E.S.
Truman), pp. 83-120, Cambridge University Press.

Clayton, R.M. (1982*b*). The molecular basis for competence,
determination, and transdifferentiation: A hypothesis.
In "Stability and Switching in Cellular Differentiation"
(Eds R.M. Clayton and D.E.S. Truman), pp. 23-38, Plenum
Press, New York.

Clayton, R.M., Campbell, J.C. and Truman, D.E.S. (1968). A
re-examination of organ specificity of lens antigens.
Exp. Eye Res., **7**, 11-29.

Clayton, R.M., Thomson, I. and de Pomerai, D.I. (1979).
Relationship between crystallin mRNA expression in retinal
cells and their capacity to re-differentiate into lens
cells. *Nature* **282**, 628-629.

Clayton, R.M. and Patek, C.E. (1982). The effects of N-methyl-
N'-nitro-N-nitrosoguanidine on the differentiation of
chicken lens epithelium *in vitro*: the cocurrence of unusual
cell types. In "Stability and Switching in Cellular Differentiation" (Eds R.M. Clayton and D.E.S. Truman), pp. 229-
238, Plenum Press, New York.

Deguchi, T. (1981). Rhodopsin-like photosensitivity of isolated
chicken pineal gland. *Nature* **290**, 706-707.

Eguchi, G. (1979). "Transdifferentiation" in pigmented epithelial cells of vertebrate eyes *in vitro*. In "Mechanisms
of Cell Change" (Eds J.D. Ebert and T.S. Okada), pp. 273-291.
John Wiley and Sons, New York.

Eguchi, G. and Okada, T.S. (1973). Differentiation of lens

tissue from the progeny of chick retinal pigment cells
cultured *in vitro*: a demonstration of a switch of cell
type in clonal cell culture. *Proc. Nat. Acad. Sci.* **70**,
1495-1499.

Eguchi, G. and Itoh, Y. (1981). Regulation of transdifferentiation by microenvironmental factors in vertebrate pigmented epithelial cells *in vitro*. In "Phenotypic Expression in Pigment Cells" Proc. of XIth Int. Pigment Cell
Conference, Japan, 1980, (Ed. M. Seiji), University of
Tokyo Press, pp. 27!-278.

Hamada, Y., Watanabe, K., Aoyama, H. and Okada, T.S. (1979).
Differentiation and dedifferentiation of rat lens epi-
thelial cells in short- and long-term cultures. *Develop.,
Growth and Differ.* **21**, 204-219.

Hoperskaya, O.A. and Zviadadze, K.G. (1981). Transdifferentiation of adult frog iris in retina or lens by exogenous
influences. *Develop. Growth and Differ.* **23**, 201-213.

Jackson, J.F., Clayton, R.M., Williamson, R., Thomson, I.,
Truman, D.E.S., and de Pomerai, D.I. (1978). Sequence
complexity and tissue distribution of chick lens crystallin mRNAs. *Develop. Biol.* **65**, 383-395.

Kodama, R. and Eguchi, G. (1982). Dissociated limb bud cells
of chick embryo can express lens specificity when re-
aggregated and cultured *in vitro*. *Dev. Biol.* **91**, 221-226.

Kondoh, H., Yasuda, K., Okada, T.S. and Clayton, R.M. (1980).
Differentiation and transdifferentiation *in vitro* of
neural retina from mutant chickens with hyperplastic lens
epithelium. *Dev. Growth and Differ.* **22**, 875-885.

Kondoh, H., Okada, T.S., Randall, C., Brodie, J., Zehir, A.
and Clayton, R.M. (1980). Intrinsic programming of neural
retina degeneration in a mutant chick. *Dev. Growth Diffn.*
22, 724.

Mikhailov, A.T. and Barabanov, V.M. (1975). Immunochemical
analysis of water-soluble antigens of chick retina in the
course of embryogenesis. *J. Embryol. exp. Morph.* **34**,
531-537.

Okada, T.S. (1980). Cellular metaplasia or transdifferentiation. *Curr. Topics in Develop. Biol.* **16**, 349-380.

Okada, T.S., Itoh, Y., Watanabe, K. and Eguchi, G. (1975).
Differentiation of lens in cultures of neural retinal cells
of chick embryos. *Dev. Biol.* **45**, 318-29.

Patek, C.E. and Clayton, R.M. (1982). The dedifferentiation of
of abnormal differentiation of chicken lens epithelium
by N-methyl-N'-Nitro-N-nitrosoguanidine *in vitro*. *Exp.
Eye Res.* (in press).

Perkins, E.S. and Wood, R.M. (1963). Antigenic components
of guinea-pig tissues. *Exp. Eye Res.* **2**, 255-264.

Reyer, R.W. (1977). The amphibian eye: development and

regeneration. In "The Visual System in Vertebrates"
(Ed. F. Crescitelli), pp. 309-90, Springer-Verlag, Berlin.
Salvini-Plawen, L.V. and Mayr, E. (1977). Evolution of photo-
receptors and eyes. In "Evolutionary Biology" (Eds M.K.
Hecht, W.C. Steene and B. Wallace), Vol. 10, pp. 207-263.
Plenum Press, New York.
Stone, L.S. (1959). Regeneration of the retina, iris, and
lens. In "Regeneration in Vertebrates", (Ed. C.S. Thorn-
ton), pp. 3-14, University of Chicago Press, Chicago.
Thomson, I., Wilkinson, C.E., Jackson, J.F., de Pomerai, D.I.,
Clayton, R.M., Truman, D.E.S., and Williamson, R. (1978).
Isolation and cell-free translation of chick lens crystallin mRNA during normal development and transdifferentiation
of neural retina. *Develop. Biol.* **65**, 372-382.
Thomson, I., Yasuda, K., de Pomerai, D.I., Clayton, R.M. and
Okada, T.S. (1981). The accumulation of lens-specific
protein and mRNA in cultures of neural retina from 3.5
day chick embryos. *Exp. Cell Res.* **135**, 445-459.
Tsunematsu, Y. and Coulombre, A.J. (1981). Demonstration of
transdifferentiation of neural retina from pigmented
retina in culture. *Dev., Growth and Differn.* **23**, 297-311.
Yasuda, K., Thomson, I., de Pomerai, D.I., Clayton, R.M. and
Okada, T.S. (1979). Changes in crystallin mRNA contents
in the course of the transdifferentiatio of lens from
neural retina. *Proc. Jap. Soc. Dev. Biol.* p. 68.

ENHANCED TRANSDIFFERENTIATION IN CULTURES OF EMBRYONIC NEURAL RETINAL CELLS BY CHINOFORM-FERRIC CHELATE INDUCED SELECTIVE ELIMINATION OF NEUROBLASTS

S.L. SHINDE and G. EGUCHI

*Institute of Molecular Biology, Faculty of Science,
Nagoya University, Nagoya 464, Japan*

SUMMARY

Transdifferentiation of 6- to 8-day-old chicken embryonic
neural retina was observed both in the complete absence of
neuroblasts, which was induced by treating cultures with
chinoform-ferric chelate, and in the presence of neuroblasts
in the corresponding untreated controls. Shortly after
treatment, some of the epithelial cells underwent precocious pigmentation in treated cultures. During the latent
growth phase, both treated and control cultures local areas
with fusiform cells or stratification of the epithelial cells
were observed. During the predifferentiation phase, lentoid
bodies appeared precociously and gradually increased in
number in treated cultures. In addition to pigmentation, the
density of the fusiform cells and the extent of epithelial
stratification was more noticeable in the controls and continued so until terminal differentiation. During the terminal phase of differentiation, lentoidogenesis and formation of pigment cell colonies continued in both control and
experimental cultures. Macroscopic observations and measurements of crystallin and melanin contents showed enhancement
of both "lentoid" and "pigment" transdifferentiation in
treated cultures, especially of lentoids. Enhanced transdifferentiation in the absence of neuroblasts suggests a
putative "inhibitory influence" and also that transdifferentiation appears to occur in this system from retinal glia
cells or undifferentiated progenitor cells. In treated
cultures, both pigmentation and lentoid differentiation are
precocious, the pigmentation of some epithelial cells appearing shortly after exposure, and lentoids appearing in the
predifferentiation phase.

INTRODUCTION

The transdifferentiation of cultured chicken embryonic neural retinal cells is now a well-established phenomenon (see reviews by Okada, 1976 and Clayton, 1979) after its discovery by Okada *et al.* (1975) and Itoh *et al.* (1975). It is already known that certain factors such as culture medium (Itoh, 1976; Okada, 1977; Clayton *et al.*, 1977; Pritchard *et al.*, 1978; Araki and Okada, 1978), embryonic age (Araki and Okada, 1978; de Pomerai and Clayton, 1978; Nomura and Okada, 1979), inoculum density (Clayton *et al.*, 1977) and serum factors (de Pomerai and Gali, 1981) control the extent and direction of this change.

   The mechanisms involved in transdifferentiation remain to be elucidated and the attempts to analyse the origin and mode of transient structural changes are limited. As to the origin of transdifferentiated cells, there are already suggestions that there are multipotent embryonic neural retina cells (Okada *et al.*, 1979), and dissociation-reaggregation culture studies suggest retinal glia as a source of lentoidogenesis (Moscona and Degenstein, 1981). Intermediate structural changes during the transdifferentation of neural retina into pigment cells have been observed by time-lapse photography, and evidence obtained that such a change occurs in response to stimulation of the tricarboxylic acid cycle (Pritchard, 1981).

   The present studies were based on the observation that chinoform induced the degeneration of neuroblasts in cultures of embryonic neural retina cells (Ohtsuka *et al.*, 1981). We were able to develop this method further as a technique for the complete elimination of neuroblasts from cultured cells of 6- to 8-day-old embryonic neural retina. Chinoform-treated cultures compared with corresponding controls showed enhancement in transdifferentiation both in time and extent. This indicates that the retinal nerve cells produce an inhibitory influence on transdifferentiation.

MATERIALS AND METHODS

Tissue Isolation

Entire eyes removed from 6- to 8-day-old chick embryos were dissected in Ca^{++}- and Mg^{++}-free Hank's saline (CMF) according to the procedure described by Okada *et al.* (1975) so as to get a clean neural retinal layer.

Cell Suspension

Cleaned pieces of neural retinae after rinsing twice with CMF were dissociated by incubating them in 0.25% trypsin (Difco, 1:250) for 30 min. A cell suspension was then prepared according to the procedure of Okada *et al.* (1975).

Cell Culture

Dissociated cells were inoculated in 55 mm plastic culture dishes (Nuncatom) at an approximate density of $5-7 \times 10^6$ cells/plate, or cells from the neural retina of one eye per plate. Most cultures were grown and maintained in 3.5 ml of medium containing Eagle's minimum essential medium (MEM, NISSUI, Tokyo) supplemented with 6% foetal calf serum (Chimera Biochemicals, USA), 0.03% L-glutamine and 0.2% sodium bicarbonate. The same batch of serum was used during the experiments. The medium was changed every 2 days in controls and during treatment by chinoform in the experimental cultures until the termination of cultures by 70 days. The culture dishes were incubated in a water-saturated atmosphere with 95% air-5% CO_2.

Chinoform Treatment

Chinoform (5-chloro-7-iodo-8-quinolinol) is insoluble in water, and was dissolved in dimethyl sulphoxide (DMSO) together with $FeFl_3$ to produce chinoform-ferric chelate. The molar ratio of chinoform to ferric ion in the solution was maintained at 10:3 according to the method of Ohtsuka *et al.* (1981). Four to six days after inoculation of embryonic neural retinal cells, the experimental cultures were treated with 50 µM of chinoform-ferric chelate and the corresponding control cultures with an equivalent volume of DMSO solvent for 4 days. It is important to note that free chinoform is known to be ineffective in bringing about degeneration of neuroblasts in culture (Ohtsuka *et al.*, 1981). Although the ferric chelate of chinoform was used in the present study, it will be referred to only as chinoform in the text for the sake of brevity.

Termination of Cultures

During the terminal phase of cultures, between 40 to 70 days, they were examined both qualitatively and quantitatively. Some of the cultures were fixed with Bouin's and stained by Mallory's method. From these, the number of macroscopically visible "lentoid bodies" and colonies of pigmented

cells were counted using a reference dish marked with iso-
diametric squares. Certain other cultures were individually
harvested at appropriate intervals, using a rubber policeman,
and then homogenizing in a fixed volume of CMF.

Quantitative Estimations

CMF homogenates were used for measurements of total protein,
melanin and crystallin contents. The protein content of the
crude homogenate was estimated by the method of Lowry *et al.*
(1951) with lyophilized bovine γ-globulin as standard. Homogenates were then centrifuged for 10 min at 3500 × g. The
melanin content of the sediment fraction was determined by
a photometric method (Oikawa and Nakayasu, 1973). The presence of δ-crystallin and its approximate amount were
assessed by performing Ouchterlony's immunodiffusion test.
The estimation of δ-crystallin content was made by quantitative immunoelectrophoresis (Laurell, 1966). The relative
amount of melanin content estimated from the sediment
fraction is expressed per culture, while the crystallin content is represented per mg protein of the individual cultures (Table 1).

RESULTS

*Initial Spreading Phase of Whole Neural Retina Culture
(4 to 6 days)*

During this phase, cultured embryonic neural retinal cells
of 6- to 8-day-old chick embryos formed a sheet of flattened
epithelial cells underlying aggregates of neuroblast cells.
The neuroblasts had long cytoplasmic processes, which may
have been axons. By the end of the spreading phase, the
aggregates of neuroblasts segregated into more compact
clumps and developed an intricate pattern of inter-aggregate
cytoplasmic connections.

Phase of Chinoform Treatment (6 to 14 days)

Almost all neuroblasts were gradually eliminated over the 4
days of chinoform treatment. Soon after the treatment was
stopped, some of the epithelial cells in the experimental
cultures showed a precocious appearance of pigmentation
(Fig. 1A) and many of them had become pigmented by only four
days after the treatment. The DMSO-treated controls, on
the other hand, remained completely unaffected and still
contained epithelial cells and neuroblasts (Fig. 1B).

TABLE 1

Quantitative variations in extent of transdifferentiation in neuro-retinal cells of 8-day-old chick embryos

Culture No.	Period of culture	Amount of δ-crystallin (µg/mg of proteins)		E/C for crystallin content	Amount of melanin (µg/culture)		E/C For melanin content
		Chinoform treated [E]	Control [C]		Chinoform treated [E]	Control [C]	
1	48	149	25	5.96	3.2	2.5	1.28
2	50	123	33	3.73	5.9	5.6	1.06
3	52	76	9	8.44	8.6	8.8	0.98
4	65	119	15	7.93	6.8	2.8	2.42

Culture medium: Eagle's minimum essential medium supplemented with 6% Foetal calf serum.

Treatment with chinoform: 60 M of chinoform ferric chelate (Experimentals) and corresponding volume of DMSO (Controls) for 4 days.

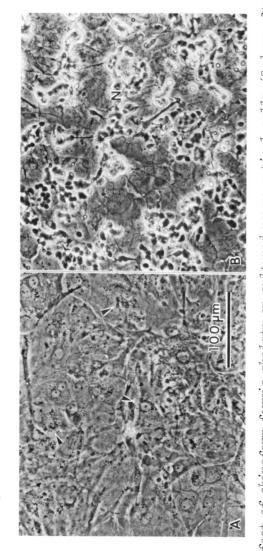

Fig. 1 Effect of chinoform-ferric chelate on cultured neuro-retinal cells (7 days after treatment). (A) Treated cells, showing complete absence of neuroblasts. Note the partially pigmented cells (arrows). (B) Corresponding control, showing aggregates of neuroblasts (N) upon a sheet of flattened epithelial cells.

Latent Growth Phase (15 to 20 days)

No major change was observed in either control or experimental cultures apart from the appearance and increase in number of fusiform cells and localized initiation of epithelial stratification. These processes were more marked in controls.

Predifferentiation Phase (20 to 40 days)

The lentoid bodies began to appear in the experimental cultures only. Initially, they were small in size and appeared singly. By the end of this phase, both individual and the composite lentoids were found sparsely distributed throughout the culture (Fig. 2A). Over this period the majority of the epithelial cells in the experimental cultures became partially pigmented. The control cultures remained devoid of lentoid bodies (Fig. 2B). However, the apparent density of the fusiform cells and the stratifying epithelial cells increased continuously so that the previously identified sites of such cells became confluent in places. The relative apparent density of these cells remained low and the areas restricted in the experimental cultures. After the onset of this phase, some of the epithelial cells in the controls underwent partial pigmentation, nearly 20 days later than in the experimental cultures. It is important to note that in control cultures of this phase, most of the neuroblast aggregates gradually diminished due to loss of neuroblasts and were then no longer seen.

Differentiation Phase (40 to 70 days)

The number of lentoid bodies increased in experimental cultures; many of them acquired composite form and showed a dense distribution (Fig. 2C). The lentoid bodies also began to appear at occasional sites in the control cultures. Although the number of lentoid bodies increased gradually in the controls, their size remained relatively small and they were sparsely distributed compared to the experimental cultures (Fig. 2D). The number of lentoid bodies counted from some of the terminal cultures was always 2 to 7 times more in the experimental than in the control cultures.

Pigment cell colonies appeared in both the cultures during the beginning of this phase as local sites of densely packed epithelial cells. They were often sharply delimited from the rest of the epithelium. Gradually, the cells of these colonies became compactly arranged and underwent pigmentation in a centrifugal direction. No significant

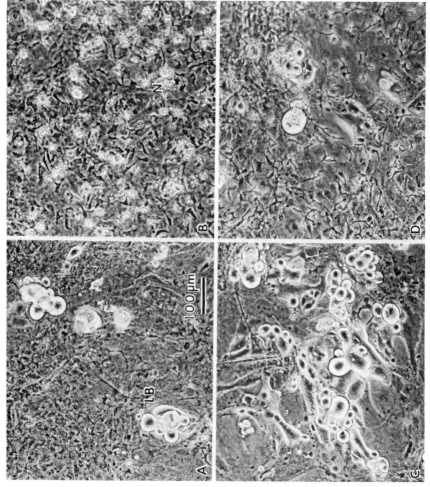

(For legend, see opposite)

difference was noticed between the morphology of pigment
cell colonies from the experimental and the control cultures.
However, the colonies in the experimental cultures were usually
much larger in size and showed a relatively compact arrangement of the constituent cells. In addition, now most of the
epithelial cells in the experimental cultures appeared partially
pigmented. The number of pigment cell colonies in the experimental cultures was usually more than in the controls. Epithelial stratification continued only in the controls at this
stage and towards the end of this phase they were much stratified and occupied a greater area with increasing confluence.

Quantitative measurements of δ-crystallin and melanin content from cultures harvested during the terminal phase evince
the enhancement of transdifferentiation in chinoform-treated
cultures as compared to controls (Table 1). The crystallin
content was found to be always higher in treated cultures
with four- to eight-fold increase over the corresponding
controls. The rise in melanin content, however, is limited
to a maximum of two-fold and occasionally, as in case of
sample 3, it was lower than in the control.

DISCUSSION

The temporal appearance and extent of transdifferentiation in
cultured embryonic neural retina cells is known to be controlled by various culture conditions. In the present study,
the elimination of neuroblasts is followed by earlier and
more extensive transdifferentiation to both "pigment" and
"lentoid" compared to the corresponding controls. Transdifferentiation appears to be controlled by neuroblasts. It
is important to note that transdifferentiation events follow
soon after elimination of the neuroblasts, not only in the
treated but also in the control cultures. The possibility is,
therefore, that the neuroblasts block the transdifferentiation pathways by some kind of inhibitory influence, which
operates optimally under *in vivo* conditions. The relative
increase of stratified epithelium in control cultures of this
study may be due to the presence of competent cells capable

Fig. 2 *Enhancement in lentoid transdifferentiation in absence
of neuroblasts killed by treatment of chinoform-ferric chelate.
(A) 27 days after treatment, composite and smaller lentoids
(LB) are seen in treated cells but not in the control cells
(B) (C) 47 days after treatment, many composite lentoids are
visible in treated cells while such lentoids are few and
smaller in control cells (D). (Scale: 100 μm).*

of entering into the transdifferentiation pathways but blocked
from doing so by the influence of neuroblasts, and hence
piling up. Work is now under progress in this laboratory
to confirm this inhibitory effect.

The specific origin of transdifferentiating structures
from cultured embryonic neuro-retinal cells remains largely
unresolved because of the complex behaviour of multispecific
cells. However, they can be broadly classified into epithelial cells and neuroblasts. The epithelial cells can be
considered as derivatives of glial cells, as in cultured
brain cells (Shein, 1965). However, the possibility of progenitor cells giving rise to both cell types can not be excluded. Okada *et al.* (1979) suggested that such multipotent
progenitor cells are able to enter the various possible pathways of normal differentiation and transdifferentiation.
The lentoidogenic cells are suggested to have neuronal origin
(de Pomerai *et al.*, 1977) or glial origin (Moscona and Degenstein, 1981) but from the present studies, neuronal cells
can be directly ruled out as precursors. In cultures showing enhanced transdifferentiation in the absence of neural
cells, the possibility of secondarily formed nerve cells is
most unlikely although we are at present examining this possibility. Therefore, it appears that transdifferentiation
originates either from retinal glial cells or from undifferentiated progenitor cells.

ACKNOWLEDGEMENT

We sincerely thank Professor K. Yakgi, School of Medicine,
Nagoya University and Dr K. Ohtsuka, Aichi Cancer Research
Institute, for their kind introduction of chinoform. G.E.
particularly thanks Dr R.M. Clayton, Institute of Animal
Genetics, University of Edinburgh, for her invaluable discussion and criticism. S.L.S. expresses particular thanks
to the Japanese Ministry of Education, Science and Culture,
who supported him financially as a visiting scientist for
the exchange programme between Nagoya University and Poona
University. This work was supported in part by a Grant-in-
Aid for Cancer Research (Project No. 5610033) from the Ministry of Education, Science and Culture to G.E.

REFERENCES

Araki, M. and Okada, T.S. (1978). Effects of culture media
    on the 'foreign' differentiation of lens and pigment cells
    from neural retina in vitro. *Devl. Growth & Differ.* **20**,
    71-78.

Clayton, R.M. (1979). Genetic regulation in the vertebrate lens cell. In "Mechanisms of Cell Change" (Eds J. Ebert and T.S. Okada), Wiley, New York.

Clayton, R.M., de Pomerai, D.I. and Pritchard, D.J. (1977). Experimental manipulation of alternative pathways of differentiation in cultures of embryonic chick neural retina. *Devl. Growth & Differ.* **19**, 319-328.

Itoh, Y. (1976). Enhancement of differentiation of lens and pigment cells by ascorbic acid in cultures of neural retinal cells in chick embryos. *Devl. Biol.* **54**, 157-162.

Itoh, Y., Okada, T.S., Ide, H. and Eguchi, G. (1975). The differentiation of pigment cells in cultures of chick embryonic neural retinae. *Devl. Growth & Differ.* **17**, 39-50.

Laurell, C.B. (1966). Quantitative estimation of proteins by electrophoresis in agarose gel containing antibodies. *Anal. Biochem.* **15**, 45-52.

Lowry, O.H., Rosebrough, N.J., Farr, R.J. and Randall, R.J. (1951). Protein measurements with the Folin phenol reagent. *J. Biol. Chem.* **193**, 265-275.

Moscona, A.A. and Degenstein, L. (1981). Lentoids in aggregates of embryonic neural retinal cells. *Cell Differ.* **10**, 39-46.

Nomura, K. and Okada, T.S. (1979). Age dependent change in the transdifferentiation ability of chick neural retina in cell culture. *Devl. Growth & Differ.* **21**, 161-168.

Ohtsuka, K., Ohishi, N., Eguchi, G. and Yagi, K. (1982). Degeneration of cultured neural retinal cells by chinoformferric chelate. *Experentia* **38**, 121-122.

Oikawa, A. and Nakayasu, M. (1973). Quantitative measurements of melanin as tyrosine equivalents and as weight of purified melanin. *Yale J. Biol. Med.* **46**, 500-507.

Okada, T.S. (1976). Transdifferentiation of cells of specialized eye tissues in cell culture. In "Tests of Teratogenicity *in vitro*", pp. 95—105, North-Holland; Amsterdam.

Okada, T.S. (1977). A demonstration of lens forming cells in neural retina in clonal cell culture, *Devl. Growth & Differ.* **19**, 47-55.

Okada, T.S., Itoh, Y., Watanabe, K. and Eguchi, G. (1975). Differentiation of lens in cultures of neural retinal cells of chick embryos. *Devl. Biol.* **45**, 318-329.

Okada, T.S., Yasuda, K., Araki, M. and Eguchi, G. (1979). Possible demonstration of multipotential nature of embryonic neural retina by clonal cell culture. *Devl. Biol.* **68**, 600-617.

de Pomerai, D.I., and Clayton, R.M. (1978). Influence of embryonic stage on the transdifferentiation of chick

neural retina cells in culture. *J. Embryol. exp. Morph.*
47, 179-193.

de Pomerai, D.I. and Gali, M.A.H. (1981). Influence of
serum factors on the prevalence of "normal" and "foreign"
differentiation pathways in cultures of chick embryo
neuroretinal cells. *J. Embryol. exp. Morphol.* **62**, 291-308.

de Pomerai, D.I., Pritchard, D.J. and Clayton, R.M. (1977).
Biochemical and immunological studies of lentoid formation in cultures of embryonic chick neural retina and
day old chick lens epithelium. *Devl. Biol.* **60**, 416-427.

Pritchard, D.J. (1981). Transdifferentiation of chicken
embryo neural retina into pigment epithelium: indication
of its biochemical basis. *J. Embryol. exp. Morphol.* **62**,
47.

Pritchard, D.J., Clayton, R.M. and de Pomerai, D.I. (1978).
"Transdifferentiation" of chicken neural retinal into
lens and pigment epithelium in culture: controlling influences. *J. Embryol. exp. Morphol.* **48**, 1-21.

Shein, H.M. (1965). Propagation of human fetal spongioblasts
and astrocytes in dispersed cell cultures. *Exp. Cell
Res.* **40**, 554-569.

ACCUMULATION OF GABA AND CHOLINE IN CULTURES OF CHICK EMBRYO NEURORETINAL CELLS

D.I. DE POMERAI

*Department of Zoology, University of Nottingham,
Nottingham NG7 2RD, UK*

SUMMARY

High levels of (^{3}H)GABA are accumulated by many neurone-like cells (but few glia) in early cultures of 9 day chick embryo neuroretinal (NR) cells. After 7 days *in vitro*, (^{3}H)GABA accumulation by these cultures declines markedly, associated with a loss of neurite processes and later disappearance of many neuronal aggregates. GABA accumulation remains sodium-dependent and highly sensitive to nipecotic acid (20 µM), even after 14 days *in vitro*. (^{3}H)choline accumulation, however, remains at a much lower and almost constant level throughout the culture period studied. Previous work has suggested that choline accumulation occurs into NR glial cells as well as a subpopulation of neurone-like cells. We suggest that choline accumulation may be largely neuronal in early NR cultures, but later becomes predominantly glial. This is supported by studies with sodium-free medium and the choline uptake inhibitor hemicholinium III (30 µM), which show that the sensitivity of (^{3}H)choline accumulation to both inhibitors declines progressively during NR culture.

INTRODUCTION

In a previous study (de Pomerai and Carr, 1982), we have shown that (^{3}H)GABA is accumulated predominantly by neurone-like cells in 8 day cultures of chick embryo neuroretinal (NR) cells. This involves a high affinity uptake process which is temperature and sodium dependent and is strongly inhibited by nipecotic acid (50 µM), but not by 2-4-diaminobutyric acid (DABA, 5 mM) nor by β alanine (5 mM).

Although the majority of neuronal cells and processes are strongly labelled by (^{3}H)GABA, a minority of unlabelled neurones and small numbers of densely-labelled glial cells are also found in autoradiographs of these NR cultures (de Pomerai and Carr, 1982).

By contrast, (^{3}H)choline is accumulated only by a minority of neurone-like cells in chick embryo NR cultures, while most glial cells also show considerable labelling. Although the uptake process again shows high affinity kinetics and is temperature dependent, it is only 40 to 50% inhibited by sodium-free medium or by hemicholinium III (20 µM; de Pomerai and Carr, 1982).

Thus GABA accumulation is predominantly neuronal in chick embryo NR cultures, while choline accumulation is partly neuronal and partly glial. The present report extends these studies to both earlier and later stages of culture.

MATERIALS AND METHODS

Fertile chick eggs were obtained from Ross Poultry Ltd (Bilsthorpe, Notts), and radiochemicals ((^{3}H)choline, 70 Ci/mmole; (^{3}H)GABA, 55 Ci/mmole) from the Radiochemical Centre, Amersham. All methods were as detailed previously (de Pomerai and Carr, 1982), and are outlined briefly in the figure legends.

RESULTS AND DISCUSSION

Figure 1 shows the accumulation of (^{3}H)GABA and (^{3}H)choline by 9 day chick embryo neuroretinal cultures after varying periods (3 to 18 days) *in vitro*. The data presented here are derived from 30 min assays, but essentially the same pattern emerges from 2 or 8 min assay periods (results not shown). Accumulation of (^{3}H)GABA is already high by 3 days *in vitro* and reaches a maximum around 7 days. The levels of GABA accumulation decrease sharply (by over 60%) between 7 and 10 days, and then decline more slowly until 18 days (by which stage total GABA accumulation is less than 15% of maximum). Similar but more detailed results have been obtained with cultures of 7 day chick embryo NR cells (Guérinot and Pessac, 1979), again showing a peak of GABA accumulation during the first week *in vitro* followed by a sharp decline in later cultures.

For (^{3}H)choline, a very different pattern emerges, with total accumulation levels changing relatively little (apart from some decrease around 14 days) throughout the culture

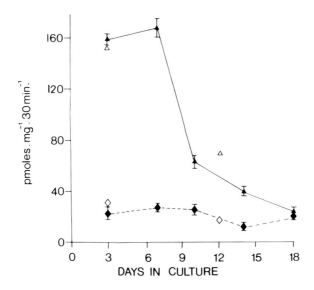

Fig. 1 *Choline and GABA accumulation by cultures of 9 day chick embryo NR cells. Cultures of 9 day embryonic NR cells were established at an initial density of 3.5 × 10⁶ cells per ml as described previously (de Pomerai and Gali, 1981a), and maintained for up to 18 days in Eagle's MEM medium with Earle's salts, containing 2 mM L-glutamine, 26 mM NaHCO₃, 100 I.U./ml penicillin, 100 µg/ml streptomycine and 10% foetal calf serum (all from GIBCO Europe Ltd, Paisley). At the indicated stages, cultures were washed 3 times in phosphate-buffered saline (PBS), then incubated for 30 min (also for 2 or 8 min; results not shown) at 27°C in PBS containing 1 µM (³H)GABA or 1 µM(³H)choline (both at 5 µCi/ml). Cultures were then rapidly washed 6 times in PBS containing excess (1mM) unlabelled GABA or choline, and the cell sheet was extracted with 0.1 ml of 1N NaOH. Duplicate 10 µl aliquots were taken for protein determinations (by the method of Lowry et al., 1951), while the remainder was neutralized with 8 µl of 10N HCl. Duplicate 30 µl aliquots were then mixed with 3 ml of a toluene-Triton-PPO-POPOP scintillant (700 ml: 300 ml: 1.0g: 0.1g) for counting on an Intertechnique SL30 scintillation counter (33% efficient when counting tritium).*

Each point gives the mean accumulation of (³H) label (as pmoles per mg protein per 30 min assay) together with the standard error (vertical bar) derived from duplicate samples of 3 separate cultures belonging to the same large batch.

▲——▲ *, GABA accumulation;* ◆---◆ *, choline accumulation. Open symbols give the mean levels of GABA (Δ)   (cont.)*

*(cont.) and choline (◇) accumulation determined in a pre-
liminary experiment comparing 3 and 12 day old cultures from
a different batch (only two cultures used per point).*

period studied. Again, the same pattern is found with 2 or
8 min assay periods as with the 30 min assay data presented
in Fig. 1.

In order to interpret these results, the following general
features of chick embryo NR cultures should be noted (see
e.g. Okada *et al.*, 1975; Clayton *et al.*, 1977).

Days 2 to 7   abundant neuronal aggregates present, with
                many interconnecting neurite processes; cell
                numbers at first declining, then static.
Days 7 to 12   total cell numbers beginning to increase; most
                neurite processes disappear; some loss of
                neuronal cells.
Days 12 to 20   rapid increase of total cell numbers, despite
                the loss of most neuronal aggregates; pre-
                sumably cell division is largely confined to
                the flattened epithelial cells (immature
                Müller glia).

Thus the marked decline in GABA accumulation after 7 days
in vitro (Fig. 1) is temporally correlated with the disappearance of neurite processes (indicative of neuronal dedifferentiation?) but precedes the stage at which most
neuronal cells detach. Since the majority of neurone-like
cells in chick embryo NR cultures can be labelled with
(^{3}H)GABA (de Pomerai and Carr, 1982), a 60% loss of neurones
after 7 days would not have escaped detection. In fact, we
find that the major decline in neuronal cell numbers occurs
only after 10 to 12 days of culture under our standard conditions (M. Gali, unpublished estimates of percentage cover
by different cell types in random culture fields), suggesting
that some degree of dedifferentiation may precede actual loss
of neuronal cells.

As shown in Fig. 2, GABA accumulation remains sodium
dependent (>95% inhibition by sodium-free medium) and sensitive to 20 μM nipecotic acid (approx. 90% inhibition, though
rather lower on day 9) until at least 14 days of culture.
By 18 days, however, there is some decline in the sensitivity
of GABA accumulation to both agents. This is consistent
either with a decrease in the number of cells actively accumulating GABA, or with a much reduced level of GABA accumulation by most such cells, over the 7 to 14 day period *in
vitro*. However, the specificity of the GABA uptake system
appears largely unaffected during this period.

By contrast, the sensitivity of choline accumulation to

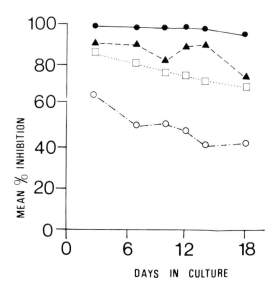

Fig. 2 *Inhibitor sensitivity of choline and GABA accumulation by cultures of 9 day chick embryo NR cells. The culture and assay methods were as detailed in the legend to Fig. 1, except that the standard assay period was 8 min. Controls used PBS for the pre-wash, incubation and post-wash steps (as for Fig. 1). Sodium-free medium (PBS containing equiosmolar Li^+ in place of Na^+; Barald and Berg, 1979a,b) was used throughout these three steps in the assays indicated. Similarly, uptake inhibitors (20 μM nipecotic acid for GABA assays; 30 μM hemicholinium III for choline assays) were present at the same concentration throughout the labelling and washing procedures where indicated. For each point, the mean accumulation of label obtained from duplicate samples of 3 separate cultures has been used to calculate the mean percentage inhibition relative to controls, as follows:*

% inhibition =

$$100 - \left(\frac{mean\ accumulation\ in\ presence\ of\ inhibitor \times 100}{mean\ accumulation\ in\ control}\right)$$

Inhibition of choline accumulation:
    ○——·——○ , *by sodium free medium;*
    □········□ , *by 30 μM hemicholinium III.*
Inhibition of GABA accumulation:
    ●————● , *by Na^+-free medium;*
    ▲-------▲ , *by 20 μM nipecotic acid.*

both sodium-free medium and hemicholinium III is high initially
(3 days) but declines progressively during the culture period.
Barald and Berg (1979a, b) have shown that high affinity
neuronal uptake of (^{3}H)choline is both sodium-dependent and
highly sensitive to hemicholinium III in culture. Thus the
results obtained with early (3 day) NR cultures are consistent with choline uptake occurring mainly into neuronal
cells. However, non-cholinergic cells with a high choline
requirement for membrane biosynthesis (e.g. retinal photoreceptors) have been shown to take up choline by a high
affinity uptake system which is partly sodium-independent and
less sensitive to hemicholinium III (Masland and Mills, 1980).
We have shown previously that 1 µM (^{3}H)choline labels the
glial cells extensively (as well as a minority of neurones)
in 8 day cultures of chick NR cells (de Pomerai and Carr,
1982). Thus the results in Fig. 2 might imply that glial
accumulation of choline gradually comes to predominante over
neuronal accumulation during the later stages of culture.
Since the total level of choline accumulation does not increase significantly during the culture period studied, the
choline-accumulating neurones present initially must presumably dedifferentiate and/or detach from the culture (as
for GABA-accumulating neurones). This interpretation is
supported by the observation that choline acetyltransferase
(CAT) activity is high in chick embryo NR cultures during
the first 5 to 8 days *in vitro*, but then falls to insignifi-
cant levels by about 12 days (de Pomerai and Gali, 1981a,b).
Thus the cholinergic (CAT-active) neuronal cells present in
early cultures of chick NR, must later dedifferentiate or
detach (see also Betz, 1981).

Alternative explanations for these results, in terms of
increased choline or GABA metabolism during the later stages
of culture, have not yet been excluded. Further studies on
the activities of GABA transaminase and acetylcholinesterase
in chick NR cultures, are currently in progress.

ACKNOWLEDGEMENTS

This work was supported by a grant from the Medical Research
Council.

REFERENCES

Barald, K.F. and Berg, D.K. (1979a). Autoradiographic
    labelling of spinal cord neurons with high affinity
    choline uptake in cell culture. *Devel. Biol.* **72**, 1-14.

Barald, K.F. and Berg, D.K. (1979*b*). Ciliary ganglion neurons in cell culture: high affinity choline uptake and auto-radiographic choline labelling. *Devel. Biol.* **72**, 15-23.

Betz, H. (1981). Choline acetyltransferase activity in chick retinal cultures: effect of membrane depolarizing agents. *Brain Res.* **223**, 190-4.

Clayton, R.M., de Pomerai, D.I. and Pritchard, D.J. (1977). Experimental manipulation of alternative pathways of differentiation in cultures of embryonic chick neural retina. *Develop., Growth and Differ.* **19**, 319-28.

Guérinot, F. and Pessac, B. (1979). Uptake of γ-amino-butyric acid and glutamic acid decarboxylase activity in chick embryo neuroretinas in monolayer cultures. *Brain Res.* **162**, 179-83.

Lowry, O.H., Rosebrough, N., Farr, A. and Randall, R. (1951). Protein measurements with the Folin-phenol reagent. *J. biol. Chem.* **193**, 265-75.

Masland, R.H. and Mills, J.W. (1980). Choline accumulation by photoreceptor cells of the rabbit retina. *Proc. natl. Acad. Sci. (USA)* **77**, 1671-5.

Okada, T.S., Itoh, Y., Watanabe, K. and Eguchi, G. (1975). Differentiation of lens in cultures of neural retinal cells of chick embryos. *Devel. Biol.* **45**, 318-29.

de Pomerai, D.I. and Gali, M.A.H. (1981*a*). Influence of serum factors on the prevalence of "normal" and "foreign" differentiation pathways in cultures of chick embryo neuroretinal cells. *J. Embryol. Exp. Morphol.* **62**, 291-308.

de Pomerai, D.I. and Gali, M.A.H. (1981*b*). Alterations in pH and serum concentrations have contrasting effects on normal and "foreign" pathways of differentiation in cultures of embryonic chick neuroretinal cells. *Develop., Growth and Differ.* **23**, 561-70.

de Pomerai, D.I. and Carr, A. (1982). Choline and GABA accumulation in cultures of chick embryo neuroretinal cells. *Exp. Eye Res.*, **34**, 553-563.

THE ROLE OF CELL CONTACTS IN THE DIFFERENTIATION OF EMBRYO RETINA CELLS

A.A. MOSCONA

*Laboratory for Developmental Biology,
Cummings Life Science Center, University of Chicago,
Chicago, Illinois, 60637, USA*

The developmental biology of two enzymes in the embryonic chick neural retina was described. Glutamine synthetase (GS) and carbonic anhydrase (CA) are found in the CNS, where they characterize different cells, GS being confined mainly to astrologlia and CA to oligo-dendroglia. Both enzymes are found in the Müller glial cells of the mature retina, but they have different developmental programmes and control mechanisms.

GS is low until the onset of functional and physiological maturation in the retina; at 16 days it rises steeply and increases 100 fold over a few days, remaining at a high level in the mature retina. This increase follows induction by adrenocorticosteroids, which increase in the systemic circulation 1 to 2 days before the rise of GS in the retina. However, the competence for inducibility by corticosteroids has been shown to arise between 5 to 7 days of development and to increase gradually. By 8 to 10 days of incubation GS in the retina is inducible within 2 h following treatment with hydroxycortisone *in vitro*. Inducibility is affected by the culture medium: it is lower in Eagles M.E.M. and higher in Medium 199. Inducibility is also dependent on cell-cell contacts. Dissociated neural retinal cells can be grown as a mono-disperse monolayer. The neuroblasts are relatively unmodified in morphology, but glial cells flatten out and attach to the plastic. Normal cell contacts and interactions are destroyed, and such cultures are not inducible for GS. Dissociation is followed by a decline in the number of steroid receptors, but these increase again following cell aggregation, and if cell aggregates are allowed to form and the cells restore histological relationships, GS is once again inducible.

It has been shown that GS induction represents enzyme
synthesis and accumulation, and requires gene activity and
expression. It is not due to activation of pre-existing
enzyme or assembly of preformed subunits into the octamer.
Titration by antisera of the nascent radio-labelled enzyme
showed a genuine increase in enzyme synthesis. Induction
is also prevented by inhibition of RNA or protein synthesis.
Immunohistology of the retina with labelled antisera has
shown that GS is always localized only in Müller glial cells
in the differentiated retina, in chick and mouse. Double
labelling with antibodies to GS and CA with two fluorochromes
confirm that these two enzymes are in the same cells. In the
early stages of development, CA is found in all retino-blasts,
but when the cells begin to differentiate into definitive
glial cells and neurons, CA becomes restricted to the former.
It is not inducible with cortisol and its expression appears
not to depend on contacts between glia and neurons as
stringently as the expression of GS.

REFERENCES

Linser, P. and Moscona, A.A. (1979). Industion of glutamine
    synthetase in embryonic neural retina: localization in
    Müller fibers and dependence on cell interactions. *Proc.
    Natl. Acad. Sci. (USA)* **76**, 6476-6480.
Linser, P. and Moscona, A.A. (1981). Carbonic anhydrase in
    the neural retina: transition from generalized to glia
    specific cell localization. *Proc. Natl. Acad. Sci. (USA)*
    78, 7190-7194.
Saad, A.D., Soh, B.M. and Moscona, A.A. (1981). Modulation
    of cortisol receptors in embryonic retina cells by changes
    in cell-cell contacts: correlations with induction of
    glutamine synthetase. *Biochem. Biophys. Res. Commun.* **98**,
    701-708.

STABILIZATION OF PIGMENT RETINAL STRUCTURE *IN VIVO* AND *IN VITRO*

GORO EGUCHI

*Institute of Molecular Biology, Faculty of Science,
Nagoya University, Nagoya 464, Japan*

ABSTRACT

In suitable culture conditions pigment retinal cells (PRCs)
can reconstitute a typical monolayer epithelium which is
structurally identical to the pigment retina differentiated
in *in vivo* eyes. The PRCs adhere tightly to each other at
their apical level to show the hexagonal cellular pattern,
and are stabilized structurally and functionally. Each PRC
bears circumferential microfilament bundles just underneath
the opposed cell membrane at the apical level, and these
bundles exhibit high contractility in the presence of MgATP.
The microfilament bundles are first organized in PRCs *in
vitro*, when the culture attains confluency. At this stage,
however, the cellular pattern is not yet stable, although
intercellular junctions at the apical level have already been
established. We assumed from the results of theoretical and
experimental analysis that the PRCs in monolayer epithelia
shorten their cell boundaries by the contractile function of
the circumferential actomyosin bundles, to stabilize the monolayer epithelial structure and to realize the hexagonal
cellular pattern. Such an assumption can be applicable to
the process of structural and functional stabilization of the
pigment retina in *in vivo* eyes.

REFERENCE

Owaribe, K., Kodama, R. and Eguchi, G. (1981). Demonstration
    of contractility of circumferential actin bundles and
    its morphogenetic significance in pigmented epithelium
    in vitro and *in vivo*. *J. Cell Biol.* **90**, 507-514.

MOLECULES THAT DEFINE A DORSAL-VENTRAL AXIS OF RETINA CAN BE USED TO IDENTIFY CELL POSITION

G.D. TRISLER, MICHAEL D. SCHNEIDER, JOSEPH R. MOSKAL
and MARSHALL NIRENBERG

*National Heart, Lung and Blood Institute,
National Institutes of Health, Bethesda, Maryland 20205 USA*

ABSTRACT

A hybridoma antibody was obtained that binds to cell membrane
molecules distributed in a gradient in chick retina.   Thirty-
five fold more antigen was detected in dorsoposterior than
ventroanterior retina.   The concentration of antigen detected
(F_x) is a function of the square of circumferential distance
(D_x) from the ventroanterior margin towards the dorsoposterior
margin of the retina; thus, the antigen can be used as a
marker of cell position along the ventroanterior-dorsoposterior
axis of the retina, i.e.,

$$D_x = D_{max}(F_x/F_{max})^{0.5}$$

where D_{max} and F_{max} are values for the dorsoposterior margin.
Immunofluorescence and autoradiography revealed the antigen
on the surface of most, or all, cell types in dorsoposterior
retina with most of the antigen found in the synaptic
layers.   The antigen was detected in the optic cup of 48 h
chick embryos, and evidence for a gradient was found with
retina from 4-day embryos, the earliest time examined, through
the adult.   The antigen was found in chick retina > cerebrum
> thalamus >> cerebellum > optic tectum and retinal pigment
epithelium.   The antigen was not detected in heart, liver,
kidney, or cells from blood.   Antigen gradients were found
in chicken, quail, duck and turkey retina, but little or no
antigen was detected in goldfish, toad, frog, or rat retina.
    The antigen was inactivated at 100°C and was converted
from a membrane bound to a soluble form by trypsin.   No
antigen was detected on trypsinized retina cells.   However,
the antigen was found on retina cells after 24 h in culture.

Antigen synthesis by cultured cells in the presence of 7 μM cycloheximide or 0.8 μM actinomycin D was 24% and 0% of control, respectively. Cells that were dissociated with trypsin from dorsal, middle, or ventral retina and were cultured separately for 10 days contained the levels of antigen expected for cells from the corresponding regions of retina *in ovo*. Cells from dorsoposterior and ventro-anterior retina dissociated with trypsin were mixed in different proportions and cocultured for 6 days; the levels of antigen were almost additive, without evidence of induction or suppression of antigen synthesis. These results show that dissociated cells in culture synthesize the amount of antigen expected for their position of origin in the retina despite the absence of other embryonic tissues.

^{35}S-Protein from retina was solubilized with 0.2% SDS and 1% Triton X-100 and fractionated by protein A-Sepharose or hybridoma antibody-Sepharose column chromatography, and by SDS-polyacrylamide gel electrophoresis. Forty per cent of the radioactivity recovered was in a single band approximately 55,000 M_r. Further work is needed to determine whether the antigen plays a role in the coding of positional information in the retina and the specification of synaptic connections.

REFERENCE

Trisler, G.D., Schneider, M.D. and Nirenberg, M. (1981). A topographic gradient of molecules in retina can be used to identify neuron position. *Proc. Natl. Acad. Sci. U.S.A.* **78**, 2145-2149.

ANGIOGENIC ACTIVITY OF A CELL GROWTH-REGULATING FACTOR DERIVED FROM THE RETINA

[+]P. THOMPSON, *[†]C. ARRUTI, [+][§]D. MAURICE, *J. PLOUET,
*[¶]D. BARRITAULT and *Y. COURTOIS

[+]*INSERM U. 86 — Laboratoire d'Opthalmologie de l'Hotel Dieu,
75001, Paris, France*
*INSERM U. 118 · CNRS ERA 842 — Unité de Recherches
Gérontologiques, 29, rue Wilhem, 75016, Paris, France*
[†]*On leave from Montevideo Faculdad de Medicina, Uruguay*
[§]*On leave from Division of Ophthalmology, Stanford University
Medical School, Stanford, CA, USA*
[¶]*University of Paris XII, UER Sciences, 94100, Créteil, France*

SUMMARY

EDGF, a partially purified growth factor present in the
retina of adult cattle eyes was tested for a presumptive
angiogenic activity by three different methods. First, it
was shown to stimulate the proliferation of bovine endothelial vascular cells *in vitro*. Second, it was able to
induce a vasoproliferative activity in chick chorioallantoic
membrane. Third, when it was infused at a controlled rate
into the rabbit cornea for 7 days, neovascularization was induced after four days and was very prominent after seven
days. EDGF was shown to be stable over this period. Histological studies demonstrated the presence of some inflammatory cells as early as 3 days after the beginning of
the experiment. It appears that EDGF is directly or
indirectly angiogenic.

INTRODUCTION

An Eye Derived Growth Factor, EDGF has been extracted
from bovine retina and vitreous, (Arruti and Courtois, 1978)
partially purified, (Barritault *et al.*, 1981; Courtois *et
al.*, 1981). Among other target cells, it stimulates the

proliferation of bovine vascular endothelium. The presence
of this factor in the retina raises the question of its possible angiogenic role in pathological conditions. Several
growth factors such as EGF and FGF have been reported to
be angiogenic in different systems (Gospodarowicz *et al.*,
1978*a*, 1979*b*), and recently two groups have found that crude
extracts of retina and vitreous (Chen and Chen, 1980), or
retina alone (Glaser *et al.*, 1980) can provoke new vessel
growth.

Several methods have been devised to assess the angiogenic
potential of such compounds. The first is to show that
vascular endothelial cells can be stimulated to proliferate
in vitro. Many compounds have the ability to control the
growth rate of cells in culture. Several criteria are
required to demonstrate that a protein extract or a purified
protein possesses a spefic growth factor activity (Gospodoro-
wics and Moran, 1976). In this work, we have chosen to
investigate whether EDGF (formerly called RE for retinal
extract) is able to increase the growth rate of bovine
endothelial vascular cells maintained in optimal culture
conditions. These experiments were performed with Adult
Bovine Aortic and Foetal Bovine Heart Endothelial cells
(ABAE and FBHE) in the laboratory of Denis Gospodarowicz
in San Francisco.

The second widely used method to demonstrate an angiogenic effect is the classic chorioallantoic membrane (CAM)
assay (Folkman, 1974; Ausprink *et al.*, 1975). This assay
was performed with numerous retinal extracts, first in
France, and lately in Dr Arruti's laboratory in Montevideo.

Finally a system that has proved valuable in assaying
the potential of neovascularization of a substance is to
introduce it into a pocket formed within the cornea, close
to the limbus. If the substance is angiogenic, new vessels
will grow in a few days (Gimbrone *et al.*, 1974). In previous reports, the substance was incorporated into either
a gel foam (Chen and Chen, 1980), acrylamide (Godpodarowicz
et al., 1978*a,b*) or Elwax 40 (Godpodarowicz, 1979). No data
are available on the rate of release of the substances
from such implants or on whether their activity was maintained throughout the duration of the experiments. To
overcome these uncertainties, we have used a perfusion
system described by Eliason and Maurice (1979, 1980), in
conjunction with a partially purified preparation of EDGF,
whose activity was precisely controlled. The angiogenic
potential of EDGF *in vivo* was confirmed by this technique.

MATERIALS AND METHODS

EDGF Purification

EDGF was extracted from freshly collected bovine retina as already described (Barritault *et al.*, 1981). Briefly, 200 retinas were suspended in 200 ml of phosphate saline buffer (PBS), homogenized in a blender, centrifuged at 30,000 g for 30 min and 100,000 g for 5 h. At this stage, the protein concentration was about 5 to 7.5 mg/ml. EDGF mitogenic activity was found to be enriched by ammonium sulphate precipitation between 20 and 60% salt concentration. The precipitated pellet was redissolved in the same volume of PBS and dialyzed at 4°C overnight against 0.1 N acetic acid. The precipitated protein was removed by centrifugation and the supernatant dialyzed against PBS. Samples were sterilized by filtration through a 0.22 μm Millipore membrane, divided into aliquots and stored at -20°C.
The dose response of each preparation was tested for its mitogenic activity on bovine lens epithelial (BEL) cells, measured by ^{3}H thymidine incorporation. A unit of stimulation was defined as the amount of protein which induces 50% of the maximal incorporation (Gospodarowicz, 1978b). This test allowed enrichment during purification procedures to be followed and comparisons to be made with other growth factors, such as FGF, for which BEL cells are a target. In a crude extract, after 100,000 g centrifugation, one unit corresponded to 50 μg of protein, and in the 0.1 N acetic acid-treated EDGF to 500 ng; in the same test almost pure FGF from brain (given by D. Gospodarowicz) gives one unit per 20 ng protein.

Thermal stability of the mitogenic activity of the crude and partially purified EDGF was tested (Barritault, Plouet, Courtois, in prep.), after a 5 day incubation at 37°C. Nine-tenths of the activity was destroyed on incubation of the non-purified extracts and 30% on incubation of the 0.1 N acetic acid partially purified preparation; therefore we used the latter preparation to perfuse the cornea.

Stimulation of Vascular Endothelial Bovine Cells

ABAE and FBHE cell cultures have been extensively described by Godpodarowicz *et al.*, 1978a). 2×10^4 cells were seeded in 33 mm diameter petri dishes, and either FGF (100 ng/ml), EDGF from retina, iris or choroid-pigment epithelium pre-

pared as in Barritault *et al.* (1981) (100 µg/ml) were added
the first day to each culture. On day 4, the cell population
was counted using a Coulter counter (Coultronics).

Choriollantoic Membrane Assay

Pieces of neutral saline agar were soaked overnight in the
retinal extract at 4°C and briefly rinsed in neutral saline
solution before implantation on CAM. In several experiments,
a defined volume of retinal extract was deposited on glass
fibre filters. In the experiments performed in Montevideo
the activity of the retinal extract was determined from its
stimulation potential on corneal endothelial cells. The glass
filters or the agar pieces were laid on the CAM of 8-day chick
embryos (Leghorn). The CAM was punctured with a 30 gauge
hypodermic needle before placing the sample at a point
located at 2 mm from a vessel. In some cases a second sample
moistened with the retinal extract or with a buffer was put
on the same CAM. After 5 days of incubation the CAMs were
fixed in neutral formalin, the membranes were excized and
dipped in a petri dish, upside down, and promptly photo-
graphed.

Perfusion System

The technique used has been reported previously (Eliason and
Maurice, 1980). The EDGF solution is delivered from an
osmotically driven pump (Alzet minipump) implanted beneath
the scalp (Fig. 1) and connected to a polyethylene tube
drawn down to a fine tip (20 to 40 µm diameter). This tube
runs subconjunctivally and passes across the cornea between
the lamellae so that the tip is located 2.5 mm from the
limbus. The system delivers the EDGF solution at a nominal
rate of 1 µl/h; its lifespan is 7 days. The addition of
dilute fluorescein to the samples allows direct visualization
of the flow by slit-lamp examination.

Experimental Animals

Ten adult rabbits of either sex, weighing 2 to 3 kg, were
divided into two groups. In the experimental group (7
rabbits), the pumps were filled with EDGF solution and in
the control group (3 rabbits) with PBS buffer. On every
alternate day the eyes were examined with a slit-lamp.

Histology

After each experiment, the whole eye was enucleated and

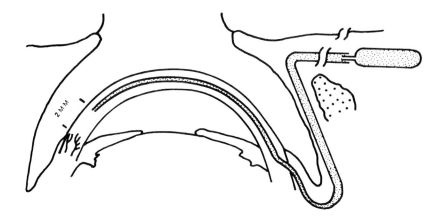

Fig. 1 *Schematic representation of the perfusion device implanted in the rabbit eye as described by Eliason and Maurice (in prep.)*

fixed in formalin solution.   Serial sections were made of the paraffin-embedded cornea and were stained with hematoxylin-eosin.

RESULTS

In Vitro *Stimulation of ABAE and FBHE Cells*

Table I represents the number of cells counted in each Petri dish on day 4 after stimulation by preparations of EDGF from iris, choroid and pigment epithelium, or retina which were compared with brain FGF and with the absence of growth factors.   The untreated ABAE cell population increased 4 fold (from 2 to 8 × 10μ), approximately two doublings, while after treatment with growth factors the cells underwent an average of 4 to 4.5 doublings.   At the doses of EDGF used, similar results were obtained with FBHE cells, although the control shows a 2.8 doubling in the same four days.   The small differences found between the various preparations of EDGF and FGF are not considered significant, and may be due to differences in dose responses of these cells

Chorioallantoic Membrane Vascularization

In the conditions described in "Material and Methods" it was observed that while the general vascular pattern of most of

TABLE 1

Comparative study of the proliferation induced by FGF and
EDGF from retina, iris and choroid-pigmented epithelium
on ABAE and FBHE cells

	Number of cells per dish at day 4 (means of triplicate experiments	
	FBHE	ABAE
Control	140,000	90,000
FGF	617,000	415,000
EDGF (iris)	520,000	414,000
EDGF (choroid+pigmented ep.)	420,000	380,000
EDGF (retina)	523,000	575,000

Cells seeded at 2×10^4 per dish were counted at day 4 100 ng
of FGF or 100 µg of EDGF were added per ml of culture medium
at day 1 and 3.

the controls was unchanged the treated samples exhibited a
modified spatial distribution of the vessels surrounding the
implanted pellets. These membranes presented a radial orientation of vessels of different diameters as is shown in Fig.
2. The samples presenting vessels of larger diameters and a
higher density than in the controls were scored as giving
a strong response. By double blind analysis we have defined
negative, weak and strong responses.

As shown in Table 2, in the results from an experiment
with 50 samples (25 controls and 25 treated) with pellets
containing 15 µl of retinal extract (100 µg of proteins),
64% of the CAMs presented a strong vasoproliferative
response. An increase in the amount of retinal extract
added to the pellets did not modify significantly these
results. The controls were all negative or gave a weak
response. The sensitivity of the technique is such that
small injuries or perhaps the onset of a small inflammation
provoked by the surgery give rise to a weak response. This
background response is characteristic of this technique
and makes it useful only as a first approach for screening
the angiogenic potential of a product. Thus, even if an
angiogenic activity is strongly suggested by these results,
which confirms the observations with a crude extract of

TABLE 2

Vascular response of chorioallantoic vessel treated by a retinal extract

Vascular response	PBS	EDGF
Strong	0	64%
Weak	44%	36%
Negative	56%	0

Two batches of 25 samples received either 15 µl of PBS or 15 µl of retinal extract.

retina recently published by other workers, it is important to confirm it with more accurate tests.

Corneal Vascularization by Diffusion

In the experiments performed with EDGF, a consistent pattern was observed in all 7 eyes (Fig. 3). After 2 days, a small edema was noted around the tip of the cannula. After 4 days, vessels started to invade the stroma and they reached the tip of the cannula in 7 to 8 days. Adjacent to this neovascularized zone, the conjunctiva was moderately inflamed. In the 3 controls, slight edema developed around the tip of the cannula, but no vascularization was observed by direct examination with a slit lamp during 7 days.

Histological examination performed on day 7 showed blood vessels extending from the adjacent limbus to the tip of the cannula in a trinagular pattern. The vessels were found across the whole thickness of the stroma but mostly at the level of the cannula (Fig. 4). There was a moderate infiltrative reaction composed of macrophages, neutrophils, eosinophils and lymphocytes. The cells had invaded as far as the cannula on the third day, although new vessels had not yet formed at the limbus. The epithelium and endothelium were normal in appearance, although inflammatory cells were found in the anterior chamber close to the endothelial layer (Fig. 5).

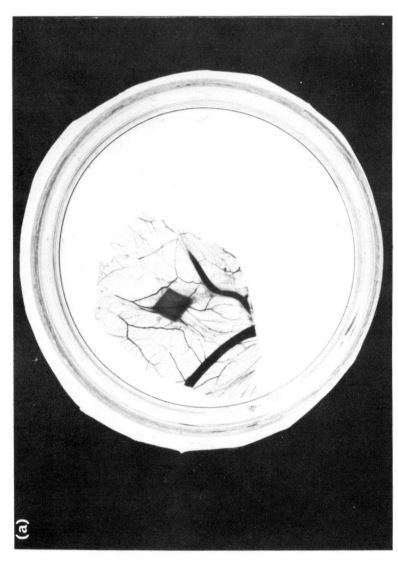

Fig. 2 Angiogenic effect of retinal extracts on chorioallantoic membranes (a) treated (b) controls

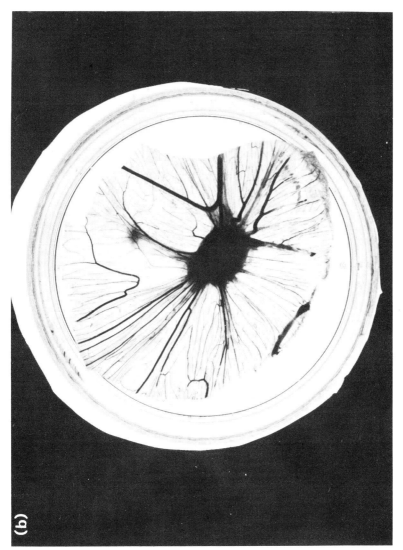

(b)

(For legend, see opposite).

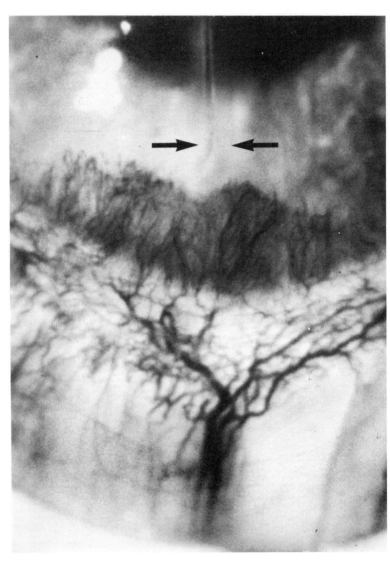

(Fig. 3 for legend see opposite)

DISCUSSION

The stimulatory activity of EDGF on vascular endothelial
cells in culture and the neovascularization obtained following EDGF administration to the cornea *in vivo* suggest that
EDGF might be angiogenic. An angiogenic activity for similar
retinal extracts has been reported by Glaser *et al.* (1980)
using a chorioallantoic membrane technique. However, in
order to compare our results with previous reports involving
similar extracts or other purified growth factors we have
evaluated the mitogenic effect of those substances on BEL
cells. 0.5 µg of our preparation had the same mitogenic
activity as 50 µg of the crude extract prepared according
to Chen and Chen (1980) or as 2 ng of pituitary FGF.
    In order to effect exact comparisons of the results of
different experiments on vasoformative factors *in vivo*, it
is desirable to be able to estimate the concentration of the
factor that is maintained at the capillaries during the
period of endothelial sprouting. This is very difficult
when the material is injected directly into the corneal
stroma or is implanted in a pocket in an impregnated matrix.
It is complicated to compute the changes in concentration at
a point distant from an extended source, and moreover the
original distribution or rate of release is not easy to
establish. Under these conditions, the concentration found
at the capillary tips is likely to undergo considerable
changes over the period of 2 to 3 days required to establish
vessel growth. Furthermore, the active material lies un-
protected within the stroma and is open to enzymic degradation from the moment of its introduction.
    On the other hand, if the active factor is steadily in-
fused into the stroma at a definite point, it establishes a
simple concentration distribution within a few hours (Maurice
et al., 1966). The concentration at any distance from the
point of introductioncan be estimated from a knowledge of
the molecular weight of the factor (Eliason and Maurice,
in prep.). In the present experiments, the most distant
point at which vascular growth was provoked at the limbus
was about 3 mm from the tip of the cannula. The injection
rate was 40 U/day. By gel filtration on AcA 34, the molecular weight of EDGF is found to be 25,000 to 40,000 daltons.

Fig. 3 *Neovascularization induced in the cornea by a slow
release of EDGF within 2.5 mm of the limbus. The two arrows
point towards the tip of the cannula. Note the slight
edema around it; the white spots on the left side are due to
artefacts of illumination during the process of photography.*

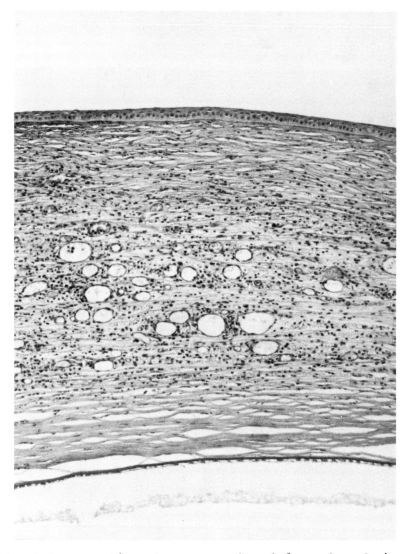

Fig. 4 *Cross section of a cornea after 8 days of perfusion. At this time inflammatory cells can be seen in the stroma as well as many new vessels.*

The concentration of albumin, a slightly larger protein, at this distance from the cannula tip can be calculated to be of the order of 500 U/ml. The question of whether EDGF plays a role in angiogenesis in any natural situation can

be answered by determining whether it is present at the growing capaillaries at a comparable concentration.

A further advantage of delivering the active extract
with a minipump is that it is protected from enzymatic degradation in the tissue except for the few hours when it is
diffusing from the cannula tip. It will be recalled that
incubation of the purified factor used here resulted only
in a small drop of activity in 7 days.

A question arises whether EDGF operates directly by inter-
acting with receptors on the capillary endothelial cells
or indirectly by means of an intermediate system. Various
intermediaries have been suggested in other contexts; for
example, the growth factor could liberate the angiogenic
agent from the corneal cells (Zauberman et al., 1969), it
could cause the invasion of inflammatory cells which release
the agent (Polverine et al., 1977), or it could activate
a plasminogen activator shown to be present at the corneal
periphery (Berman et al., 1980). As regards the first possibility, both corneal endothelium (Arruti and Courtois,
1979, 1980, 1982) and epithelium (Thompson et al., 1982)
have been shown to be target cells for EDGF. Observations
on the natural history of capillary invasion at threshold
levels of EDGF may eliminate some of these hypotheses, but
a full understanding will probably have to come from other
experiments; thus it has been shown that the invasion of
leucocytes is not necessary for corneal vascularization to
occur (Eliason, 1978).

The results presented in this work tend to show that the
retina contains its own angiogenic factor. How such an
activity is confined in the normal tissue and is involved
in the hypervascularization of the tissue in various pathological conditions remains to be solved.

ACKNOWLEDGEMENTS

This work was supported by an INSERM grant number 78-100
and by an NIH Grant (EY 00431) and a Guggenheim Fellowship
awarded to one of us (D.M.). It was presented in part
at the IVth International Congress for Eye Research, New
York, September 1980.

We wish to thank Prof. Y. Pouliquen for his continuous
support during this study, and M. Saldovelli for histological
preparation. The experiments with vascular endothelial
cells in culture were performed first by one of us (D.B.) in
D. Gospodarowicz's laboratory. We wish to thank him also
for helpful discussion.

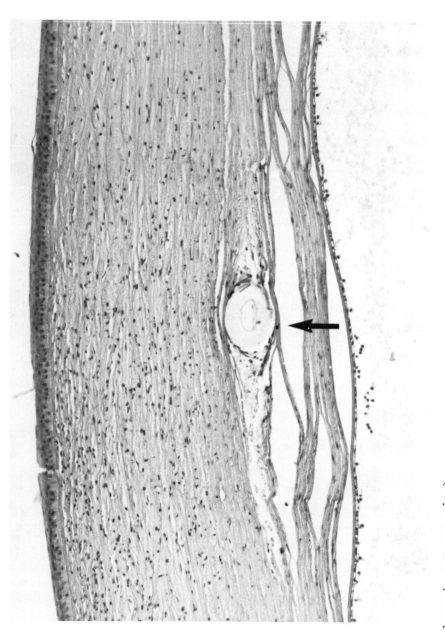

(For legend, see opposite).

REFERENCES

Arruti, C. and Courtois, Y. (1978). Morphological changes
   and growth stimulation of bovine epithelial lens cells by
   a retinal extract *in vitro*. *Exp. Cell Res*. **117**, 283–292.
Arruti, C. and Courtois, Y. (1979). Retinotrophic stimulation of proliferation of bovine corneal endothelial cells
   in vitro. *20th Meeting Eur. Assoc. Eye Res*., Paris, Sept.
Arruti, F. and Courtois, Y. (1980). The *in vitro* control
   of proliferation and cell interaction of bovine corneal
   endothelial cells by a retinal growth factor. *Eur. J. Cell
   Biol*. **22**, 386.
Arruti, C. and Courtois, Y. (1982). Monolayer Organization by
   serially cultured bovine corneal endothelial cells: Effects
   of a retina derived growth promoting activity. *Exp. Eye Res*.
   (in press).
Barritault, D., Arruti, C. and Courtois, Y. (1981). Is
   there an ubiquitous growth factor in the eye?
   Differentiation, **18**, 29–42.
Ausprunk, D.H., Knighton, D.R. and Folkman, J. (1975). Vascularization of normal and neoplastic tissues grafted
   to the chick chorioallantoic membrane. *Am. J. Pathol*.
   79, 597–628.
Berman, M., Winthrop, M., Ausprunk, D., Rose, J., Langer, R.
   and Gage, J. (1980). Plasminogen activators cause neovascularization of the cornea. *Proc. Int. Soc. Eye Res*.
   1, 75.
Chen, C.H. and Chen, S.C. (1980). Angiogenic activity of
   vitreous and retinal extract. *Invest. Ophthalmol*. **19**,
   596–602.
Courtois, Y., Arruti, C., Barritault, D., Tassin, J.,
   Olivier, M. and Hughes, R.C. (1981). Modulation of the
   shape of epithelial lens cells *in vitro* directed by a
   retinal extract factor. A model of interconversion and
   the role of actin filaments and fibronectin.
   Differentiation, **18**, 11–27.
Eliason, J. (1978). Laucocytes and experimental corneal
   vascularization. *Invest. Ophthal*. **17**, 1087–1095.
Eliason, J.A. and Maurice, D. (1979). Angiogenesis by the
   corneal epithelium. *ARVO Abs*. p. 141.
Eliason, J.A. and Maurice, D. (1980). An ocular perfusion
   system. *Invest. Ophthalmol. Vis. Sci*. **19**, 102–104.

Fig. 5 *Cross section of the cornea after 3 days of perfusion.
Note the tip of the cannula (arrow) and the presence of some
inflammatory cells in the stroma and in the anterior chamber
in the total absence of new vascularization. Both epithelium
and endothelium cells seem well preserved.*

Folkman, J. (1974). Tumour angiogenesis factor. *Cancer Res.* **34**, 2109—2113.

Gimbrone, M.A., Cotran, R.S., Leapman, S.B. and Folkman, J. (1974). Tumour growth and neovascularization: an experimental model using the rabbit cornea. *J. Natl, Cancer Inst.* **52**, 413—427.

Glaser, B., d'Amore, P., Michels, R.G., Patz, A. and Fenselan, A. (1980). Demonstration of vasoproliferative activity from mammalian retina. *J. Cell Biol.* **84**, 298—304.

Gospodarowicz, D. and Moran, J. (1976). Growth factors in mammalian culture. *Ann. Rev. of Biochemistry*, **45**, 531—558.

Gospodarowicz, D., Greenburg, G., Bialecki, H. and Zetter, R.R. (1978*a*). Factors involved in the modulation of cell proliferation *in vivo* and *in vitro*. The role of fibroblast and epidermal growth factor in the proliferative response of mammalian cells. *In Vitro* **14**, 85—118.

Gospodarowicz, D., Mescher, A.L. and Birdwell, C.R. (1978*b*). The control of cellular proliferation by the fibroblasts and epidermal growth factor. In "Gene Expression and Regulation in Cultured Cells." pp. 109—130. Third Decennial Review Conference. Nat. Canc. Inst. (1978*b*).

Gospodarowicz, D., Bialecki, H. and Thakral, T.K. (1979). The angiogenic activity of the fibroblast and epidermal growth factor. *Exp. Eye Res.*, **28**, 501—514.

Maurice, D.M., Zauberman, H. and Michaelson, I.C. (1966). The stimulus to neovascularization in the cornea. *Exp. Eye Res.* **5**, 168—173.

Polverine, P., Cotran, R., Gimbrone, M. and Uname, E. (1977). Activated macrophages induce vascular proliferation. *Nature* **269**, 804—806.

Thompson, P., Debordes, J.M., Giraud, J., Pouliquen, Y., Barritault, D. and Courtois, Y. (1982). The effect of an eye derived growth factor (EDGF) on rabbit corneal epithelial regeneration. *Exp. Eye Res.* **34**, 191—199.

Zauberman, H., Michaelson, I.C., Bergmann, F., and Maurice, D.M. (1969). Stimulation of neovascularization of the cornea by biogenic amines. *Exp. Eye Res.* **8**, 77—82.

Properties of retina cells in culture, and retinal molecular species were discussed. MOSCONA, answering questions from CHADER on the appearance of enzymes, and from LOLLEY on evidence for the requirement for neurone-glial cell interaction for GS induction, replied that GS (glutamine synthetase) appeared at 8 days and CA (carbonic anhydrase) at 12. No GS was induced in aggregates of almost pure retina neuronal cells, nor from retinal neurones aggregated with neurones from other sources. He said, in answer to a further question from LOLLEY, that corticosteroid-containing medium did not prevent loss of receptors. SANYAL asked whether CA might be an indicator of functional differentiation between PE cells and Müller cells. Only the latter contained CA in the mouse. MOSCONA replied that there were several CA isomers, and he had failed to confirm CA in Müller cells using antibody to CA_c.

Replying to ARDEN, TRISLER said they had not yet found other molecular retinal gradients, and replying to HOLLY-FIELD, that binding occurred in the 4 day optic cup; earlier stages had not yet been tested. CHADER asked about the high binding in the cerebrum; and TRISLER replied that the histological location had not been determined. Replying to OSBORNE he reported that binding of monoclonal antibody or control sera was measured by radio-iodinated rabbit anti-mouse IgG.

EGUCHI, replying to several speakers, said that medium and culture conditions determined the morphology of pigment cells and their organization, which in some conditions closely resembled the *in vivo* pigment epithelium.

READING asked PESSAC whether the proportion of neural retina cells in culture positive for a specific marker resembled that of retina in *in vivo*. PESSAC replied that between 60 to 80% of cells were positive; clonal culture was a selective procedure. Replying to OSBORNE he said that GFAP-positive cells did not react with tetanus toxin.

LOLLEY asked BEALE whether he had assessed the characteristics of different types of normal cells obtained before

culture. **BEALE** said he had not yet done so; membrane markers
might be readily detectable but aminoacid uptake could be
measured only on undamaged cells. **HOLLYFIELD** said that
GABA and muscimol might be taken up by neurones but not by
glia in culture. **MOSCONA** and **LAVAIL** both discussed a consequence of the vascularization of mammalian retinas; the
release of endothelial cells and monocytes into the culture,
which can become pleiomorphic. **BEALE** agreed, but considered
that he could definitely identify astrocytes, and Müller
cells. **LAVAIL** asked about separation of PE cells from
neural retina, since these cells may adhere, although apical
processes might be broken. **IKEDA** commented that they can be
separated from dark-adapted retinas. **BEALE** did not dark
adapt, but found less admixture in preparations from younger
animals. He replied to questions from **ANDERSON** that he had
not yet tried cholera toxin binding, and to **PESSAC** that he
had not yet examined cells by EM for synapse formation. The
problems of synapse formation and response of neuronal cells
to signals was discussed further. **LOLLEY** asked **PESSAC**
whether ribbon synapses were found in his cultures, and
PESSAC replied that their absence might be due to the rapid
growth in culture rather than a failure to be able to form
them. **READING** pointed out that neuronal function could not
be studied without stimulation, even in culture, and cultured
retina fragments could continue to respond to light for some
time. **MOSCONA** said that ERG recordings could be obtained
from embryonic retina, and **IKEDA** mentioned that neurones
from the CNS develop recording potentiality in culture.
BEALE said that cells starting to differentiate cannot trans-
duce. **MOSCONA** commented that cultured retina cells respond
to a hormonal stimulus before the response appears in the
intact retina.

   The transformation of iris or retina to lens was discussed.
LOLLEY asked which iris quadrant in the normal and the
rotated eye could regenerate lens. **McDEVITT** replied that
in vivo, it was the mid-dorsal region; the capacity falling
off both laterally, and towards the limbus, but Eguchi had
shown that ventral iris could form lens if cells were disrupted and cultured, or after treatment with MNNG (a mutagen/
carcinogen) *in vivo*. **LAVAIL** asked if cell junctions of
dorsal and ventral iris differed. **EGUCHI** replied that there
was no critical ultrastructural data but 30 hr after lentectomy electrical coupling dropped in the dorsal region only.
MOSCONA suggested that retinal dorso-ventral gradients such
as that described by **TRISLER**, might be regulatory. **TRISLER**
commented that gradients had also been reported for cell
adhesion, the number of amacrine cells, of receptors, and of
coloured oil droplets. **MOSCONA** raised the problem of species

differences between amphibia — as to whether regeneration could
occur, and in its site, and **EGUCHI** reported that the loach
(a fish) could regenerate lens from all of the iris periphery.
COURTOIS asked whether regeneration could take place after
damage to the retina, and **ARDEN** asked whether it could take place
after removal of the dorsal region. **EGUCHI** replied that it could
not. He said that eyes reversed through 180° at an early
stage regenerated lens from the new dorsal position, and
McDEVITT commented that rotation of the pupil led to depigmentation in the area nearest to the retina. **LOLLEY**
commented that a regulatory agent must come from the neural
retina. **McDEVITT** suggested that Courtois' retinal mitogenic
factor (EDGF) might be a regulator. Mitosis occurred in the
iris only after lentectomy; ventral iris cells, which had a
longer cycle than dorsal cells, merely partially depigmented
and repigmented when mitosis stopped. **ARDEN** asked if EDGF
affected retina as well as lens; **COURTOIS** said that this was
under test. It had angiogenic properties.

CLAYTON asked Courtois whether mutant retinas lacked or
had different levels of EDGF. **COURTOIS** replied that only
large differences would be detected at present, but they
hoped to prepare specific antisera to EDGF, which was distinct from other growth factors. An inhibitor had to be
removed during purification.

VOADEN asked about the role of the cornea in lentectomy.
McDEVITT said cornea showed a normal repair response and
EGUCHI said that lens regeneration still took place if lentectomy was via the back of the eye. **LOLLEY** said that while
retina was involved in lens development, the development of
cataract in retinal degenerative diseases in rodents pointed
to a continuing role in maintenance. General discussion
between **LOLLEY, LAVAIL, BERMAN** and **READING** indicated that
there were differences in the size of the opacity, and also
between strains and age groups, and the detection of cataract
might also depend on instrumentation. **CLAYTON** said that the
finding of three different protein profiles specific to RP
cataracts suggested the existence of some other factors
besides the retinal maintenace of lens.

COURTOIS and **McDEVITT** asked Clayton about the characteristics of the antiserum to lens which bound to retina cell
membranes. **CLAYTON** replied that the experiment, (done 10
years ago) used an antiserum to the total insoluble fraction,
which reacted with both crystallins and membranes. However
the reaction was not species specific, and was strongest
with photoreceptors. **CHADER** asked whether the crystallin
mRNAs in the retina were for particular crystallins, and
CLAYTON replied that total crystallin cDNA had been used,
but they were now using recombinant cDNA probes. They

thought that the specific representation might depend on the
stage of development, since transdifferentiated lentoids from
early retina expressed mainly δ crystallin but from later
retinas mainly α and β crystallin. **CHADER** asked if lentoids
could be cataractous and **CLAYTON** said that lentoids never
had the organized structure of a lens. **LOLLEY** asked whether
crystallin mRNA was always translated in retina; **CLAYTON**
replied that the level of hybridizable crystallin RNA was
highest in 3.5 day embryo retina but crystallins were only
found in eight day retina. Unprocessed nuclear, and post-
polysomal hnRNA would be hybridized but not translated.

CELLULAR AND MOLECULAR BIOLOGY OF THE RETINA: SUMMING UP

T.S. OKADA

*Department of Biophysics, Faculty of Science,
University of Kyoto, Kyoto 606, Japan*

The subject matter of this session is "Molecular and Cellular
Biology of the Retina". It is extremely broad, and an almost
limitless variety of topics could come under such a heading.
Nevertheless, it is rather surprising, at least to me, that
there seems to be coherence between all the communications.
That is, all the topics discussed here are related with the
developmental biology, in the broadest sense, of this most
interesting tissue, the retina. We have discussed mainly the
dynamics of several interesting patterns of behaviour of
retinal cells, sometimes using the terminology of biochemistry
and of molecular biology, but there has been little about the
morphological characteristics of the mature retinal tissue.
This trend may reflect the current research interests in the
topics covered by the title of the session.

The dynamics of the cellular behaviour of the retina seem
to be understood from two different aspects; on the one hand,
the interactions between retinal and other cell types, and
on the other, events which occur inside the retinal cells.
As to the first aspect, Dr Trisler described a promising and
pioneering approach for understanding the most intriguing
problem of the specificity of the retino-tectal relationship
in terms of the function of specific molecule(s). Dr Courtois
described several new molecules secreted from neural retina
which are certainly related with the interaction between
this and other ocular tissues.

As to the second aspect, it is hoped that the introduction
of techniques of cell culture of neural retina cells as
described by Drs Pessac and Beale, will open new systems for
studying many problems related to the biology of the retina in
in vitro conditions. However, the most remarkable property
of retinal cells is their unusual instability in cell differentiation. The property is the capacity for *transdif-*

ferentiation. It is natural that this is one of the important
subjects in discussing the dynamics of retinal cells.   Drs
Clayton, Eguchi and McDevitt contributed much to this problem
by presenting new meaningful data.

Finally it must be emphasized that these two aspects of
retinal research do not remain separate; the synthesis
between them has been started.   Dr Moscona showed that disruption of the normal cell-interactions between different
cell types in the retinal can be a cue which causes the
*intra*cellular changes leading to transdifferentiation.

RETINAL BIOCHEMISTRY — A HOLISTIC VIEW

G.J. CHADER

*Laboratory of Vision Research, National Eye Institute,
National Institutes of Health, Bethesda, MD, USA*

In trying to best define retinal biochemistry, one can only think of the story of the blind men who are asked to touch and then describe an elephant. The blind man touching the tail describes it as a rope, the man touching the ear feels a fan while the man touching the trunk feels a snake. Similarly, retinal biochemistry can be thought of in many ways.

To a large number of retinal biochemists, the retina begins at the photoreceptor cilium and ends at the outer segment tip. Most of these biochemists subclassify themselves mainly as chemists or biophysicists and concentrate on studying the visual cycle in the photoreceptor unit with all its fascinating low temperature kinetics, absorption spectral changes and short-lived intermediates. Those with a predilection towards protein or carbohydrate biochemistry have also not had to look further than the outer segment (Hargrave, 1982). Nature has provided in the rod outer segment a perfect model system for studying membranes since the organelle is relatively easy to isolate, consists in greatest part of only one protein, opsin, and has an extremely well-defined physiological function. Most of these people spend their time stringing together various permutations and combinations of amino acids and sugar moieties into a rhodopsin chain that itself can be twisted and turned in innumerable ways as one attempts to examine its position in the membrane or its conformational changes during the visual cycle (Fig. 1).

The retina has been quite useful to those who classify themselves as neurochemists since it is a simple and readily accessible part of the CNS composed of neuronal and glial elements as is the brain. Developmental biochemists view the retina as a series of ascending steps or plateaus which allows them to investigate and perhaps even to attain the fully differentiated state. Sometimes, to a developmental

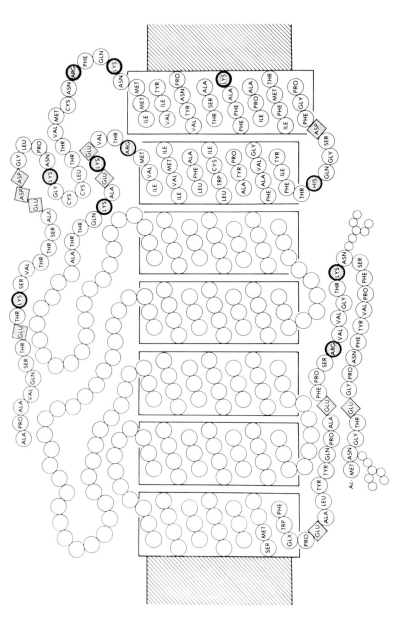

Fig. 1 Model for organization of the rhodopsin chain in the lipid bilayer of the outer segment disc membrane (from Hargrave, 1982).

biologist, the retina is ephemeral and elusive and changes
before one's eyes. In the pineal of lower vertebrates like
the lizard, retinal-like cells are quite apparent (Eakin,
1970). In mammalian embryos, the pineal actually goes
through stages which are quite parallel to ocular development except that the retinal-like cells differentiate into
pinealocytes usually by the time of birth (Zimmerman and
T'so, 1975).

I would prefer however to take a more holistic view of the
retina and admire it as more than the sum of its parts. Ad-
mittedly, it is easy to think of the retina in parts or
layers. This stratification has led to a most profitable
line of investigation for Drs Lowry, Passonneau and their
collaborators as discussed below. In fact, functionally,
the retina *is* composed of two distinct parts. First, a
photoreceptor unit comprised of photoreceptor cells and
attendant pigment epithelial cells whose function is to
capture the photic stimulus and convert it into a chemical
signal (Fig. 2). The other part of the retina can be considered as a more integral part of the CNS, beginning the
long series of processing steps seen in the neural "wiring
diagram" (Fig. 2B) which ultimately results in a visual
image in the brain.

Recently, study of the visual process has brought the

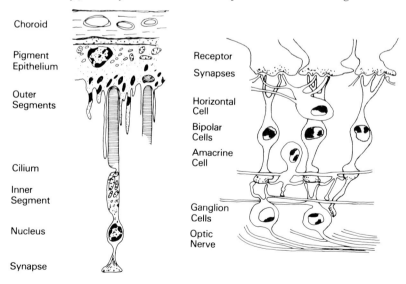

Choroid

Pigment
Epithelium

Outer
Segments

Receptor
Synapses

Horizontal
Cell

Bipolar
Cells

Amacrine
Cell

Cilium

Inner
Segment

Ganglion
Cells

Nucleus

Optic
Nerve

Synapse

A   B

Fig. 2 *Schematic diagram of the two functional parts of the
retina. (A) The Photoreceptor-Pigment Epithelial-Choroidal
Unit. (B) Inner layers of the retina.*

retina into the forefront of cyclic nucleotide research. In
the visual process itself, the calcium theory of Hagins
(1982) proposes that this cation is released from the discs
by a light stimulus, blocking sodium channels, causing hyper-
polarization and thus modulation of the electrical (neural),
impulse. Cyclic GMP has now been implicated in rod photoreceptor function as well (Bitensky et al., 1975). Although
its precise role is not clear, there certainly is a large
light-dark difference in cyclic GMP in isolated ROS (Table 1).
In rods, a high level of cyclic GMP in the dark could maintain
open sodium channels. In the light, phosphodiesterase (PDE)
is activated, and after an amplification process (Stryer et al.,

TABLE 1

*Effect of Light and Dark on Cyclic Nucleotide
Content in Isolated Rod Outer Segments (ROS)*

Condition	Cyclic Nucleotide Concentration (pmol/mg protein)	
	cyclic GMP	cyclic AMP
A - *in vivo* adaptation		
- dark	29.3 ± 4.3	1.8 ± 0.8
- light	3.1 ± 1.2	3.4 ± 1.9
B - *in vitro* adaptation		
- dark	23.4 ± 4.1	2.2 ± 0.4
- light	3.2 ± 1.6	1.9 ± 1.2

A - ROS prepared from frogs dark- or light-adapted *in vivo*.
B - ROS prepared from dark-adapted animals; a portion of the
    ROS was subsequently bleached (from Fletcher and Chader,
    1976).

1981), cyclic GMP levels fall and sodium channels may close.
The analogy made by Dr Mark Bitensky's laboratory (Stein,
Rasenick and Bitensky, 1982) comparing the control of ROS-
PDE activity with Rodbell's generalized scheme for control
of adenylate cyclase activity is striking. Kinetic evidence
from Liebman's laboratory (Yee and Liebman, 1978) demonstrates that the great speed of PDE activation and the high
gain in cyclic GMP hydrolysis are compatible with a role
for the nucleotide in the visual process. Individually, the
calcium and cyclic nucleotide models are probably too sim-
plistic, but studied together they may lead to a final
understanding of the chain of events in the visual cascade.
    Similar light-dark differences in cyclic GMP are not

observed in cone-dominant retinas, although there is evidence
that cyclic AMP could function in cones in an analogous manner to that of cyclic GMP in rods (Farber *et al.*, 1982).
Parenthetically, cyclic AMP has been implicated in the process of phagocytosis of outer segments by cultured pigment
epithelial cells (Edwards and Bakshian, 1980) and in fluid
transport across the pigment epithelium (Miller *et al.*,
1982). Burnside (Burnside *et al.*, 1982) has found that
cyclic AMP can control photomechanical movement in teleost
fish both in retina and PE. Thus, the two nucleotides may
subserve several different functions in the photoreceptor
unit.

Cyclic nucleotides could also be involved in at least
some types of hereditary retinal degeneration. In the early
onset type seen in the C3H mouse (Farber and Lolley, 1975),
Irish Setter dog (Aguirre *et al.*, 1978) and Collie (Woodford
et al., 1982), extraordinarily high cyclic GMP concentrations
are found in the photoreceptor cell due to abnormally low
phosphodiesterase activity (Fig. 3). Pathology in this

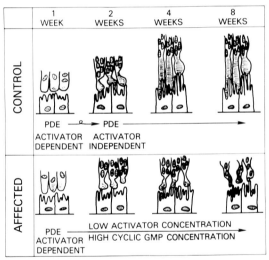

Fig. 3 *Model for rod-cone dysplasia in the Irish Setter
dog: biochemical and morphological correlates in early
onset retinal degeneration (from Liu* et al., *1979).*

disease is delimited to the photoreceptor organelle in the
early stages making this an interesting model for studying
localized inborn errors of metabolism.

Since Young and his associates (Young, 1976) elucidated
the process of ROS disc shedding and phagocytosis, many
new ideas of molecular and cell biology have been melded

with more conventional and traditional studies of retinal
metabolism. This renewal process could very well be referred
to as the "UCLA Marching Band" (Fig. 4). in accordance
with the movement of the bands of radioactive tracer substances from their point of incorporation in the cilial area

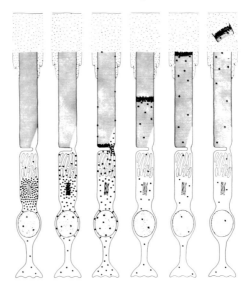

Fig. 4 *Renewal process in the rod outer segment (from Young,
1976).*

to their shedding into phagosomes at the outer segment tip.
Moreover, LaVail's discovery of the circadian nature of the
shedding process (LaVail, 1976) links retinal homostatic
processes with the systemic endocrine organs albeit in a
yet unknown manner (Fig. 5). In the past, only Moscona and
a few others have looked at the retina as a hormonal target
tissue (Moscona, 1971). This has mainly been from a developmental viewpoint, although it is interesting to note that
even the adult retina exhibits the same type of glucocortoid
receptor Gordon Tompkins described in cultured hepatoma cells,
as well as classical induction of a specific enzyme (glutamine synthetase). The role of retinoids (retinol, retinoic
acid) in retinal physiology must also be re-examined. They
could very well play a much more generalized role in retinal
biochemistry, controlling nuclear events in early development
and/or maintenance of differentiated function as do the
steroid hormones in their specific target tissues (Chader
et al., 1981). In a manner analogous to the steroid hormones, specific intracellular bindng proteins for retinol

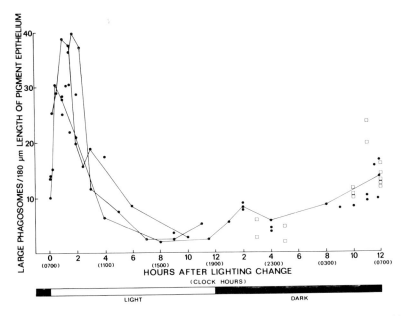

Fig. 5 *Phagosomal pattern in rat pigment epithelium at different times of the lighting cycle (from LaVail, 1976).*

(CRBP) and retinoic acid (CRABP) are present in retina; perhaps they facilitate movement of retinoid between cytoplasm and nucleus (Fig. 6).

One cannot forget the PE cell in discussing the photoreceptor, since the two truly do form a functional unit.

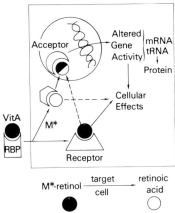

Fig. 6 *Model for the uptake, metabolic conversion, intracellular binding, translocation and possible action(s) of vitamin A (from Chader et al., 1981).*

The PE cell could perhaps be thought of as a "wet-nurse" for
the photoreceptor cell, responsible for its feeding and also
for removal of photoreceptor "garbage" i.e. spent or cast-off
outer segment tips. For these purposes, the PE cell is rich
in organelles and is distinctly polarized into apical and
basal portions. This is reflected biochemically in several
ways. Only the basal surface, for example, exhibits receptors for the serum RBP-retinol complex (Bok and Heller, 1976)
while the apical surface has high ATPase activity (Ostwald
and Steinberg, 1980). Enzymes of melanin biosynthesis and
lysosomal enzymes are also in high concentration; the former
necessary for light-screening in the eye and the latter of
course necessary for degradation of ingested ROS. The cycle
of phagosome uptake, fusion with lysosomes and ultimate
digestion of the ROS components (Fig. 7) is important in both

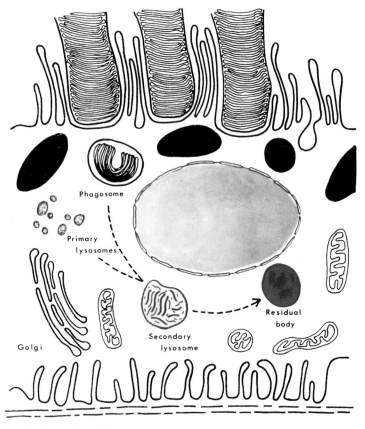

Fig. 7 *Schematic diagram of a typical pigment epithelial
cell showing the steps involved in the digestion of shed outer
segment membranes (diagram courtesy of Dr W.G. Robison, Jr.).*

normal and pathological functioning of the pigment epithelial
cell. Glucose transport, critical in ROS feeding and care,
has been "actively" studied in the PE cell (Miller and Steinberg, 1976; Zadunaisky and Degnan, 1976) although the actual
transport appears to be facilitated rather than active (Pascuzzo *et al.*, 1980; Masterson and Chader, 1981). Last but
not least, the PE acts as a main supply depot for vitamin A.
More than this though, there is active participation with
the ROS in movement and chemical transformations of the
retinoids. It is now clear that a specific protein (m.w.
about 140,000)is present in the subretinal space (or peripherally bound at the membrane surfaces) which binds retinol
with great avidity and whose apparent binding characteristics
are dependent on the state of light- and dark-adaptation of
the photoreceptor membranes (Lai *et al.*, 1982). This protein
could act as a transport vehicle, facilitating the movement
of retinoid between retina and PE cell and even perhaps
catalysing one or more of the chemical and conformational
changes that the retinoid molecule undergoes during the
visual process (Fig. 8).

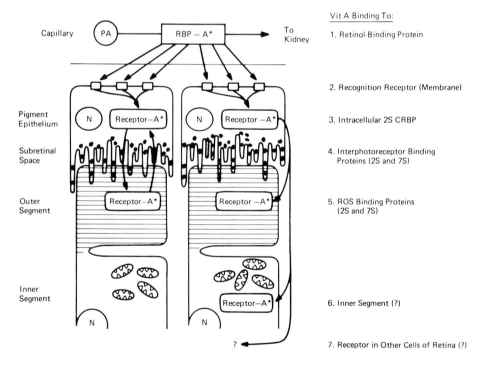

Fig. 8 *Model for the pathway(s) of uptake of vitamin A into
the PE cell and movement between PE and retina (from Chader,
1982).*

Much less is known about the biochemistry of the inner,
more neural strata of the retina although it is again a
perfect tissue for investigation due to its relatively simple
structure, stratified morphology and directed function. One
discipline that has used these characteristics to good
advantage is that of neurochemistry. Many types of neurotransmitters and neuromodulators are now known to function
in the various synaptic layers of the inner retina e.g.
catecholamines (Laties and Jacobowitz, 1966) and indolamines
(Hauschild and Laties, 1973). Synaptic receptors for acetylcholine (Vogel *et al.*, 1977) and GABA have also been identified (Brandon, Lam and Wu, 1979; Yazulla and Brecha, 1981)
as well as cells that take up several other putative amino
acid neurotransmitters (Lam and Hollyfield, 1980). Neuropeptides such as TRH (Schaeffer *et al.*, 1978) and somatostatin (Rorstad *et al.*, 1979) are also present in the retina;
specific peptide-containing amacrine cells have been identified for several of these including glucagon, somatostatin, enkephalin and neurotensin (Torngvist *et al.*, 1981).
As in other research areas cited above, the retina offers
one of the best model systems for studying neurotransmitter
and neuromodulator action.

Several lines of present investigation indicate future
breakthrough areas in retinal research. Some of the most
exciting and potentially important information on functioning
of both inner and outer portions of the retina will undoubtedly come from a delicate and difficult grouping of techniques put together several years ago by Lowry and Passonneau
(1972) and recently reapplied to the retina by Drs Lowry,
Cohen and Ferrendelli in St. Louis (Orr *et al.*, 1976)
and Dr Janet Passonneau at NIH (deAzeredo *et al.*, 1981). This
method combines the techniques of microdissection and biochemical cycling to measure substrates and metabolites or
enzyme levels in microgram amounts of tissue. Similar
studies using quick freeze techniques will not only give us
a comparative picture of the biochemical situation in the
different layers of the retina under any particular static
condition but ultimately be able to give us a "freeze-frame"
sequence of the dynamic changes induced in retinal metabolism in response to light or other stimuli. Moreover, the
retina offers a perfect opportunity for application of the
newly emerging techniques of molecular biology. Cloning
the rhodopsin gene or those for phosphodiesterase, opsin
kinase, etc. offers a unique opportunity for important contributions to both basic and clinically-oriented research.
The process of "transdifferentiation" as first described by
Eguchi and Okada (1973) is also ripe for biochemical investigation particularly at the molecular level. Understanding,

controlling and possibly redirecting ocular tissue development would have startling biological and clinical ramifica-
tions.

In sum, then, as beauty is in the eye of the beholder,
so retinal biochemistry is whatever one considers it to be.
I hope I have convinced you that the retina is the perfect
model system for membrane biochemistry, developmental biochemistry, neurochemistry and virtually every other sub-
discipline of biochemistry. I hope I have also convinced
you that the only study more interesting and productive than
these is the integration of all of them, resulting in the
study of retinal biochemistry for its own sake.

REFERENCES

Aguirre, G., Farber, D., Lolley, R., Fletcher, R. and Chader,
    G. (1978). Rod-cone dysplasia in Irish Setters: A defect
    in cyclic GMP metabolism in visual cells. *Science* **201**,
    1133-1134.
Bitensky, M., Miki, N., Keirns, J., Kerns, M., Baraban, J.,
    Freeman, J., Wheeler, M., Lacy, J. and Marcus, F. (1975).
    Activation of photoreceptor disc membrane phosphodiesterase
    by light and ATP. In "Adv. Cyclic Nucleotide Res."
    (Eds G. Drummond, P. Greengard and G. Robison). Vol. 5,
    Raven Press, New York, NY. pp. 213-240.
Bok, D. and Heller, J. (1976). Transport of retinol from
    the blood to the retina: an autoradiographic study of the
    pigment epithelial cell surface receptor for plasma
    retinol-binding protein. *Exp. Eye Res*. **22**, 395-402.
Brandon, C., Lam, D. and Wu, J.-Y. (1979). The γ-aminobutyric
    acid system in rabbit retina: localizationby immuno-
    chemistry and autoradiography. *Proc. Natl. Acad. Sci*.
    (USA) **76**, 3557-3561.
Burnside, B., Evans, M., Fletcher, R. and Chader, G. (1982).
    Induction of dark-adaptive retinomotor movement (cell
    elongation) in teleost retinal cones by cyclic adenosine
    3',5'-monophosphate. *J. Gen. Physiol*. **79**, 759-774.
Chader, G. (1971). Hormonal effects on the neural retina.
    1. Glutamine synthetase development in retina and liver
    of the normal and triiodothyronine-treated rat. *Arch.
    Biochem. Biophys*. **144**, 657-662.
Chader, G. (1982). Retinoids in ocular tissues: binding
    proteins, transport and mechanism of action. In "Cell
    Biology of the Eye (Ed. D. McDevitt) Academic Press, New
    York, NY pp. 377-433.
Chader, G., Wiggert, B., Russell, P. and Tanaka, M. (1981).
    Retinoid-binding proteins of retina and retinoblastoma

cells in culture. *Ann. N.Y. Acad. Sci.* **359**, 115–134.

deAzeredo, F., Lust, D. and Passonneau, J. (1981). Light-induced changes in energy metabolites, guanine nucleotides and guanylate cyclase within frog retinal layers. *J. Biol. Chem.* **256**, 2731–2735.

Eakin, R. (1970). A third eye. *Am.Scientist* **58**, 73–79.

Eguchi, G. and Okada, T. (1973). Differentiation of lens tissue from the progeny of chick retinal pigment cells cultured *in vitro*: A demonstration of a switch of cell type in clonal cell culture. *Proc. Natl. Acad. Sci. (USA)* **70**, 1495–1499.

Edwards, R. and Bakshian, S. (1980). Phagocytosis of outer segments by cultured rat pigment epithelium. *Invest. Ophthalmol. Vis. Sci.* **19**, 1184–1188.

Farber, D., Souza, D., Chase, D. and Lolley, R. (1981). Cyclic nucleotides of cone-dominant retinas: reduction of cyclic AMP levels by light and by cone degeneration. *Invest. Ophthalmol. Vis. Sci.* **20**, 24–31.

Fletcher, R. and Chader, G. (1976). Cyclic GMP: Control of concentration by light in retinal photoreceptors. *Biochem. Biophys. Res. Commun.* **70**, 1297–1302.

Hagins, W. (1972). The visual process: excitatory mechanisms in the primary receptor cell. *Annu. Rev. Biophys. Bioeng.* **1**, 131–158.

Hargrave, P. (1982). Rhodopsin Chemistry Structure and Topography in "Progress in Retinal Research" (Eds N. Osborne and G. Chader) Vol. 1, Pergamon Press, Oxford, UK (in press).

Hauschild, D. and Laties, A. (1973). An indolamine-containing cell in chick retina. *Invest. Ophthalmol.* **12**, 537–540.

Lai, Y., Wiggert, B., Liu, Y. and Chader, G. (1982). Inter-photoreceptor retinol binding proteins: possible transport vehicles between compartments of the retina. *Nature (London)* **298**, 848–849.

Lam, D. and Hollyfield, J. (1980). Localization of putative amino acid neurotransmitters in the human retina. *Exp. Eye Res.* **31**, 729–732.

Laties, A. and Jacobiwitz, D. (1966). A comparative study of the autonomic innervation of the eye in monkey, cat and rabbit. *Anat. Rec.* **156**, 383–398.

LaVail, M. (1976). Rod outer segment disc shedding in rat retina: relationship to cyclic lighting. *Science* **194**, 1071–1074.

Liu, Y.P., Krishna, G., Aguirre, G. and Chader, G. (1979). Involvement of cyclic GMP phosphodiesterase activator in an hereditary retinal degeneration. *Nature (London)* **280**, 62–64.

Lowry, O. and Passonneau, J. (1972). A Flexible System of

Enzymatic Analysis. Academic Press, New York.

Masterson, E. and Chader, G. (1981). Characterization of glucose transport by cultured chick pigment epithelium. *Exp. Eye Res*. **32**, 279-289.

Miller, S., Hughes, B. and Machen, T. (1982). Fluid transport across retinal pigment epithelium is inhibited by cyclic AMP. *Proc. Natl. Acad. Sci. USA* **79**, 2111-2115.

Miller, S. and Steinberg, R. (1976). Transport of taurine, L-methionine and 3-0-methyl-D-glucose across frog retinal pigment epithelium. *Exp. Eye Res*. **23**, 177-189.

Moscona, A. (1971). Control mecahnisms in hormonal induction of glutamine synthetase in the embryonic retina. In "Hormones in Development" (Eds M. Hamburgh and E. Barrington) pp. 169-189. Appleton, New York.

Ostwald, T. and Steinberg, R. (1980). Localization of frog retinal pigment epithelium Na^+-K^+ ATPase. *Exp. Eye Res*. **31**, 351-360.

Orr, H., Lowry, O., Cohen, A. and Ferrendelli, J. (1976). Distribution of 3':5'-cyclic AMP and 3':5'-cyclic GMP in rabbit retina *in vivo*: selective effects of dark and light adaptation and ischemia. *Proc. Natl. Acad. Sci. (USA)* **73**, 4442-4445.

Pascuzzo, G., Johnson, J. and Pautler, E. (1980). Glucose transport in isolated mammalian pigment epithelium. *Exp. Eye Res*. **30**, 53-58.

Schaeffer, J., Brownstein, M. and Axelrod, J. (1977). Thyrotropin-releasing hormone-like material in rat retina: changes due to environmental lighting. *Proc. Natl. Acad. Sci. (USA)* **74**, 3579-3581.

Stein, P., Rasenick, M. and Bitensky, M. (1982). Biochemistry of the cyclic nucleotide-related enzymes and rod photoreceptors. In "Progress in Retinal Research" (Eds N. Osborne and G. Chader) Vol. 1. Pergamon Press, Oxford, UK (in press).

Stryer, L., Hurly, J. and Fung, B. (1981). Transducin: an amplifyer protein in vision. *Trends Biochem. Sci*. **6**, 245-247.

Torngvist, K., Loren, I., Hakanson, R. and Sundler, F. Peptide-containing neurons in the chicken retina. *Exp. Eye Res*. **33**, 55-64.

Vogel, Z., Maloney, G., Ling, A. and Daniels, M. (1977). Identification of synaptic acetylcholine receptor sites in retina with peroxidase-labelled α-bungarotoxin. *Proc. Natl. Acad. Sci. (USA)* **74**, 3268-3272.

Woodford, B., Liu, Y., Fletcher, R., Chader, G., Farber, D., Santos-Anderson, R. and T'so, M. (1982). Cyclic nucleotide metabolism in inherited retinopathy in collies: a biochemical and histochemical study. *Exp. Eye Res*. **34**, 703-714.

Yazulla, S. and Brecha, N. (1981). Localized binding of ^{3}H-
    muscimol to synapses in chick retina. *Proc. Natl. Acad.
    Sci.* **78**, 643-647.
Yee, R. and Liebman, P. (1978). Light-activated phosphodie-
    sterase of the rod outer segment. Kinetics and parameters
    of activation and deactivation. *J. Biol. Chem.* **253**,
    8902-8909.
Young, R. (1976). Visual cells and the concept of renewal.
    Invest. Ophthalmol. Vis. Sci. **15**, 700-725.
Zadunaisky, J. and Degnan, K. (1976). Passage of sugars and
    urea in isolated retina pigment epithelium of the frog.
    Exp. Eye Res. **23**, 191-196.
Zimmerman, B. and T'so, M. (1975). Morphologic evidence of
    photoreceptor differentiation of pinealocytes in the
    neonatal rat. *J. Cell Biol.* **66**, 60-75.

CHEMICAL MESSENGERS IN THE RETINA

NEVILLE N. OSBORNE

*Nuffield Laboratory of Ophthalmology,
The University of Oxford, Walton Street, Oxford OX2 7AW, UK*

INTRODUCTION

The retina is part of the central nervous system and offers
several advantages for neurochemical, histological and
neuropharmacological studies. It can be isolated rapidly
without being injured and kept for hours in a viable condition (Ames and Gurian, 1960; Gouras and Hoff, 1970). The
responses of the tissue can be monitored by recording intra-
cellularly from specific cells or the electroretinogram.
Different areas of the retina corresponding to specific cell-
types or parts of cell-types are well defined, which facilitates the necessary correlation of neurochemical, morphological, histological, autoradiographical and neurophysiological findings. Furthermore, the retina is very thin with
short diffusion pathways; the extracellular fluid therefore
equilibrates rapidly with the bathing fluid. This is an
obvious advantage in the use of the retina to study release
mechanisms of putative transmitter substances, and the
absence of a barrier in the diffusion pathways also makes
the preparation useful for pharmacological studies. Specific
populations of nerve endings can be isolated from the retina
(Redburn, 1977), which is enormously helpful for studies
designed to establish the types of chemicals involved in
neurotransmission.
   Despite the advantages offered by the retinal preparation
over other nervous tissue (brain, spinal cord, various
ganglia), the identification of the various transmitters
employed at the different synapses has proved to be a difficult task. Analysis of recent reviews by Graham (1974),
Starr (1979) and Bonting (1976) revealed that no substance
has been unambiguously established as a positive transmitter at the cellular level in the retina. Gerschenfeld
and Piccolino (1979) in their article suggest that dopamine

may now qualify as a positive transmitter for certain interplexiform cells. In reality, it is difficult to establish
beyond doubt that a certain substance is a transmitter. The
evidence for serotonin being a neurotransmitter at certain
synapses in the snail CNS (Osborne, 1978; Cottrell, 1977) is,
for example, many times greater than for dopamine utilization
by certain retinal interplexiform cells (Dowling, 1979a, b).

Within the vertebrate CNS the rigorous criteria for identifying chemical transmitters are not easily satisfied.
Werman (1966) suggests that the following criteria have to
be fulfilled:

(1) The compound should be present in the nerve endings.
(2) the corresponding synthesizing enzymes should be present.
(3) there should be a mechanism for terminating the action
of the compound on the postsynaptic membrane.
(4) stimulation of the neurone should lead to its release
into the extracellular fluid.
(5) the action of the suspected transmitter should be identical in every way to the natural transmitter.

The complexity of the vertebrate CNS, which includes the
retina, makes it almost impossible to satisfy the fifth
criterion. Uncertainties about the status of a substance
have led to the unattractive designation "putative transmitter".

POSSIBLE TRANSMITTER CANDIDATES

Since the vertebrate retina is derived embryologically from
the brain, it would not be unreasonable to assume that substances which are proposed chemical messengers in the brain
have similar functions in the retina. Table 1 lists a number
of substances which, it has been suggested, could be involved
in the communication between neurones and might therefore
have such roles in the retina.

AMINO ACIDS AS CHEMICAL MESSENGERS IN THE RETINA

There is evidence that glutamate, aspartate, glycine,
γ-aminobutyrate (GABA) and taurine are potential retinal
transmitters (see Graham, 1974; Neal, 1976; Bonting, 1976;
Voaden, 1978; Voaden et al., 1980). It would appear that
glutamate and/or aspartate may be transmitters released
from photoreceptors and possible bipolar cell terminals.
The inhibitory amino acid GABA is thought to be a transmitter and to be released from terminals of the horizontal

TABLE 1

Substances which have been proposed to be involved in the communication between neurones
(from Osborne, 1981c)

Dopamine	Aspartate
Norepinephrine	Glutamate
Epinephrine	Prostaglandins
Tyramine	Corticosteroids
Octopamine	Estrogens
Phenylethylamine	Enkephalin
Phenylethanolamine	Testosterone
Dimethoxyphenylethylamine (DMPEA)	Thyroid hormone
Tetrahydroisoquinolines	Bombesin
Serotonin (5-hydroxytryptamine)	Cholecystokinin (CCK)
Malatonin	β-Endorphin
Tryptamine	Gastrin
Dimethyltryptamine (DMT)	Glucagon
5-Methoxytryptamine	Neurotensin
5-Methoxydimethyltryptamine	Proctolin
5-Hydroxydimethyltryptamine (bufotenin)	Prolactin
Tryptolines	Oxytocin
ATP	Substance P
Acetylcholine	Somatostatin
Carnosine	Angiotensin
Histamine	Lutenizing hormone releasing hormone (LHRH)
γ-Aminobutyric acid (GABA)	Vasopressin
γ-Hydroxybutyrate (GHB)	Vasoactive intestinal polypeptide (VIP)
Glycine	Adrenocorticotropic hormone (ACTH)
Taurine	Thyrotropin releasing hormone (TRH)
Purine	Sleep factor delta

and amacrine cells. It is also possible that glycine and
taurine have similar functions at terminals of amacrine cells.
The latter two amino acids have also been proposed as transmitter candidates for photoreceptors, even though they are
inhibitory and not excitatory, as one would suspect the
photoreceptor transmitters to be.

AMINES AS CHEMICAL MESSENGERS IN THE RETINA

There is now good reason to suppose that dopamine is a transmitter of certain interplexiform cells (Dowling, 1979*a*, *b*)
and amacrine neurones (Kramer, 1971; Ehinger, 1976) of the
vertebrate retina. Recent studies (Osborne, 1981*a*) have also
provided data strongly suggesting that noradrenaline is a
transmitter employed by certain amacrine neurones.

Since it has been reported that adrenaline exists in the
amphibian retina (Ehinger, 1976), it may well be that the
catecholamines dopamine, noradrenaline and adrenaline all
have transmitter functions in the retina as they appear to
have in the brain. The evidence for serotonin being a
retinal transmitter was questionable until recently (see
Ehinger and Florèn, 1980; Florèn, 1979). The latest experiments have produced data, however, which indicate quite
clearly that serotonin is the transmitter substance of certain amacrine neurones (see Osborne, 1980; Osborne and
Richardson, 1980; Osborne *et al.*, 1981a; Osborne, 1982).

ACETYLCHOLINE AS A CHEMICAL MESSENGER IN THE RETINA

The results of neurophysiological studies, in particular,
have shown that acetylcholine is a likely excitatory transmitter of selective populations of amacrine and bipolar cells
(Graham, 1974; Neal, 1976; Masland, 1980). The observation
by Lam (1975) that isolated cones of the turtle are able to
synthesize acetylcholine has also led to speculation that it
might be an excitatory photoreceptor neurotransmitter.
Further experiments to test this hypothesis (see Gerschenfeld
and Precolini, 1979) have proved contradictory and tend to
suggest that the photoreceptors do not utilize acetylcholine
as a neurotransmitter (see Masland and Mills, 1980).

PEPTIDES AS CHEMICAL MESSENGERS IN THE RETINA

The use of specific antibodies labelled with fluorescent
dyes has shown that the following peptides occur in specific

populations of amacrine cells: bombesin (unpubl. data), thyro-
tropin releasing hormone, somatostatin, neurotensin, enkephalin, substance P, vasoactive intestinal polypeptide (VIP),
glucagon, β-endorphin and cholecystokinin (see Stell *et al.*,
1980; Karten and Brecha, 1980; Eskay *et al.*, 1980; Jackson
et al., 1980; Osborne *et al.*, 1981*b*). Studies by Karten and
collaborators (Stell *et al.*, 1980, Karten and Brecha, 1980)
showed that groups of amacrine cells showing particular
physical characteristics were always associated with the
same peptides. Neurones could be classified according to
the size and spacing of their cell bodies or whether their
outgrowing nerve fibres branched into one, two or more levels
in the inner plexiform layer of the retina.

Whether the peptides are involved in classical types of
neurotransmission remains to be discovered. Their distinctive localization would suggest that they have specific roles
to play. They have generally been described as "neuromodulators", agents which are thought to attenuate or enhance the
passage of a nerve impulse set off by neurotransmitters. It
is of interest to note in this respect that all the peptide-
containing neurones so far described as occurring in the
retina belong to the amacrine neurones, and while the critical functions of these cells are poorly understood, they
are thought to modify spatial, temporal, intensive and
chromatic information by lateral interactions among bipolar,
ganglion and other amacrine neurones.

CONCLUSION

Many of the compounds which were assumed to be involved in
neuronal communication in the brain (see Table 1) are now
thought to have the same function in the retina. It is impossible to discuss in detail here the evidence for specific
chemicals having transmitter functions in certain neurones
in the retina. However it is clear that the retina, with
its inherent advantages enumerated in the introduction, allows
the experimental study of the roles of specific chemicals in
a defined cell-type (see Table 2). It is equally clear that
not all morphologically similar-type cells in the retina
e.g. amacrine cells, are biochemically identical. As pointed
out in a recent review by Osborne (1981*b*), nervous system
functions cannot be understood simply in terms of neurones
acting as relay stations, but rather by a variety of complex cellular mechanisms. The retina may function in certain
areas almost entirely without the need for any propagated
action potentials where "local circuits", both electrical
and chemical, may be important. Other synapses in the retina

TABLE 2

Summary of suspected chemical messengers in retinal neurones

Chemical	Neurones utilizing substance	Evidence for transmitter function
GABA	Horizontal and amacrine cells	Good
Glycine	Amacrine cells	Fairly good
Taurine	Amacrine cells	Questionable
Glutamate	Photoreceptors, bipolar cells	Fairly good
Aspartate	Photoreceptors, bipolar cells	Fairly good
Acetylcholine	Amacrine and bipolar cells	Excellent
Dopamine	Amacrine and inter-plexiform cells	Excellent
Noradrenaline	Amacrine cells	Fairly good
Serotonin	Amacrine cells	Good
Substance P	Amacrine cells	Questionable
Thyrotropin releasing hormone	Amacrine cells	Questionable
Somatostatin	Amacrine cells	Questionable
Neurotensin	Amacrine cells	Questionable
Enkephalin	Amacrine cells	Questionable
Bombesin	Amacrine cells	Questionable
Vasoactive Intestinal polypeptide	Amacrine cells	Questionable
Glucagon	Amacrine cells	Questionable
β-Endorphin	Amacrine cells	Questionable
Cholecystokinin	Amacrine cells	Questionable

may only be "activated" by modulation of a continuous release
of transmitter and not a triggering of release of a burst of
transmitter. We still have to discover how the chemicals
function precisely, which are specifically restricted to
certain cell types in the retina and thought to be chemical
messengers. Our present definitions of "neurotransmission",
"neuroregulation" or "neuromodulation" (see Osborne, 1981*c*)
are perhaps too narrow.

ACKNOWLEDGEMENTS

The author is grateful to the Stiftung Volkswagenwerk for
financial support.

REFERENCES

Ames, A. and Gurian, B. (1960). Measurement of function in
an *in vitro* preparation of mammalian central nervous tissue.
J. Neurophysiol. **23**, 676-691.

Bonting, S.L. (1976). Transmitters in the Visual Process.
Pergamon Press, Oxford.

Cottrell, G.A. (1977). Identified amine-containing neurones
and their synaptic connections. *Neuroscience* **2**, 1-18.

Dowling, J.E. (1979*a*). Information processing by local
circuits: the vertebrate retina as a model system. In
"The Neurosciences. Fourth Study Program" (Eds F.O.
Schmitt and F.G. Worden) pp. 163-181. MIT Press,
Cambridge, Mass.

Dowling, J.E. (1979*b*). A new retinal neurone — the interplexiform cell. *Trends in Neuroscience* **2**, 189-191.

Ehinger, B. (1976). Biogenic monoamines as transmitters in
the retina. In "Transmitters in the Visual Process"
(Eds S.L. Bonting) pp. 145-163. Pergamon Press, Oxford.

Ehinger, B. and Florèn, I. (1980). Retinal indoleamine
accumulating neurones. *Neurochem. Int.* **1**, 209-229.

Eskay, R.L., Long, R.T. and Iuoone, P.M. (1980). Evidence
that TRH, Somatostatin and substance P are present in
neurosecretory elements of the vertebrate retina.
Brain Res. **196**, 554-559.

Florèn, I. (1979). Arguments against 5-hydroxytryptamine
as a transmitter in the rabbit retina. *J. Neural. Trans.*
46, 1-15.

Gerschenfeld, H.M. and Piccolino, M. (1979). Pharmacology
of the connections of cones and L-horizontal cells in
the vertebrate retina. In "The Neurosciences; Fourth
Study Program" (Eds F.O. Schmitt and F.G. Worden)

pp. 213-226. MIT Press, Cambridge, Mass.

Gouras, P. and Hoff, M. (1970). Retinal function in an
isolated perfused mammalian eye. *Invest. Ophthalmol.*
9, 388-399.

Graham, L.T. Jr (1974). Comparative aspects of neurotrans-
mitters in the retina. In "The Eye" (Eds H. Dawson and
L.T. Graham, Jr) Vol. 6 pp. 283-342. Academic Press,
New York.

Jackson, I.M.D., Bolaffi, J.L. and Guillemin, R. (1980).
Presence of immunoreactive -endorphin and enkephalin —
like material in the retina and other tissues of the frog
Rana pipiens. *Gen. Comp. Endocrinol.* **42**, 505-508.

Karten, H.J. and Brecha, N. (1980). Localization of substance P immunoreactivity in amacrine cells of the
retina. *Nature (Lond)*. **283**, 87-88.

Kramer, S.B. (1971). Dopamine: a retinal transmitter. I.
Retinal uptake, storage and light stimulated release
of ^{3}H-dopamine *in vivo*. *Invest. Ophthalmol.* **10**, 438-452.

Lam, D.M.K. (1975). Synaptic chemistry of identified cells
in the vertebrate retina. Cold Spring Harbor *Symp.*
Quant. Biol. **40**, 571-579.

Masland, R.H. (1980). Acetylcholine in the retina. *Neurochem. Int.* **1**, 501-518.

Masland, R.H. and Mills, J.W. (1980). Choline accumulation
by photoreceptors of the rabbit retina. *Proc. Nat. Acad.*
Sci. **77**, 1671-1675.

Neal, M. (1976). Amino acid transmitter substances in the
vertebrate retina. *J. Gen. Pharmacol.* **1**, 321-332.

Osborne, N.N. (1978). The neurobiology of a Serotenergic
Neuron. In "Biochemistry of Characterized Neurons"
(Ed. N.N. Osborne) pp. 47-80. Pergamon Press, Oxford.

Osborne, N.N. (1980). *In vitro* experiments on the metabolism, uptake and release of 5-hydroxytryptamine in the
bovine retina. *Brain Res*. **184**, 283-297.

Osborne, N.N. (1981*a*). Noradrenaline — a transmitter
candidate in the bovine retina. *J. Neurochem*. **36**, 17-27.

Osborne, N.N. (1981*b*). Communication between neurones:
current concepts. *Neurochem. Int.* **3**, 3-16.

Osborne, N.N. (1982). Binding of ^{3}H-serotonin to membranes of the retina. *Exp. Eye Res*. **34**, 639-649.

Osborne, N.N. and Richardson, G. (1980). Specificity of
Serotonin uptake by bovine retina: Comparison with
tryptamine. *Exp. Eye Res*. **31**, 31-39.

Osborne, N.N., Nesselhut, T., Nicholas, D.A. and Cuello,
A.C. (1981*a*). Serotonin: a transmitter candidate in
the vertebrate retina. *Neurochem. Int.* **3**, 171-176.

Osborne, N.N., Nicholas, D.A., Cuello, A.C. and Dockray,
G.J. (1981*b*). Localization of Cholecystokinin immuno-

reactivity in amacrine cells of the retina. *Neuroscience Letters* **26**, 31-35.

Redburn, D.A. (1977). Uptake and release of ^{14}C-GABA from rabbit retina synaptosomes. *Exp. Eye Res.* **25**, 265-275.

Starr, M.S. (1979). Prospective neurotransmitters in vertebrate retina. In "Essays in Neurochemistry and Neuropharmacology" (Eds M.B.H. Yondim, W. Lovenberg, D.F. Sharman and J.R. Lagnado). Vol. 2. pp. 151-174. John Wiley & Sons, Chichester.

Stell, W., Marshak, D., Yamada, T., Brecha, N. and Karten H. (1980). Peptides are in the eye of the beholder. *Trends in Neuroscience* **3**, 292-295.

Voaden, M.J. (1978). Localization and metabolism of neuro-active amino acids in the retina. In "Amino Acids as Transmitters (Ed. F. Forman) pp. 257-274. Plenum Press, New York.

Voaden, M.J., Morjaria, B. and Oraedu, A.C.T. (1980). The Localization and metabolism of glutamate, aspartate and GABA in the rat retina. *Neurochem. Int.* **1**, 151-166.

Werman, R. (1966). Criteria for identification of a central nervous transmitter system. *Comp. Biochem. Physiol.* **18**, 745-766.

FERROUS ION-MEDIATED RETINAL DEGENERATION: ROLE OF ROD OUTER SEGMENT LIPID PEROXIDATION

LAURENCE M. RAPP, REX D. WIEGAND and ROBERT E. ANDERSON

Cullen Eye Institute, Baylor College of Medicine
Houston, Texas 77030, USA.

SUMMARY

The degenerative changes that follow an intravitreal injection of ferrous sulphate into the frog eye were examined.
ERG a- and b-wave amplitudes were reduced by 50% within 1 h
post-injection and were extinguished by 24 h. Light microscopy revealed a progressive degeneration of the photoreceptor
cells and their subsequent death. Chemical analyses showed
that injection of ferrous sulphate leads to the production of
lipid peroxides and the disappearance of long chain polyunsaturated fatty acids from the retina.

INTRODUCTION

A variety of experimental models have been utilized to study
retinal degenerations which specifically affect photoreceptor
cells (reviewed by Botermans, 1972). Among the more recent
of these investigations, there has been growing evidence
that lipid peroxidation may be directly involved in photoreceptor destruction. Surgical implantation of an iron nail
into the rabbit vitreous (Hiramitsu *et al.*, 1979) or X-
irradiation (Hiramitsu *et al.*, 1978) reduced ERG amplitude
over a time course that followed the production of lipid
peroxides in the retina. These treatments further caused
the progressive deterioration of the photoreceptor cells.
Similarly, exposure of chick embryos (Yagi *et al.*, 1977) or
rabbits (Hiramitsu *et al.*, 1976) to high concentrations
of oxygen led to photoreceptor degeneration and increased
levels of retinal lipid peroxides. Indeed, the intravitreal injection of lipid peroxides into the rabbit eye
causes ERG loss and structural alterations in the retina

(Hiramitsu *et al.*, 1978; Armstrong *et al.*, 1981).

We have begun a series of experiments to test the hypothesis that lipid peroxidation may be the first step in a
chain of events that leads to retinal degenerations. In the
present study, we have investigated the degenerative changes
resulting from intravitreal injections of ferrous sulphate.
For several years now, clinical case reports have shown that
an iron-containing foreign body retained in the eye may
result in a retinal degeneration resembling retinitis pigmentosa (Cogan, 1969). Furthermore, a number of studies
have documented the degenerative retinal changes associated
with experimental ocular siderosis (e.g. Declercq *et al.*,
1977; Masciulli *et al.*, 1972). Our experiments demonstrate
that the intravitreal injection of ferrous sulphate leads
to the production of lipid peroxides, disappearance of long
chain polyunsaturated fatty acids, loss of amplitude of
both the a- and b-wave of the ERG, and a progressive photoreceptor degeneration.

METHODS

Frogs (*Rana pipiens*) were dark-adapted overnight, and im-
mobilized with an intraperitoneal injection of d-tubocurarine
chloride (9µg/g body weight). Using a 32 gauge needle, frogs
were then injected intravitreally at the pars plana with 10
µl of an aqueous solution of 20 mM ferrous sulphate into one
eye and sham-injected with 10 µl solution of 20 mM sodium
sulphate into the contralateral eye. The pH of the ferrous
sulphate solution was found to be 4.0. Accordingly, the
sodium sulphate solution was adjusted to this pH with HCl.

Electroretinography was performed before intravitreal
injections and at various times thereafter. When ERG monitor-
ing was carried out for longer than 4 h post-injection, frogs
were returned to their normal 12L:12D cycle. Any subsequent
ERG analyses were preceded by 2 h dark-adaptation. An
Ag-AgCl cotton wick electrode was placed on the eye to be
stimulated and a reference on the animal's tongue. Signals
from the electrodes were coupled to a PAR model 113 preamplifier with a time constant to 1.6 seconds. The output of
the preamplifier was displayed on a storage oscilloscope.
Intensity response curves were generated with 20 millisecond
flashes of white light from a Xenon lamp (maximum intensity
= 10^6 µW/cm^2). Calibrated neutral density filters were placed
in the light path to control intensity and a Melles Griot
KG-1 water filter was permanently installed in the optical
system to eliminate heat.

At various times, frogs were killed by decapitation and

retinas taken for either morphological or biochemical
evaluation. Retinas were fixed in 0.09 M sodium phosphate
(pH 7.4) containing 2.5% glutaraldehyde and 1% paraformaldehyde. After postfixation in 1% OsO_4, tissues were dehydrated, embedded in Epon-Araldite, and sectioned for
light microscopy. Purified rod outer segments (ROS) were
prepared from retinas taken for biochemical analysis. The
ROS were made to a known volume in water and aliquots were
removed for protein assay, polyacrylamide gel disk electrophoresis, and lipid extraction. The lipid extract was
evaporated to dryness under a stream of nitrogen, and redissolved in cyclohexane:ethanol (1:1, v/v). Lipid peroxide
content of this solution was determined by scanning on a
Cary 219C from 320 nm to 210 nm, the absorbance at 233 nm
being taken as peroxides containing conjugated dienes. After
spectrophotometry, aliquots were removed for determination
of lipid phosphorus, and the remaining lipid was trans-
methylated with boron trifluoride-methanol for gas-liquid
chromatographic analysis.

RESULTS

The intravitreal injection of ferrous sulphate caused a
dramatic deterioration of the electroretinogram. Figure 1
shows the normal appearance of the ERG pattern of the pre-
injection control (PC). However, within 1 h of injection
of ferrous sulphate, there was a marked loss in amplitude
of both the a- and b-waves. By 4 h both a- and b-waves had
been nearly extinguished, and were not detectable 24 h
after injection. A slow potential (implicit time ≃ 2 sec)
which may have been the c- or the e-wave of the ERG,
could be recorded even after 24 h. In contrast, sham-injection
with sodium sulphate caused no differences in the ERG in
comparison to pre-injection controls. Figures 2 and 3 show
the time course of loss of amplitude of the a- and b-waves
of the ERG, respectively, for the 24 h period following the
injection of ferrous sulphate or sodium sulphate. Although
it would be difficult from our data to speculate whether the
loss of amplitude is exponential or bimodal, it is apparent
that the amplitude of both a- and b-waves is reduced by 50%
or greater within 1 h after injection of the ferrous ion.
     Histological changes also were observed soon after the
injection of ferrous ion. Figure 4a is a light micrograph
of a retina 24 h following injection of sodium sulphate.
There are no apparent differences between this retina and non-
injected controls. Four hours after the injection of ferrous
sulphate, however, there is obvious disruption of the orderly

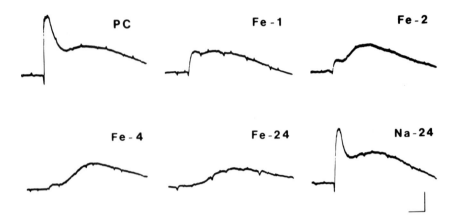

Fig. 1 *ERG waveforms recorded at various intervals following intravitreal injections of ferrous sulphate or sodium sulphate. All responses were elicited with saturating flashes. Stimulus duration was 20 milliseconds. The small spikes superimposed on the ERG are due to the frog's heartbeat. Calibration bars denote an amplitude of 200 μV and a duration of 0.5 seconds. PC: pre-injection control; Fe-1, -2, -4, -24,: 1, 2, 4, 24 h following FeSO₄ injection; Na-24, 24 h following Na₂SO₄ injection.*

arrangement of the rod outer segment disks, and the nuclei of most (if not all) of the photoreceptor cells are pyknotic (Fig. 4b). The retinal pigment epithelium (RPE) is somewhat swollen, but otherwise appears intact. After 8 days (Fig. 4c), there are no detectable rod nuclei. A layer of debris exists between the outer limiting membrane and the RPE, which appears to be made up of photoreceptor remnants and invading macrophages which may contain melanin. Also to be noted, at this advanced stage of degeneration, is the presence of oil droplets in the subretinal space and their increase in size and number in the RPE (Fig. 4c). The degenerative changes described above were predominantly restricted to photo-receptor cells and RPE, with the exception of an occasional darkening of inner nuclear layer cells.

Chemical changes were observed in the ROS following ferrous sulphate injection. The data in Table 1 are comparisons of pre-injection controls with those injected with sodium sulphate or ferrous sulphate. The yield of ROS from ferrous sulphate-injected retinas was always less than from pre-injection or sham-injected controls. At 4 h, the protein-

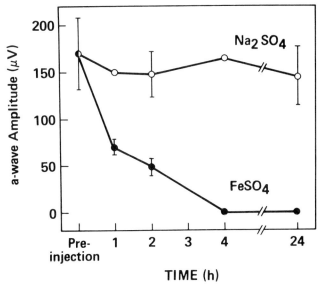

Fig. 2 *Time course for changes in a-wave amplitude following intravitreal injections of ferrous sulphate or sodium sulphate into the frog eye. Amplitudes represent the saturation level of the a-wave. Standard deviations are drawn upon mean values for groups of 4 or more frogs.*

to-phospholipid ratio was not drastically different between the sham-injected and experimental groups, although an increase in this ratio did become pronounced after 24 h. Polyacrylamide gel disk electrophoresis of experimental and control ROS did not show any significant differences, indicating that our ROS preps were of equal purity (data not shown). The presence of lipid peroxides, determined by increased absorbance at 233 nm in the experimental group, confirmed that injection of ferrous ion had resulted in an increase in lipid peroxidation. The peroxide levels were 3 to 4 times higher in the ferrous-injected eyes than in the control. Concomitant with the increase in peroxide was a loss of long chain polyunsaturated fatty acids from total ROS phospholipids. This was observed as a selective decrease in docosahexaenoic acid (22:6ω3). Palmitic acid (16:0), a saturated fatty acid which is not subject to peroxidation reactions, was essentially unchanged over the 24 h time course.

DISCUSSION

The data we have presented in this paper clearly implicate

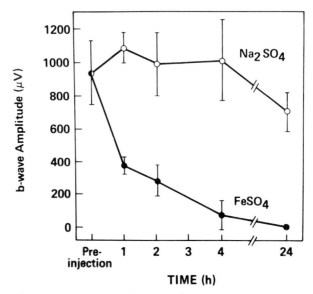

Fig. 3 *Time course for changes in b-wave amplitude following intravitreal injections of ferrous sulphate or sodium sulphate into the frog eye. Amplitudes and standard deviations were determined in the same manner as in Fig. 2.*

lipid peroxidation in photoreceptor degenerations. Shortly after the injection of ferrous sulphate, a known stimulant for the production of oxygen radicals, there was a rapid and reproducible loss of both the a- and the b-wave of the electroretinogram. As early as 4 h after injection, morphological changes in the photoreceptor outer segments had already taken place. Chemical analysis of these membranes at 4 h showed a loss of long chain polyunsaturated fatty acids and the appearance of products of lipid peroxidation (conjugated dienes). In a related study by Shvedova (1979), frog retinas were incubated with Fe^{++} and ascorbate for up to 20 minutes. A progressive decrease in ERG amplitude correlated with the appearance of lipid peroxides, although no ultrastructural changes were apparent after this short time. At the present, we have not examined enough early time points to determine the temporal relationship between loss of ERG amplitude, appearance of lipid peroxidation, loss of polyunsaturated fatty acids, and morphological changes. These studies are currently underway in our laboratory.

In another paper in this volume (Wiegand *et al.*, 1981), data were presented on the chemical changes associated with

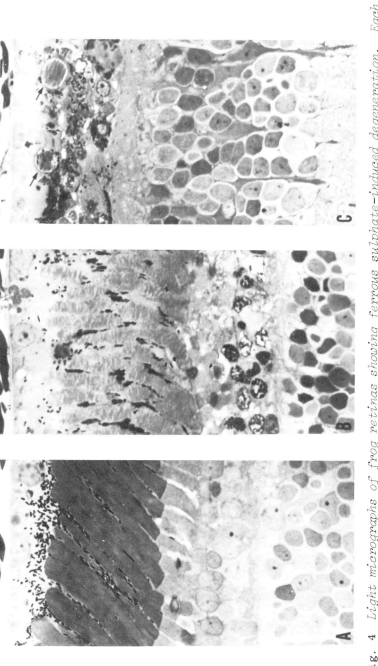

Fig. 4 *Light micrographs of frog retinas showing ferrous sulphate–induced degeneration. Each section was taken from a region of the nasal retina approximately 2 mm from the optic nerve along the horizontal meridian. (A) 24 h sham–injected retina. (B) 4 h FeSO₄⁻ injected retina. (C) 8 d FeSO₄⁻injected retina. Note enlarged oil droplets (arrows) and compaction of the retina at 8 days (all micrographs × 540).*

TABLE 1

Protein, lipid and peroxide content of frog rod outer segments

GROUP*	INJECTION	ROS YIELD (μg protein/retina)	PROTEIN/ PHOSPHOLIPID (wt/wt)	PEROXIDE LEVELS**	FATTY ACIDS (nmol/mg protein)	
					$16:0$***	$22:6$****
Preinjection	none	215	1.13	0.56	364	950
Preinjection	none	228	1.12	0.33	363	958
4 hours	Na_2SO_4	301	1.15	0.55	344	902
4 hours	$FeSO_4$	154	1.19	1.98	351	798
24 hours	Na_2SO_4	214	1.19	0.59	327	1012
24 hours	$FeSO_4$	72	1.39	1.53	354	684

* In each group analyses were performed on ROS membranes isolated from 3 pooled retinas. Injected frogs received 10 μl of 20 mM Na_2SO_4 in the left eye and 10 μl of 20 mM $FeSO_4$ in the right eye.

** Absorbance/mg phospholipid dissolved in 1 ml cyclohexane-ethanol (1:1, v/v) at $\lambda = 233$ nm (1 cm optical path).

*** Palmitic acid.

**** Docosahexaenoic acid.

light-induced retinal degeneration in the albino rat. These
data share many common features with those reported here for
frogs. For example, in both studies there is a progressive
loss of recovery of ROS, an increase in protein-to-phos-
pholipid ratios in the ROS, and a progressive loss of a
specific long chain polyunsaturated fatty acid ($22:6\omega3$).
Also, the morphological changes showing early ROS damage and
specific loss of rod cells are similar. In our frog studies,
we observed lipid peroxides, but this analysis has not yet
been carried out on light-damaged rats. However, it has
been reported that lipid peroxides are produced in the retina
of frogs (Kagen *et al*., 1973) and rats (Organisciak *et al*.,
1981) exposed to relatively short periods of light.

   Although the etiologic agents for the light- and ferrous
ion-induced retinal degenerations are different, the mechanism of retinal degeneration may be quite similar. In the
case of ferrous ion, lipid peroxides could be generated
from hydroxyl radicals, which are produced by the oxidation of ferrous ion with hydrogen peroxide (Hashstein *et al*.,
1964). Hydrogen peroxide is formed in the ROS by the dis-
mutation of superoxide radicals (Hall and Hall, 1975).
Hydroxyl radicals rapidly initiate the chain reactions of
lipid peroxidation, ultimately leading to the formation of
malonaldehyde. This bi-functional compound cross-links
amino groups of both lipids and proteins in biological membranes (Nielson, 1981; Dillard and Tappel, 1973). In the
photoreceptors, this could result in loss of cellular com-
partmentalization and eventual cell death.

ACKNOWLEDGEMENTS

This research was supported in part by grants from the
Retina Research Foundation (Houston, Texas), National
Retinitis Pigmentosa Foundation, Research to Prevent Blindness, Inc., and the National Eye Institute (EY 07001, EY
02520, EY 00871, EY 1406 and EY 05493). We are grateful
to Dr Scott F. Basinger for his contributions to the electroretinographic study. We thank Jo Ann Garcia and Alexander
Kogan for their technical assistance.

REFERENCES

Armstrong, D., Wehling, C. and Wilson, C. (1981). Lipid
    peroxide-mediated retinal dystrophy in the rabbit: A
    model for human and canine ceroid-lipofuscinosis (Batten
    Disease) Association for Research and Vision and Oph-

thalmology (Abstract) p. 41.

Botermans, C.H.G. (1972). Primary pigmentary retinal de-
generation and its association with neurological diseases
In "Handbook of Clinical Neurology", Vol. 13, Chapter 8,
North-Holland Publ. Co., Amsterdam.

Cogan, D.G. (1969). Pseudoretinitis Pigmentosa: Report of
two traumatic cases of recent origin. Arch. Ophthalmol.
81, 45—53.

Declercq, S., Meridith, P. and Rosenthal, R. (1977). Experimental siderosis in the rabbit. Arch. Ophthalmol.
95, 1051—1058.

Dillard, C. and Tappel, A. (1973). Fluorescent products
from reaction of peroxidizing polyunsaturated fatty acids
with phosphatidyl ethanolamine and phenylalanine. Lipids
8, 183—189.

Hall, M. and Hall, D. (1975). Superoxide dismutase of bovine
and frog rod outer segments. Biochem. Biophys. Res.
Commun. 67, 1199—1204.

Hashstein, P., Nordenbrand, K. and Ernster, L. (1964). Evidence for the involvement of iron in the ADP-activated
peroxidation of lipids in microsomes and mitochondria.
Biochem. Biophys. Res. Commun. 14, 323—328.

Hiramitsu, T., Hasegawa, Y., Hirata, K., Nishigaki, I. and
Yagi, K. (1976). Formation of lipoperoxide in the retina
of rabbit exposed to high concentration of oxygen.
Separatum Experientia 32, 622—623.

Hiramitsu, T., Majima, Y., Hasegawa, Y. and Hirata, K. (1978).
Role of lipid peroxide in the induction of retinopathy
by x-irradiation. Acta Soc. Ophthalmol. Jap. 9, 819—725.

Hiramitsu, T., Majima, Y., Hasegawa, Y. and Hirata, K. (1979).
Role of lipid peroxide in the induction of the retinal
siderosis. Acta Soc. Ophthalmol. Jap. 10, 1468—1473.

Kagan, V., Shvedova, A., Novikov, K. and Kozlov, Y. (1973).
Light-induced free radical oxidation of membrane lipids
in photoreceptors of frog retina. Biochim. Biophys.
Acta. 330, 76—79.

Masciulli, L., Anderson, D. and Charles, S. (1972). Experimental ocular siderosis in the squirrel monkey. Am. J.
Ophthalmol. 74, 638—661.

Nielson, H. (1981). Covalent binding of peroxidized phospholipid to protein: III. Reaction of individual phospholipids with different proteins. Lipids 16, 215—222.

Organisciak, D., Lake, J. and Wang, H. (1981). The enzymatic determination of hydroperoxides in the ROS of cyclic
light and dark reared rats. Association for Research
in Vision and Ophthalmol. (Abstract) p. 166.

Shvedova, A., Sidorov, A., Novikov, K., Galushchenko, I. and
Kagan, N. (1979). Lipid peroxidation and electric activity

of the retina. *Vision Res*. **19**, 49—55.

Wiegand, R.D., Giusto, N.M., and Anderson, R.E. (1982). Lipid changes in albino rat rod outer segments following constant illumination. (this volume).

Yagi, K., Matsuoka, S., Onkawa, H., Ohishi, N., Takeuchi, Y. and Sakai, H. (1977). Lipoperoxide level of the retina of chick embryo exposed to high concentration of oxygen. *Clin. Chim. Acta* **80**, 355-360.

LIPID CHANGES IN ALBINO RAT ROD OUTER SEGMENTS FOLLOWING CONSTANT ILLUMINATION

REX D. WIEGAND, NORMA M. GIUSTO and ROBERT E. ANDERSON

*Cullen Eye Institute, Baylor College of Medicine,
Houston, Texas 77030, USA*

SUMMARY

Constant illumination is known to cause degeneration of rod outer segment (ROS) membranes in the albino rat. In rats exposed to 100 to 125 foot-candles illumination for 3 days, we observed a concomitant reduction in the levels of 22:6ω3, the major polyunsaturated fatty acid in ROS phospholipids. The progressive loss of 22:6ω3 is due primarily to selective loss from those phospholipid species containing two of these polyunsaturated fatty acids.

INTRODUCTION

It is well known that continuous exposure of the albino rat to light results in progressive destruction of retinal photo-receptor cells (Noell *et al.*, 1966; Anderson *et al.*, 1972; Rapp and Williams, 1980; reviewed by Lanum, 1978). The first ultrastructural changes appear to be vesiculations of ROS disks which, with increasing time of exposure, progress to total disruption of the orderly packing of these structures. Cell death quickly follows, as evidenced by the loss of rod nuclei (O'Steen *et al.*, 1974). Loss of retinal function measured by electro retinography parallels the ultrastructural alterations (Noell *et al.*, 1966).

The biochemical mechanism of light-induced retinal degenerations is not known, although, several recent preliminary reports have implicated lipid peroxidation (Joel *et al.*, 1981; Wiegand *et al.*, 1981*a*; Wiegand *et al.*, 1981*b*; Organisciak *et al.*, 1981). Clearly the ROS are ideal substrates for peroxidative reactions since their phospholipids contain large amounts of long-chain polyunsaturated fatty acids

(reviewed by Anderson and Andrews, 1982) and the retina has
a very high consumption of molecular oxygen (Warburg, 1924).
Also, superoxide dismutase, an enzyme that destroys damaging
oxygen radicals is present in high concentrations in the
retina (Hall and Hall, 1975) as is the anti-oxidant Vitamin
E (Dilley and McConnell, 1970). In this paper we present
evidence that light-induced degeneration of albino rat
retinas is accompanied by the specific loss of 22:6ω3, the
major polyunsaturated fatty acid of ROS, and the fatty acid
in these membranes most susceptible to peroxidation (Witting,
1965).

EXPERIMENTAL

Female albino rats weighing between 180 to 230 g were maintained in a metabolic chamber (25°C) with VITA–LITE Fluorescent (Duro-Test Corporation) cyclic light (12L:12D) of 10
to 15 foot-candles (ft-c). After one week of acclimatization,
the experiment was begun by exposing the rats at the usual
time of light onset to 100 to 125 ft-c at the side of the
cage nearest the light. At various times following the onset of constant illumination, rats were sacrificed by decapitation and retinas removed for the preparation of ROS
membranes. Aliquots of ROS were taken for polyacrylamide
gel disk electrophoresis, protein determination, and lipid
quantitation.
    In some experiments, animals were anaesthetized with
ether and eyes were enucleated and fixed for light and
electron microscopy. Preliminary microscopic evaluation
showed a progressive destruction of the ROS with duration
of constant illumination, evidenced by the shortening and
swelling of the ROS and vesiculation of disk membranous
material.

RESULTS AND DISCUSSION

The yield of ROS protein declined with the length of time of
constant illumination (Table 1) and by three days was approximately 50% of that obtained from retinas exposed to 10 to
15 ft-c for 1 h. The reduced yield of ROS may have been
due to the loss of lipids from the ROS membranes, resulting
in an increased density and subsequent alteration of their
flotation patterns on the sucrose gradient. The protein-
to-phospholipid ratio increased with the length of time of
constant illumination (Table 1), lending support to this
notion.

TABLE 1

Protein and lipid content of rat rod outer segments following constant illumination

Light status*	ROS yield microgram/retina	Weight ratio protein/phospholipid**
L-1 h	60.2 ± 13.6(7)***	1.24 ± 0.07(3)
H-1 d	57.3 ± 21.3(4)	1.31 ± 0.06(3)
H-3 d	29.8 ± 10.4(8)	1.32 ± 0.11(5)

*L-1 h, 10—15 ft-c for 1 h; H-1 d, 100—125 ft-c for 1 d; H-3 d, 100—125 ft-c for 3 d.

**Phospholipid calculated by multiplying 25 times the mass of phosphorus.

***Mean ± S.D., Value in parenthesis is the number of independent determinations.

The ROS membranes isolated after the various times of constant illumination were examined by polyacrylamide gel disk electrophoresis. We found no evidence that the membranes isolated after three days of constant illumination and identified as ROS were significantly contaminated with other membranes. The opsin band routinely accounted for 85 to 90% of the protein in a typical polyacrylamide gel. The purity of our various preps was an important point to establish, since we are comparing lipid compositions of ROS membranes at various stages of degeneration.

The phospholipid class composition of ROS at various times following the onset of constant illumination is given in Table 2. There appears to be a slight decrease in the relative mole % of phosphatidylethanolamine and phosphatidylserine. However, the levels of lysophospholipids, 1, 2-diglycerides and free fatty acids from the ROS were not affected (the neutral lipid data are not shown). The possibility exists that photoreceptor degeneration in constant illumination results from the activation of phospholipases, which hydrolyse membrane phospholipids to free fatty acids and 1,2-diglycerides. These fusogenic lipids could then promote membrane vesiculation and degeneration. However, the constant levels of lysophospholipids, diglycerides and free fatty acids argue against this possibility.

One of the chemical changes we observed in light-induced retinal degeneration was the loss of a specific long-chain

TABLE 2

Phospholipid class distribution of rat rod outer segments following constant illumination

Light status*	PI**	SPH	PC (MOLE %)	PS	PE	SF
L-1 h	2.0	1.5	37.0	13.7	44.1	0.9
H-1 d	1.5	1.7	37.8	13.8	44.5	0.3
H-3 d	1.8	3.0	40.3	12.8	41.3	0.4

*Refer to legend of Table 1 for explanation of light status.

**PI-phosphatidylinositol; SPH-sphingomyelin; PC-phosphatidylcholine; PS-phosphatidylserine; PE-phosphatidylethanolamine; SF-solvent front of the thin-layer chromatogram.

polyunsaturated fatty acid from the ROS. As shown in Table 3, 22:6ω3 in the total lipids was reduced at day three, while arachidonic acid (20:4ω6), the other long-chain polyunsaturated fatty acid in rat ROS, was not affected. When the major phospholipid classes were examined individually, the level of 22:6ω3 was strikingly reduced at 3 days in each by roughly 10% (absolute) compared to the level of the low-intensity control (L-1 h).

Wiegand *et al.* (1979), Miljanich *et al.* (1979), and Aveldano de Calidironi and Bazan (1977) have shown that ROS phospholipids contain high levels of dipolyunsaturated fatty acid species, which appear to be relatively unique to ROS phospholipids, since the usual phospholipid molecular species contain polyunsaturates at position-2. Table 4 contains the relative mole % distribution of the carbon number of ROS total phospholipid species for 1 h of low light and for 3 days of constant illumination. Briefly, isolated total lipids from the ROS membranes were reacted with phospholipase C, which removes the phosphate-base portion from the phospholipid molecules, leaving a 1,2-diglyceride. The mixture of 1,2-diglycerides was then acetylated, hydrogenated, and subjected to high temperature gas-liquid chromatography. The data shown as mole % of the total phospholipid molecular species are defined by a carbon number of the two long-chain fatty acids present in the unhydrolysed phospholipid molecule. For example, a carbon number 36 (C-36) species is composed of two 18-carbon fatty acids or one 16-carbon and one 20-carbon fatty acid. Those species containing two polyunsaturated fatty acids, namely, C-42 (one 20-carbon and one 22-carbon fatty acid), C-44 (two 22-carbon fatty acids), and C-46 (one 22-carbon and one 24-carbon fatty acid) were decreased after three days of constant illumination. Since these values are expressed as relative mole %, there is an apparent increase in the lower molecular weight species.

The selective loss of 22:6ω3 from photoreceptor membranes exposed to constant illumination of 3 days (Table 3), together with the data shown in Table 4, indicates that phospholipid molecular species most susceptible are those that contain two of these polyunsaturated fatty acids. This selective loss is apparently not mediated by lipolytic enzymes, since the levels of lysophospholipids, fatty acids and 1,2-diglycerides remain constant. A possible explanation is the free radical-induced peroxidation of 22:6ω3. Joel *et al.* (1981) have reported a decrease in the levels of Vitamin E in whole retinas of rats under constant illumination, which preceded the loss of 22:6ω3. Organisciak *et al.* (1981) have shown an increase in lipid peroxides in

TABLE 3

Composition of the major fatty acids of total lipids of rat rod outer segments following constant illumination

Light status*	Fatty acids** (MOLE %)				
	16:0	18:0	18:1ω9	20:4ω6	22:6ω3
L-1 h	14.9	28.0	4.0	5.1	42.0
H-1 d	13.6	30.0	3.5	4.2	42.7
H-3 d	16.9	29.5	5.4	5.7	35.9

*Refer to legend of Table 1 for explanation of light status.

**16:0-palmitic acid; 18:0-stearic acid; 18:1ω9-oleic acid; 20:4ω6-arachidonic acid; 22:6ω3-docosahexaenoic acid.

TABLE 4

Carbon number distribution in the diglyceride acetates derived from total lipids of rat rod outer segments following constant illumination

Light status*	Carbon number (MOLE %)							
	32	34	36	38	40	42	44	46
L-1 h	6.3	8.7	6.8	15.9	46.7	1.7	11.4	1.7
H-3 d	7.6	10.5	7.6	16.3	45.9	0.9	9.3	1.2

*Refer to legend of Table 1 for explanation of light status

retinas of rats maintained in light of 195 ft-c for one hour
compared to dark maintained controls. Kagan *et al.* (1973)
reported that peroxides accumulated in frog retinas exposed
to light. These data strongly suggest that lipid peroxidation is associated with retinal degeneration secondary to
constant illumination, but do not establish a causal relationship. Clearly additional studies are needed to determine
the initial biochemical insult.

ACKNOWLEDGEMENTS

This research was supported in part by grants from the Retina
Research Foundation (Houston, Texas), National Retinitis
Pigmentosa Foundation, Research to Prevent Blindness, Inc.,
and The National Eye Institute (EY 07001, EY 02520, and EY
00871). We thank Maureen B. Maude and Jo Ann Garcia for
their assistance.

REFERENCES

Anderson, K., Coyle, F. and O'Steen, W. (1972). Retinal
    degeneration produced by low intensity light. *Exp.
    Neurol.* **35**, 233—238.
Anderson, R. and Andrews, L. (1982). Biochemistry of
    retinal photoreceptor membranes in vertebrates and in-
    vertebrates. In "Visual Cells in Evolution". (Ed. J.
    Westfall), pp. 1-22, Raven Press, New York.
Aveldano de Caldironi, M. and Bazan, N. (1977). Acyl groups,
    molecular species and labeling by ^{14}C-glycerol and ^{3}H-
    arachidonic acid of vertebrate retina glycerolipids.
    In "Functions and Biosynthesis of Lipids" (Eds N. Bazan,
    R. Brenner and N. Giusto), pp. 397—404. Plenum Press,
    New York.
Dilley, R. and McConnel, D. (1970). Alpha-tocopherol in the
    retinal outer segment of bovine eyes. *J. Membrane Biol.*
    2, 317—323.
Hall, M. and Hall, D. (1975). Superoxide dismutase of
    bovine and frog rod outer segments. *Biochem. Biophys.
    Res. Commun.* **67**, 1199—1204.
Joel, C., Briggs, S., Gaal, D., Hannan, J., Kahlow, M.,
    Stein, M., Tarver, A. and Yip, A. (1981). Light causes
    early loss of retinal tocopherol *in vivo*. Association
    for Research in Vision and Ophthalmology (Abstract)
    p. 166.
Kagan, V., Shvedova, A., Novikov, K. and Kozlov, Y. (1973).
    Light-induced free radical oxidation of membrane lipids

in photoreceptors of frog retina. *Biochim. Biophys. Acta* **330**, 76–79.

Lanum, J. (1978). The damaging effects of light on the retina. Empirical findings, theoretical and practical implications. *Survey Ophthal.* **22**, 221–249.

Miljanich, G., Sklar, L., White, D. and Dratz, E. (1979). Disaturated and dipolyunsaturated phospholipids in the bovine retinal rod outer segment disk membrane. *Biochim. Biophys. Acta* **552**, 294–306.

Noell, W., Walker, V., Kang, B. and Berman, S. (1966). Retinal damage by light in rats. *Invest. Ophthalmol.* **5**, 450–473.

Organisciak, D., Lake, J. and Wang, H. (1981). The enzymatic determination of hydroperoxides in the ROS of cyclic light and dark reared rats. Association for Research in Vision and Ophthal. (Abstract) p. 166.

O'Steen, W., Anderson, K. and Shear, C. (1974). Photoreceptor degeneration in albino rats: dependency on age. *Invest. Ophthalmol.* **13**, 334–339.

Rapp, L. and Williams, T. (1980). A parametric study of retinal light damage in albino and pigmented rats. In "The Effects of Constant Light on Visual Processes". (Eds T. Williams and B. Baker) pp. 135–159. Plenum Press, New York.

Warburg, O. (1924). Verbesserte methode zur messung der atmung und glykolyse. *Biochem.* **152**, 51–63.

Wiegand, R., Guisto, N., Andrews, L., Monaco, W. and Anderson, R. (1981*a*). Chemical changes in albino rat rod outer segments following constant illumination. Association for Research in Vision and Ophthalmology. (Abstract) p. 4.

Wiegand, R., Giusto, N., Maude, M. and Anderson, R. (1981*b*). Molecular species changes in albino rat rod outer segments following constant illumination. *Fed. Proc.* **40**, 1803.

Wiegand, R., Maude, M. and Anderson, R. (1979). Phospholipid molecular species of photoreceptor membranes. Association for Research in Vision and Ophthalmology (Abstract) p. 117.

Witting, L. (1965). Lipid peroxidation *in vivo*. *Am. Oil Chemists' Soc.* **42**, 908–913.

CHLOROQUINE AND THIORIDAZINE-INDUCED RETINOPATHIES

CAROLYN A. CONVERSE

Department of Pharmacy, University of Strathclyde, Glasgow, G1 1XW, UK

INTRODUCTION

Chloroquine and thioridazine (Fig. 1) are drugs which can produce retinopathy in humans if administered at high doses and/or for long periods. Although these drugs have been the subjects of many studies (Rubin, 1968), the biochemical basis for their ocular toxicity is still unclear. Such drug induced retinopathies may serve as models for Retinitis Pigmentosa, by indicating which biochemical processes are most susceptible to disruption, and what the consequences may be.

The first process examined was the renewal of photo-receptor outer segments, since precise control of the synthesis of new rhodopsin-containing discs, and the disposal of old ones, appears essential for maintaining the health of the retina. Both chloroquine and thioridazine appeared to inhibit the renewal process, but in addition, thioridazine disrupted the structure of the membrane, causing aggregation of rhodopsin, and in higher concentrations, removal of some of the lipid. Chlorpromazine, which is not retinotoxic, showed similar effects. The possible significance of these observations in drug retinopathy is discussed below.

METHODS

Cattle eyes, obtained from Glasgow Meat Market, were used within 2 to 3 h of death. The bleached retinas were incubated in the medium of O'Brien *et al.* (1972) for 3 h at 37°C with 40 μCi L-[4,5-^{3}H] leucine (58 Ci/mol; Radiochemical Centre, Amersham) in each 2 retina flask, as described (Converse, 1979). In addition, some flasks contained 1.0 or

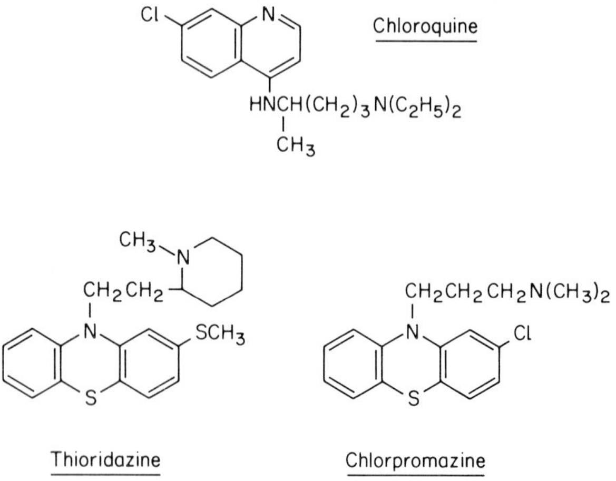

Fig. 1 *The structures of chloroquine and two phenothiazines, thioridazine and chlorpromazine.*

0.01 mM chloroquine diphosphate (Sigma) or thioridazine hydrochloride (Sandoz). Photoreceptor outer segments (ROS) were prepared according to Papermaster and Dreyer (1974) and Converse (1979), analysed by sodium dodecyl sulphate-polyacrylamide gel electrophoresis (Fairbanks *et al.*, 1971; Papermaster *et al.*, 1975) and the gels scanned with a Joyce-Loebl Chromoscan 200-201 to measure protein. Radioactivity was determined in entire ROS fractions and in rhodopsin bands cut from the gels and dissolved in NCS/PCS (Amersham-Searle).

To examine the effect of phenothiazines on ROS integrity, ^{3}H-labelled ROS were incubated at 37°C for 3 h or at 4°C for 18 h in Microfuge tubes (Beckman Instruments) with varying concentrations of drug in phosphate buffered saline (PBS: 0.01 M Na phosphate, 0.14 M NaCl, pH 7.4). After 7 min centrifugation in the Microfuge, pellets (washed with PBS) and supernatants (plus washes) were dissolved in 2% sodium dodecyl sulphate and counted in PCS, with correction for quenching.

In further studies, ^{3}H-ROS were incubated with chloro-quine or thioridazine in PBS or 10 mM tris acetate pH 7.4, at 37°C for 140 min and 4°C for 18 h, then layered on discontinuous sucrose density gradients (Papermaster and Dreyer, 1974; Converse, 1979) and centrifuged for 40 min at 4°C and 129,500 × g (MSE Prepspin 50). Tubes were examined visually, and fractions analysed by scintillation counting (for ^{3}H-rhodopsin) and by spectroscopy in 1% v/v Ammonyx LO

(Millmaster-Onyx International, Inc., Fairfield, N.J., USA)
(for phenothiazines). In addition, fractions were extracted
with 2:1 CHCl$_3$:MeOH and phosphate determined according to
Chen *et al*. (1956) (for lipids).

RESULTS

The *in vitro* system of O'Brien *et al*. (1972) is useful for
studying the renewal of rhodopsin and other ROS proteins
(Converse, 1979). These preliminary studies reveal that both
thioridazine and chloroquine inhibit the appearance of
newly synthesized proteins in the outer segment (Table 1).

TABLE 1

Inhibition by drugs of protein renewal in
photoreceptor outer segments

Drug	Concentration	% Inhibition of Total Protein Renewal*[a]	% Inhibition of Opsin Renewal*[b]
Chloroquine	1 mM	21 (±1)%	42 (±10)%
	0.01 mM	19 (±11)%	32 (±15)%
Thioridazine	1 mM	59 (±24)%	n.d.
	0.01 mM	15 (±5)%	n.d.

*Renewal measured as (a) cpm in ROS and (b) cpm in opsin
band, divided by protein (from scanned gel) and referred to
incubation in absence of drug.

The effects of preincubation with these drugs, and their
effects upon individual steps in the uptake of radiolabelled
amino acids, synthesis of proteins, and transport to the
outer segment have not yet been examined.
    One chance obervation made during these experiments, that
incubation with 1 mM thioridazine led to a decrease in ROS
yield, prompted further investigations into the effects of
thioridazine on the structure of ROS. When ROS were pre-
incubated with thioridazine then pelleted in a Microfuge
(Fig. 2), the amount of protein in the pellet was actually
greater than the control: thioridazine did not dissolve
the ROS, as was first suspected. The behaviour of thioridazine-treated ROS analysed on discontinuous sucrose density
gradients (Fig. 3) depended upon incubation buffer, as well
as drug concentration. The most extreme effects were

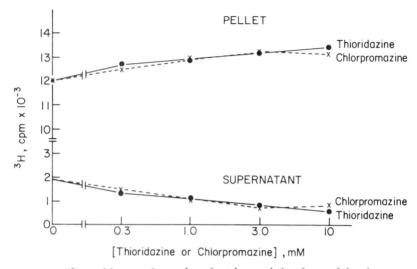

Fig. 2 *The effect of preincubation with phenothiazines on the distribution of ^3H-leucine-labelled photoreceptor outer segments after centrifugation.*

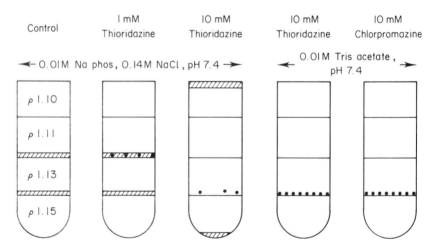

Fig. 3 *The effect of preincubation with phenothiazine on the distribution of photoreceptor outer segments on sucrose density gradients. The densities of the various sucrose layers are shown on the far left tube, and the buffer systems for preincubation above the tubes. Hatched areas indicate dense white cloudy material, and dots show clumping.*

observed after incubation in 10 mM thioridazine in PBS: lipid was extracted and appeared at the top of the gradient, and the lipid-depleted (but not lipid-free) ROS now pelleted to the bottom. About 91% of the tritium label (primarily rhodopsin) was in the pellet. But even in tris buffer, or with 1 mM thioridazine in PBS, extensive clumping was observed. Similarly thioridazine-treated ROS examined on sodium dodecyl sulphate-polyacrylamide gels (Fig. 4) showed a dose-dependent diminution of the rhodopsin band, and an

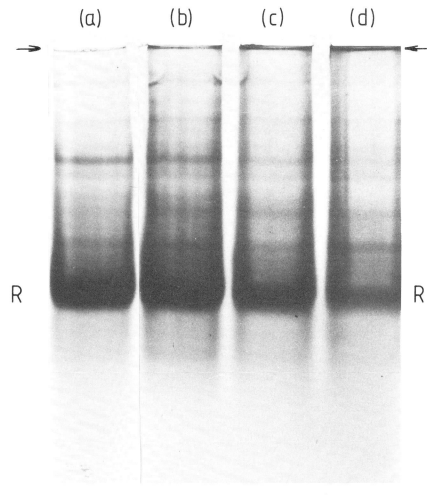

Fig. 4 *Photoreceptor outer segments analysed on SDS-poly-acrylamide gels after preincubation 18h at 4°C with (a) 0, (b) 1 mM, (c) 3 mM, (d) 10 mM thioridazine in phosphate buffered saline. The arrow indicates the top of the gel, and R, the rhodopsin band.*

increase in aggregated material on top of the gel. This
aggregation occurred in both PBS and tris buffers, even if
the ROS were washed to remove thioridazine before electrophoresis. Such aggregation and changes in density may explain the decreased ROS yield after thioridazine treatment
in the ROS renewal experiments.

DISCUSSION

The ability of chloroquine to inhibit rhodopsin renewal may
be due to its inhibition of protein synthesis (Schellenberg
and Coatney, 1961; Gonasum and Potts, 1974), and may be
part of the explanation for the retinopathy observed clinically
after h gh and prolonged chloroquine dosage. However,
other possible mechanisms must be investigated further.
Although chloroquine binds strongly to melanin (Potts,
1964), this may not be related to its mechanism of action,
as Gregory *et al.* (1970) have shown, in the rat, that both
pigmented and albino animals can develop retinopathy.
    Thioridazine appears to inhibit rhodopsin renewal,
cause aggregation of ROS proteins, and, in high concentrations, to extract ROS lipids (perhaps because phenothiazines
are surfactants: Seeman and Bialy, 1963; Attwood *et al.*,
1974). Before deciding whether these biochemical effects
may be related to the retinopathy, we must explain the
observation that chlorpromazine produces similar effects
but no clinical retinopathy.
    Clinically, retinopathy seems to be associated with the
N-methyl piperidine side chain; only phenothiazines with
this structure (thioridazine and NP-207 piperidylchloro-
phenothiazine) can produce retinopathy (Weekly *et al.*,
1960). All phenothiazines, retinotoxic or not, can exist
as free radicals and serve as electron donors in charge
transfer complexes (Forrest *et al.*, 1958; Karreman *et al.*,
1959; Pardo and Ferandez-Alonso, 1975) so it would appear
that these chemical properties are not related, at least
directly, to retinopathy.
    The key to the variable retinotoxicity of phenothiazines
may be the fact that chloropromazine binds more strongly
to melanin than does either thioridazine or NP-207 (Weekley
et al., 1960; Potts, 1964). That is, for a given drug
dosage, less chlorpromazine will be released from the
pigment epithelium and choroid and therefore less will be
free to interact with the retina. This may explain the
report that chlorpromazine produces a decrease in the
electroretinogram only in albino animals (Legros *et al.*,
1973), where presumably the concentration of free drug is

greater than in pigmented animals. Similar phenomena are
seen with mydriatics and cycloplegics, which often have a
greater effect in light-skinned than in dark-skinned
patients, where the drug is, however, often longer-lasting
(Seidehamel *et al.*, 1970; Havener, 1978). Thus, the
damage produced by retinotoxic drugs is a function not only
of their chemistry, but of their effective concentration.
To understand their mechanism of action, we require an
understanding of the melanin-binding and pharmacokinetic
properties of these drugs.

ACKNOWLEDGEMENTS

I am grateful to Professor A.T. Florence and Dr. O. Singh
for advice, and the British Retinitis Pigmentosa Society
and the W.H. Ross Foundation (Scotland) for the Study of
Prevention of Blindness for financial support. Thioridazine
hydrochloride was a gift of Sandoz Products Limited, Leeds.

REFERENCES

Atwood, D., Florence, A.T. and Gillan, J.M.N. (1974).
    Micellar properties of drugs: Properties of micellar
    aggregates of phenothiazines and their aqueous solutions.
    J. Pharm. Sci. **63**, 988-993.
Chen, P.S., Jr., Toribara, T.Y. and Warner, H. (1956).
    Microdetermination of phosphorus. *Anal. Chem.* **28**,
    1756-1758.
Converse, C.A. (1979). The large intrinsic membrane protein
    in rod outer segments: *in vitro* synthesis in cattle, and
    comparison in humans and rabbits. *Exp. Eye Res.* **29**,
    409-416.
Fairbanks, G., Steck, T.L. and Wallach, D.F.H. (1971).
    Electrophoretic analysis of the major polypeptides of
    the human erythrocyte membrane. *Biochemistry.* **10**,
    2606-17.
Forrest, I.S., Forrest, F.M. and Berger, M. (1958). Free
    radicals as metabolites of drugs derived from pheno-
    thiazine. *Biochem. Biophys. Acta.* **29**, 441-2.
Gonasun, L.M. and Potts, A.M. (1974). *In vitro* inhibition
    of protein synthesis in the retinal pigment epithelium
    by chloroquine. *Invest. Ophthalmol.* **13**, 107-115.
Gregory, M.H., Rutty, D.A. and Wood, R.D. (1970). Differences
    in the retinotoxic action of chloroquine and phenothiazine
    derivatives. *J. Path.* **102**, 139-150.

Havener, W.T. (1978). *Ocular Pharmacology* 4th edition, p. 277. C.V. Mosby Company, St. Louis.

Karreman, G., Isenberg, I. and Szent-Györgyi, A. (1959). On the mechanism of action of chlorpromazine. *Science* 130, 1191-2.

Legros, J., Rosner, I. and Berger, C. (1973). Retinal toxicity of chlorpromazine in the rat. *Toxicol. Appl. Pharmacol.* 26, 459-465.

O'Brien, P.J., Muellenberg, C.G. and Bungenberg de Jong, J.J. (1972). Incorporation of leucine into rhodopsin in isolated bovine retina. *Biochemistry* 11, 64-70.

Papermaster, D.S. and Dreyer, W.J. (1974). Rhodopsin content in the outer segment membranes of bovine and frog retinal rods. *Biochemistry* 13, 2438-44.

Papermaster, D.S., Converse, C.A. and Siu, J. (1975). Membrane biosynthesis in the frog retina: opsin transport in the photoreceptor cell. *Biochemistry* 14, 1343-52.

Pardo, A. and Fernandez-Alonso, J.I. (1975). Molecular interactions of phenothiazine drugs and biochemical acceptors, I. Electronic transitions. *An. Quim.* 71, 281-84.

Potts, A.M. (1964). The reaction of uveal pigment *in vitro* with polycyclic compounds. *Invest. Ophthalmol.* 3, 405-416.

Rubin, M. (1968). The antimalarials and the tranquilizers. *Dis. Nerv. Syst.* 29, (Suppl.) 67-76.

Schellenberg, K.A. and Coatney, G. R. (1961). The influence of ant-malarial drugs on nucleic acid synthesis in *Plasmodium gallinaceum* and *Plasmodium berghei*. *Biochem. Pharmacol.* 6, 143-152.

Seeman, P.M. and Bialy, H.S. (1963). The surface activity of tranquilisers. *Biochem. Pharmacol.* 12, 1181-1191.

Seidehamel, R.J., Tye, A. and Patil, P.N. (1970). An analysis of ephedrine mydriasis in relationship to iris pigmentation in the guinea pig eye *in vitro*. *J. Pharm. Exp. Ther.* 171, 205-213.

Weekley, R.D., Potts, A.M., Reboton, J. and May, R.H. (1960). Pigmentary retinopathy in patients receiving high doses of a new phenothiazine. *Arch. Ophthal.* 64, 65-75.

AN IONTOPHORETIC STUDY IN THE RETINA
IN OPTICALLY INTACT CAT EYE: A POSSIBLE TRANSMITTER
MEDIATING GANGLION CELL EXCITATION

HISAKO IKEDA and M.J. SHEARDOWN

Vision Research Unit, The Rayne Institute,
St. Thomas' Hospital, London SE1 7EH, UK

INTRODUCTION

Previous neuropharmacological studies in the mammalian
retina have so far been done on either isolated retina in
buffered and oxygenated media (Ames and Pollen, 1969; Masland
and Ames, 1976) or perfused eye cup (Nelson *et al.*, 1978)
or arterially perfused eyes (Niemeyer, 1977) in which a single
recording electrode was inserted in or near a cell and a drug
was introduced into the media or in the perfusion system.
However, with drugs introduced in the media or perfusion
system, it is difficult to know where the drugs acted to
cause a change in a specific cell within the retina and thus
results on cells beyond the first order synapse are difficult to interpret.

Our major interest is in synaptic transmission from the
bipolar or amacrine cells to the retinal ganglion cells, and
in such circumstances, only microiontophoresis on the retinal
ganglion cells is capable of providing the required degree
of localization of drug action. The only previous micro-
iontophoretic study on the mammalian retina is that of
Straschill and Perwein (1969), who introduced multi-barrelled
electrodes into an open eye. A further step would be to do
a detailed receptive field study which enables the precise
classification of ganglion cells. Here the stimulation by
well-controlled stimuli projected on a screen or a TV tube
sharply focused on the retina of an optically intact eye in
an anaesthetized animal provides the most ideal optical,
physiological and pharmacological experimental conditions.
These considerations led us to develop the technique of
microiontophoresis in the optically intact eye of an anaesthetized cat. We report here the first study which we have

carried out using this technique. In this study, we asked
two questions:

(1) Are the amino acids, L-aspartate and L-glutamate, which
    are present in large quantities in the retinal sites
    where the bipolar and amacrine cells make synaptic con-
    tracts with retinal ganglion cells, involved in synaptic
    transmission?
(2) Do the four major physiological classes of retinal
    ganglion cells, "sustained" and "transient" cells
    (correlated with X and Y cells) and "on-centre" and "off-
    centre cells" receive the same excitatory transmitter?

METHODS

The methods for preparation of cats and intraretinal microiontophoresis have already been described in detail (Ikeda
and Sheardown, 1981). Three- to four-barrelled electrodes
were introduced into the retina using a specially constructed
electrode advancer. One barrel was the recording electrode
and another was used for balancing net current at the electrode tip. The remaining barrel or barrels each contained
one of the following drugs made up in aqueous solution:
L-aspartate, 0.2 M, pH 7.5; *L-glutamate*, 0.2 M, pH 7.5;
2-amino-5-phosphonovalerate (2 APV), 50 mM, pH 7.0 which is
a selective antagonist of N-methyl-D-aspartate (NMDA)
receptors (Davies *et al.*, 1980); and γD-*glutamylglycine* (γDGG),
0.2 M, pH 7.0, which is an antagonist of NMDA and kainate
receptors. A Neurophore BH-2 (Digitimer Ltd.) was used for
iontophoretic application of drugs.
    Retinal ganglion cells encountered were classified using
an optimal spot for the cell located at the receptive field
centre at 0.05 Hz, i.e. 20 seconds on and 20 seconds off,
as described in Ikeda and Wright (1972). Only those cells
which produced well isolated action potentials at least 500
μv above the noise level, and whose classification was certain
with a high degree of confidence are included in the study.
Those cells classified as "sustained" cells are those which
did not show the return of the firing to the spontaneous
level within the total 20 seconds of stimulation, whereas
those cells classified as "transient" cells gave a sharp
transient firing, returning to spontaneous firing level
within 3 seconds. Furthermore, all cells which showed
changes in spike height or waveform, and those which did not
show a complete recovery from any drug effects, were excluded
from analysis.

RESULTS

Detailed results of the effects of aspartate, glutamate, 2-
APV and γDGG have been described elsewhere (Ikeda and Sheardown, 1981). We found that the excitatory response to visual
stimulation at the receptive field centre of all "sustained"
cells (16 on-centre, 10 off-centre) was significantly enhanced
by aspartate (mean current used 17.3 nA) whereas those of
"transient" cells (9 on-centre, 11 off-centre mean current
used 28.5 nA) were not.

Similarly, the excitatory response of all "sustained"
cells (23 on-centre, 19 off-centre) at the receptive field
centre was significantly reduced by 2 APV (mean current
used 15.3 nA) but that of "transient" cells (10 on-centre,
15 off-centre) was not, despite the use of higher currents
(mean current used, 30.7 nA).

Figure 1 illustrates the effects of aspartate and 2 APV
on the response of different classes of retinal ganglion cells
to a repetitive flashing spot at the receptive field centre.
Each of the left and the right columns of Fig. 1 shows four
pen recorder traces obtained from "sustained-on", "sustained-
off", "transient-on" and "transient-off" cells responding to
a flashing spot. In the response of the "sustained-on" or
"transient-on" cells, each upward deflection of the pen is
the spike count during the spot "on". The left traces show
the effect of L-aspartate, whereas the right traces show that
of 2 APV. The bar underneath each trace indicates the time
and the current used for the drug application. Aspartate produced a profound increase in the response of both on- and off-
"sustained" cells but no such effect can be seen for "transient" cells. Similarly 2 APV suppressed the responses of both
types of "sustained" cells, but not those of "transient" cells.
The time course of the effects of aspartate and 2 APV was very
rapid, ranging from immediate, to reaching the optimal effect
within 30 seconds of iontophoretic drug application. The
speed of the effects is in favour of these drugs being involved in synaptic transmission.

The upper left trace in Fig. 2 shows the response of a
"sustained" on cell to a spot of light at the receptive field
centre for 3 seconds followed by a 10 second pulse of 15 nA
aspartate given 10 seconds after the spot was switched off.
The cell gave a rigorous sustained firing of 60 spikes/
second after an initial transient phase to the spot. The
excitation is followed by a period of inhibition (post-
excitatory inhibition) when the spot was switched off but the
firing returned to the spontaneous firing level, i.e. about
10 to 12 spikes/second, within 5 seconds after the spot was
switched off. The aspartate pulse also produced an immediate

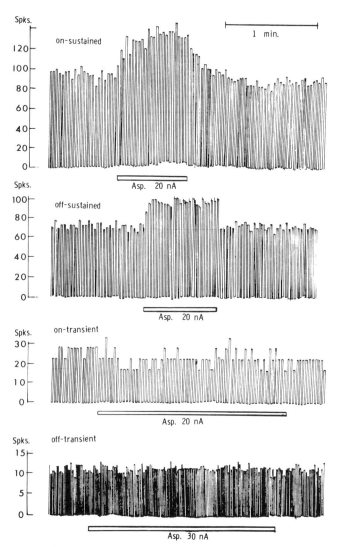

Fig. 1 *Pen recorder tracings illustrating the effect of L-aspartate (left) and that of 2 APV, a selective antagonist of NMDA receptors (right) on the responses of on-centre and off-centre "sustained" and on-centre and off-centre "transient" retinal ganglion cells to repetitive visual stimulation. The visual stimulus was an optimal spot located at the receptive field centre (spot luminance, 20 cd/m^2; background luminance, 10 cd/m^2; spot size chosen so that it produced optimal response from the cell, i.e. for the cells showing aspartate effects (left), from the top, 0.5^o, 0.5^o, 1° and 1° and for*

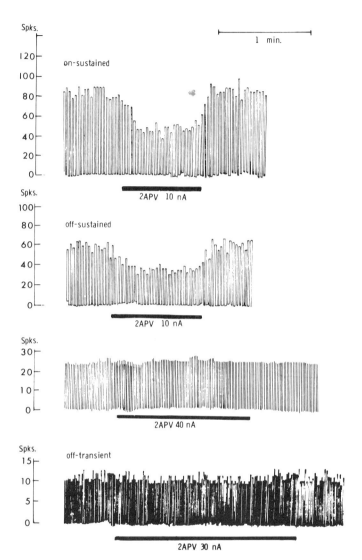

Fig. 1 (cont) *the cells showing 2 APV effects (right), from the top, 0.3°, 0.5°, 1° and 1°; stimulation rate, 0.5 Hz for all "sustained" cells and the "on-transient" cell on the left but 1 Hz for the remaining three "transient" cells. Each of the upward pen deflections shows the number of spikes during the spot "on" for the on-centre, and during "off" for the off-centre cells. The period of aspartate application is indicated by the open bars, and that of 2 APV application by the black bars. The ejection currents used are stated below the bars.*

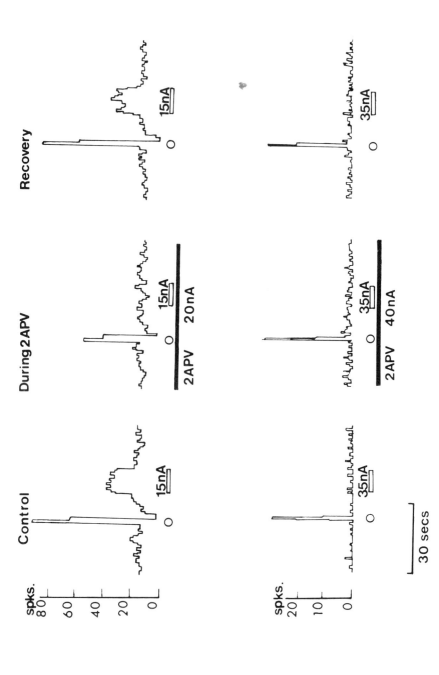

(For legend, see opposite).

and sustained increase in firing, mimicking a light stimulation. Both the cell response to the spot and the aspartate pulse were suppressed when 2 APV was applied iontophoretically, as shown by the upper middle trace.

The cell responses to the spot and the aspartate pulse returned to the original level when the 2 APV current was switched off, as the upper right-hand trace in Fig. 2 shows. Similarly, all "off-sustained" cells also responded to an aspartate pulse with a significant increase in firing, as if it mimicked the light spot "off" and this excitation was blocked by 2 APV. Recently, we have built a black spot generator on background illumination. As we already know, on-centre cells responded to a spot brighter than background, whereas off-centre cells to a spot darker than background. Here, then, all retinal ganglion cells are "on" cells, and iontophoretically applied L-aspartate mimics visual stimulation by stimuli both brighter or darker than the background, in all "sustained" retinal ganglion cells.

The three lower traces in Fig. 2 illustrate the non-responsiveness of "transient" cells to the aspartate pulse, as well as 2 APV, though it was responding transiently to the spot. (The response returned to the spontaneous firing level (0 to 2 spikes/second) within 2 seconds, although the spot was presented for 3 seconds.) The response of "transient" cells to a spot was also uninfluenced by 2 APV, as illustrated by the lower middle trace.

In contrast to the clear cut effect obtained for L-aspartate, L-glutamate (tested on 14 "sustained" and 8 "transient" cells) produced unconvincing results. It often produced changes in spike height or waveform during application, suggesting some membrane change may have been produced. The effect on the firing rate, if present, was again an enhancing effect and was only found in "sustained" and not in "transient" cells.

Fig. 2 *Pen recorder tracings illustrating the effect of 2 APV on the visually driven (open circles) and L-aspartate-induced (open bars) excitations of on-centre "sustained" and on-centre "transient" retinal ganglion cells. The visual stimulus was an optimal spot located at the receptive field centre (spot luminance, 20 cd/m ; background luminance, 10 cd/m; spot size was chosen so that it produced optimal response from the cell, i.e. 0.5° for the "sustained" and 1° for the "transient" cell; stimulus duration, 3 seconds). The control traces were obtained before the application of 2 APV, the traces in the middle column 1 minute after the beginning of 2 APV application, and the traces in the right hand column 1 minute after the termination of 2 APV applications.*

We applied DGG, which has been shown to be both a NMDA
and kainate receptor antagonist (Davies and Watkins, 1981),
to check if "transient" cells may be mediated by Kainic acid
receptors. However, no effects were found for "transient"
cells, although "sustained" cell excitation was suppressed
as expected from our results with 2 APV.

DISCUSSION AND CONCLUSIONS

We can summarize the results as follows:

(1)   Visually driven excitation of "sustained" retinal
      ganglion cells is enhanced by iontophoretically applied
      L-aspartate, and blocked by iontorphoretically applied
      2-amino-5-phosphonovalerate, a selective antagonist for
      NMDA receptors, but "transient" cells' excitation was
      neither influenced by L-aspartate nor by 2 APV.
(2)   Iontophoretically applied aspartate pulses mimicked
      visual stimulation at the receptive field centre in both
      on- and off-centre "sustained" cells, i.e. it caused
      rapid and sustained increase in firing. The aspartate-
      induced excitation was blocked by 2 APV. "Transient"
      cells' visual excitation was not mimicked by an L-
      aspartate current pulse.
(3)   Glutamate showed a minor enhancing effect but this was
      accompanied by spike height or waveform change in "sus-
      tained" cells. Here again "transient" cells differ,
      being completely unaffected by L-glutamate.
(4)   γD-Glutamylglycine,an antagonist for both NMDA and
      kainate receptors, suppressed the visual excitation
      of "sustained" cells but not that of "transient" cells.

   Visually driven excitation of "sustained" retinal ganglion
cells at the receptive field centre is mediated by NMDA
receptors and the transmitter is probably aspartate. Since
glutamate and γDGG, as well as aspartate and 2 APV, did not
influence "transient" cells, it is unlikely that the visual
excitation of "transient" cells is mediated by NMDA, quis-
qualate (which is used by glutamate) or kainate receptors.
This makes it also unlikely that an amino acid is a transmitter for "transient" cells.
   It was our concern that the absence of the drug effect in
"transient" cells may be due to the fact that the drugs did
not reach the receptors in "transient" cells which may have
larger dendritic fields than "sustained" cells (Boycott and
Wässle, 1974). Thus we applied a higher dose for a longer
time for "transient" cells in general. The results were,
however, negative in all "transient" cells.

Since both on-centre and off-centre "sustained" cells are excited by aspartate and inhibited by 2 APV, it may be that both depolarizing (on-centre) and hyperpolarizing (off-centre) bipolar cells, which make synaptic contact with on-centre and off-centre ganglion cells, release the same excitatory transmitter, i.e. aspartate. This is also interesting since it suggests that the differentiation of "on" and "off-centre" dichotomy is already decided at a stage earlier than the bipolar-ganglion synaptic site but "sustained" and "transient" class dichotomy is decided at the bipolar-amacrine-ganglion synaptic site.

ACKNOWLEDGEMENT

We are grateful to Dr J.C. Watkins for a gift of 2 APV and γDGG, and the MRC for financial support.

REFERENCES

Ames III, A. and Pollen, D.A. (1969). Neurotransmission in central nervous tissue: a study of isolated rabbit retina. *J. Neurophysiol*. **32**, 424–442.

Boycott, B.B. and Wässle, H. (1974). The morphological types of ganglion cells of the domestic cat retina. *J. Physiol*. **240**, 397–419.

Davies, J., Francis, A.A., Jones, A.W. and Watkins, J.C. (1980). 2-amino-5-phosphonovalerate (2 APV), a highly potent and specific antagonist at spinal NMDA receptors. *Brit. J. Pharmacol*. **70**, 52–53P.

Davies, J. and Watkins, J.C. (1981). Pharmacology of glutamate and aspartate antagonists on cat spinal neurones. In "GABA and Glutamate as Transmitters" (Eds G. Di Chiara and G.L. Gessa), pp. 275–284. Raven Press, New York.

Ikeda, H. and Sheardown, M.J. (1981). Aspartate may be an excitatory transmitter, mediating visual excitation of "sustained" but not "transient" cells in the cat retina: iontophoretic studies *in vivo*. *Neuroscience* **7**, 25–36.

Ikeda, H. and Wright, M.J. (1972). Receptive field organization of sustained and transient retinal ganglion cells which subserve different functional roles. *J. Physiol*. **227**, 769–800.

Masland, R.H. and Ames II, A. (1976). Responses to acetylcholine of ganglion cells in an isolated mammalian retina. *J. Neurophysiol*. **39**, 1220–1235.

Nelson, R., Famiglietti, E.V. and Kolb, H. (1978). Intracellular staining reveals different levels of stratification

for on- and off-centre ganglion cells in the cat retina.
J. Neurophysiol. **41**, (2) 472–483.

Niemeyer, G. (1977). The perfused cat eye: a model in neuro-
biologic research. *Albrecht v. Graefes Arch. Klin exp.
Ophthal*. **203**, 209–216.

Straschill, M. and Perwein, J. (1969). The inhibition of
retinal ganglion cells by catecholamines and γ aminobutyric
acid. *Pflügers Arch. ges physiol*. **312**, 45–54.

SEROTONIN, CHOLECYSTOKININ AND SUBSTANCE P AMACRINE NEURONES IN THE FROG RETINA

NEVILLE N. OSBORNE

*Nuffield Laboratory of Ophthalmology,
University of Oxford, Oxford OX2 6AW, U.K.*

INTRODUCTION

Neuropeptides such as substance P (Mroz and Leeman, 1977) and cholecystokinin (Rehfeld, 1980) and the indoleamine serotonin (Welsh, 1968) are found throughout the central nervous system of many species. Recently the retina, an outgrowth of the diencephalon, has been shown to contain all three of these substances in certain vertebrate species (Karten and Brecha, 1980; Osborne, 1980; Osborne *et al*; 1981*a*; Osborne *et al.*, 1981*b*). Consequently we addressed ourselves to the following questions: (a) What are the differences between the morphology and distribution of cells containing the various substances? (b) Does continuous light or dark adaptation influence the content of any of these substances? (c) Do any neurones contain one or more of these substances?

In order to investigate these problems, we chose to use the retina of the frog, *Rana pipiens*, because amphibians are known to contain more serotonin in their central nervous system than animals from other vertebrate phyla (Welsh, 1968). All attempts to locate serotonin in specific cells in the retina had failed (Ehinger and Florén, 1980) until the recent study by Osborne *et al.* (1981*a*) on the frog retina.

Distribution of Serotonin, Cholecystokinin and Substance P Neurones

By using a monoclonal antibody (Cuello and Milstein, 1981; Consolazione *et al.*, 1981) specific for serotonin, immuno-reactive sites were observed only in some amacrine cell bodies situated in the inner nuclear layer and processes throughout the inner plexiform layer (Fig. 1) (Osborne *et al.* 1981*a*). No immunoreactivity was observed in the outer nuclear

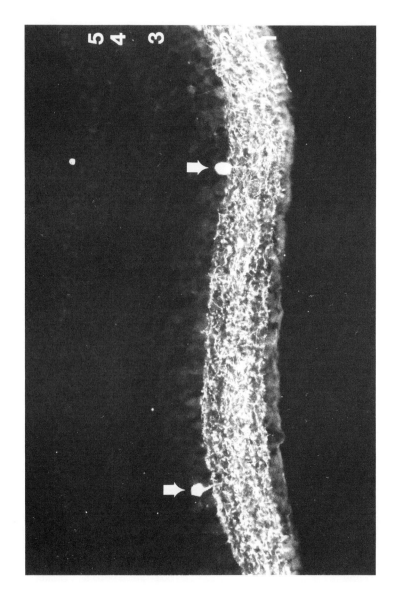

(For legend, see opposite).

layer, outer plexiform layer or Müller cells. (Fig. 1). Immunoreactive amacrine cells have only a single process which
descends directly into the inner plexiform layer where it
ramifies into a very broad band. On occasions, a few of these
cells were also situated in the ganglion cell layer. They
may well be displaced amacrine cells.

A monoclonal antibody towards substance P (Cuello *et al.*,
1980) was also used to localize neurones which reacted positively towards it. Immunoreactive material was associated
with a specific population of amacrine neurones which send
processes directly into the inner plexiform layer (Fig. 2).
The processes did not, however, ramify throughout the whole
of the inner plexiform layer as in the case of the serotonin-
containing processes, but more to the distal half, which would
correspond to lamina 3 to 5 as designated by Cajal (1893).
The number of substance P-like amacrine neurones was greater
than that of serotonin amacrines and the cells were slightly
smaller. Substance P-like immunoreactive material was not
found in any other areas of the retina.

The distribution of cholecystokinin-like immunoreactive
material within the frog retina was also studied by immunofluorescence using an antiserum raised against the synthetic
C-terminal tetrapeptide (Dockray *et al.*, 1981). Unlike the
vast populations of amacrines containing serotonin and substance P-like material, the number of amacrine cells showing
immunoreactivity was very small (Osborne *et al.*, 1981*b*).
These cells were situated at the border between the inner
nuclear and plexiform layers and sent their processes into a
narrow band in the more proximal part of the inner plexiform
layer (Fig. 3), the area corresponding to that designated
lamina 1 by Cajal (1893). Cholecystokinin-like immunoreactive
material was not associated with other areas of the retina.

Fig. 1. *Serotonin immunofluorescence in a transverse section*
of the frog retina. Somata are seen throughout the inner
nuclear layer (large arrows) and processes ramify throughout
the inner plexiform layer. Retinas were immersed in 4% para-
formaldehyde in 0.1M phosphate buffer for 1 to 3 h and 10µm
frozen sections cut. The sections were incubated overnight
at 4°C with rat × rat monoclonal antibody (YC5/45 HL) which
recognizes serotonin in formaldehyde tissue sections. The
rat antibody was developed by an anti-rat IgG FITC-conjugated
immunoglobulin incubated for 1 h at 37°C. Both antibodies
contained 0.2% Triton X-100.
1 = ganglion cell layer; 2 = inner plexiform layer; 3 = inner
nuclear layer; 4 = outer plexiform layer; 5 = outer nuclear
layer.

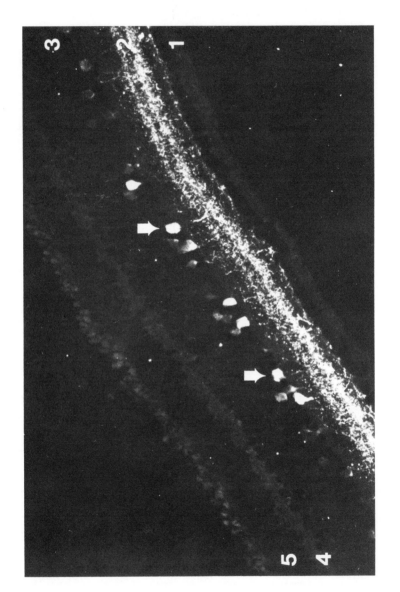

(For legend, see opposite).

Effect of Light- and Dark-Adaptations

Frogs were kept for 36 h either in continuous light or dark
and the retinas were then analysed. High performance chromatography and electrochemical detection were used to determine the serotonin content. This procedure allowed dopamine
to be measured simultaneously. Analysis showed that the
dopamine content of light-adapted retinas was four times that
of dark-adapted retinas. In contrast, the serotonin content
of the light-adapted tissue was half that found in dark-
adapted retinas (Nesselhut and Osborne, 1981). Figure 4
shows chromatograms of light- and dark-adapted retinas,
illustrating the variations in the dopamine and serotonin
levels.

Using immunochemical techniques the normal frog retina
was found to contain 23 ± 3 pmol/g wet weight cholecystokinin
(Osborne *et al.*, 1981*b*), while the substance P content was
ten times greater. No obvious differences were observed
in retinas which were dark- or light-adapted for the 36 h
period.

*Do Any of the Amacrine Neurones Contain One or More of the
Substances?*

A number of studies have revealed that certain neurones
situated in both vertebrate and invertebrate nervous systems
contain more than one transmitter-type molecule, e.g.,
serotonin and substance P (see Osborne, 1979; 1981). These

Fig. 2. *Substance P-like immunoreactivity in a transverse
section of frog retina. Retinas were fixed in 4% paraformaldehyde in 0.1M phosphate buffer for 1 to 2 h and 10μm frozen
sections cut. The sections were incubated in monoclonal
anti-substance P (NC1/34 HL) containing 0.2% of Triton X-100
for 30 to 40 min at 37°C. The antibody was developed with
an anti-rat IgG, from rabbit, and conjugated to FITC
(fluorescein isothiocyanate). The incubation was for 1 h
at 37°C and Triton X-100 (0.2%) was present. A large number
of somata staining positively for substance P-like immunoreactivity is observed throughout the inner nuclear layer
(arrows), and processes of these cells are seen in the inner
plexiform layer especially in the areas designated laminae
3, 4 and, to a lesser extent, 5.*
*1 = ganglion layer; 2 = inner plexiform layer; 3 = inner
nuclear layer; 4 = outer plexiform layer; 5 = outer nuclear
layer.*

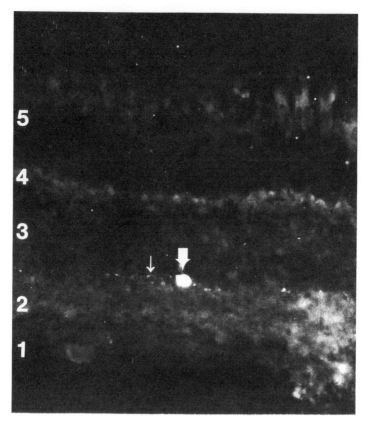

Fig. 3. *Transverse section of the frog retina to show cholecystokinin-like immunoreactivity. Retinas were rapidly dissected and fixed in 4% paraformaldehyde with 0.1M phosphate
buffer pH 7.4 for 1 h. Sections 10μm were cut on a cryostat
and then incubated with an antiserum (L-112) raised against
synthetic C-terminal tetrapeptide of cholecystokinin in the
presence of 0.2% Triton X-100. After rinsing, sections were
incubated with fluorescein isothiocyanate (FITC)-conjugated
goat anti-rabbit antiserum, rinsed and mounted. Immunoreactive somata were very sparsely located in the inner
nuclear layer (large arrow) and immunoreactive processes
within lamina 1 (small arrow).*
*1 = ganglion cell layer; 2 = inner plexiform layer; 3 = inner
nuclear layer; 4 = outer plexiform layer; 5 = outer nuclear
layer.*

findings have challenged the validity of Dale's principle,
which states that each neurone utilizes only a single transmitter substance. To date, no study has suggested that

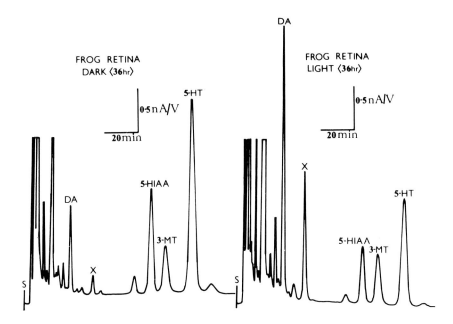

Fig. 4. *Two traces showing HPLC separations of various substances in perchloric acid extracts of frog retinas from animals maintained in dark or light for a period of 36 h. The apparatus was from DuPont, equipped with a C-18 reverse phase column and an LC-4 amperometric detector. The electrochemical detector was set at 2nA/V with a potential of 0.8V. The mobile phase was 0.02 M sodium citrate buffer pH 3.5 containing 0.2mM octane-1-sulphonic acid and 6.5% methanol. Peaks corresponding to dopamine (DA), 5-hydroxyindoleacetic acid (5-HIAA), serotonin (5-HT), methoxytyramine (MT) and an unknown substance (X) were repeatedly identified. In the case of the known substances this was confirmed by adding standards to the extracts. The amount of retinal extract analysed was always constant. The results clearly show that the amount of dopamine and an unknown substance X is greater in retinas exposed to light than those kept in the dark. In contrast, the serotonin level in the light-adapted retinas is less than that in the dark-adapted.*
S = start. (from Nesselhut and Osborne, 1981).

neurones in the retina contain more than one transmitter-type molecule.

Analysis of more than one hundred serial sections processed for serotonin, substance P and cholecystokinin-like immunoreactivity revealed that no neurone contained more than one of these substances.

GENERAL CONCLUSIONS

The general conclusion from this study is that specific
amacrine neurones of the frog retina contain either cholecystokinin, substance P, or serotonin. Cells containing any
of these substances send their terminals to particular layers
in the inner plexiform layer, as shown diagrammatically in
Fig. 5. They may therefore be classified on this basis.

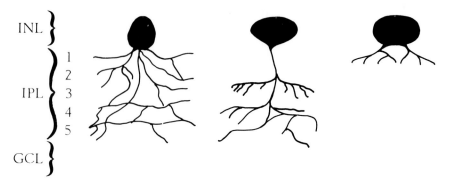

Fig. 5. *Schematic representation of amacrine neurones in
the frog retina which contain either cholecystokinin, substance P or serotonin-like substances.*

Neurones containing any of these substances were never found
to have one of the other substances. These data suggest
that there are specific groups of amacrine neurones which
have particular physical characteristics and are associated
with certain transmitter-like molecules, namely neuropeptides
and serotonin.

REFERENCES

Cajal, S.R. (1893). La Retine des vertebres. *La Cellule* **9**,
    17–257.
Consolazione, A., Milstein, C., Wright, B. and Cuello, A.C.
    (1981). Immunocytochemical detection of serotonin with
    monoclonal antibodies. *J. Histochem. Cytochem*. **29**,
    1425–1430.
Cuello, A.C., Milstein, C. and Priestley, J.V.C. (1980).
    Use of monoclonal antibodies in immunocytochemistry with
    special reference to the central nervous system. *Brain
    Res. Bull*. **5**, 575–587.
Cuello, A.C. and Milstein, C. (1981). Monoclonal antibodies
    against neurotransmitter substances. In "Monoclonal
    Antibodies to Neural Antigens". Cold Spring Harbour
    Workshop (in press).

Dockray, G.J., Vaillant, C. and Hutchinson, J.B. (1981). In "Cellular basis of chemical messengers in the digestive system" (Eds M.I. Grossman, M.A.B. Brazier and J. Lechago, Academic Press, New York, pp. 215-230.

Ehinger, B. and Florén, I. (1980). Retinal indoleamine accumulating neurons. *Neurochem. Int.* **1**, 209—229.

Karten, H.J. and Brecha, N. (1980). Localization of substance P immunoreactivity in amacrine cells of the retina. *Nature* **283**, 87—88.

Mroz, E. and Leeman, S. (1977). Substance P. In "Vitamins and Hormones, Advances in Research and Application" (Eds P. Munson, E. Diczfalusy, J. Glover and R. Olson) Vol. 35 pp. 209—281. Academic Press, New York.

Nesselhut, T. and Osborne, N.N. (1981). Serotonin and dopamine fluctuations in the frog retina in response to dark and light adaptations. *Trans. Biochem.* **9**, 418-419.

Osborne, N.N. (1979). Is Dale's Principle Valid? *Trends in Neuroscience* **2**, 73—75.

Osborne, N.N. (1980). *In vitro* experiments on the metabolism, uptake and release of 5-hydroxytryptamine in bovine retina. *Brain Res.* **184**, 283—297.

Osborne, N.N. (1981). Communication between neurones: current concepts. *Neurochem. Int.* **3**, 3—16.

Osborne, N.N., Nesselhut, T., Nicholas, D.A. and Cuello, A.C. (1981*a*). Serotonin: A transmitter candidate in the vertebrate retina. *Neurochem. Int.* **3**, 171-176.

Osborne, N.N., Nicholas, D.A., Cuello, A.C. and Dockray, G.J. (1981*b*). Localization of cholecystokin immunoreactivity in amacrine cells of the retina. *Neuroscience Letters* **26**, 31-35.

Rehfeld, J.F. (1980). Cholecystokinin. *Trends in Neurosciences* **3**, 65—67.

Welsh, J.H. (1968). Distribution of serotonin in the nervous systems of various animal species. *Advance Pharmacol* **6**A, 171—188.

THE POSSIBLE ROLE OF TRH AND OTHER PEPTIDES IN THE RETINA

H.W. READING

MRC Brain Metabolism Unit, Department of Pharmacology, University of Edinburgh, Edinburgh EH8 9JZ, UK

Dopamine (DA) is the principal catecholamine of the mammalian retina and is reasonably well established as a transmitter. Interaction between DA and TRH systems is well recognized (Kerwin and Pycock, 1979); they are both present in retina, both are released and have their synthesis stimulated by the action of light, although there is a 4 hour lag period in sustained light in the case of TRH (Ehinger 1976; Schaeffer *et al.*, 1977). I found that TRH up to a concentration of $5 \times 10^-$ M had no effect on high affinity uptake of DA into bovine retina. Using a superfusion technique following preincubation of bovine or rat retina with high specific activity [^{3}H]DA, release of DA was monitored. In dark, but not in light-adapted retina a flashing light stimulus (2 to 3 Hz) evoked Ca^{++}-dependent [^{3}H]DA release. TRH $5 \times 10^-$ M, also evoked Ca^{++}-dependent DA release only from dark-adapted retina (Fig. 1). The same concentration of TRH prevented and to some extent reversed the light-evoked release from dark-adapted retina (Fig. 2). These complex effects can be taken as evidence that the mammalian retina possesses pre-synaptic dopaminergic autoreceptors which form part of an inhibitory feed-back loop controlling the release of DA from nerve-endings. In this respect retina is similar to the caudate nucleus of the nigro-striatal system (Langer *et al.*, 1980). TRH appears to be acting as a partial DA agonist by producing a small and transient release of DA from dark-adapted retina (Fig. 1). On the other hand TRH can antagonize the light-evoked release of DA by stimulation of the presynaptic inhibitory autoreceptors. Support for this concept was obtained by demonstrating that L-Sulpiride, a selective dopaminergic D_2 receptor antagonist (Stoof and Kebabian, 1981) not only releases DA from dark-adapted retina, but produces a markedly

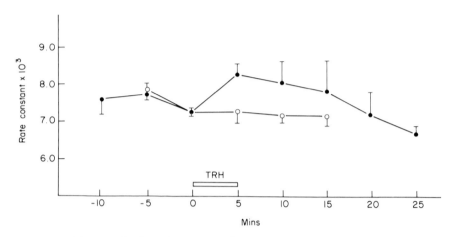

Fig. 1 *TRH evoked release of* ^3H *Dopamine from dark adapted bovine retina; Ca^{++} dependence. Dark adapted bovine retina, pre-incubated with high specific activity* ^3H *dopamine, was perfused with oxygenated Kreb's bicarbonate buffer pH 7.4 at 37°C until equilibrium release was obtained (about 40 to 45 min). TRH 5 × 10^{-4}M was then introduced for 5 min into the perfusion fluid. This produced a maximum increase in* ^3H *dopamine release of 14 ± 3% P = 0.01 lasting up to 15 min after introduction of TRH. In the absence of CA^{++} no increase in release occurred.*

Rate Constant $\dfrac{d.p.m. \ released \ mg^{-1} \ tissue}{d.p.m. \ left \ in \ tissue \ at \ each \ interval}$

●——● *Plus Ca^{++} 2.5 mM* ○——○ *No Ca^{++}*

enhanced release (Fig. 3). Final proof of the existence of
two classes of dopaminergic receptor was shown by radioligand
binding with [^{3}H] Spiperone using different competitors (D_1D_2
and D_2) in which the Scatchard analyses can be resolved into
two distinct slopes, one of which appears to be associated
with a D_2 type of receptor. Preliminary experiments using
high specific activity radiolabelled TRH have shown that
there is a high affinity binding site in rat retina for this
peptide. However, it does not appear that this specific site
is dopaminergic since neither the agonist dopamine nor the
antagonist spiperone will displace [^{3}H] TRH from this binding
site. It can be concluded therefore, that the action of TRH
in influencing DA release is a modulatory one, probably
serving to "set" the dopaminergic system at different levels
of responsivity.

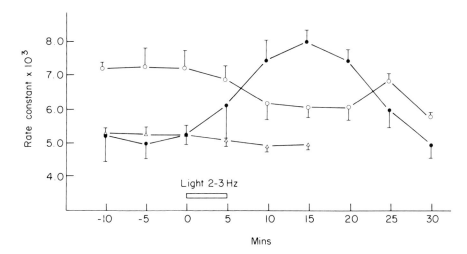

Fig. 2 *Light-evoked release of ³H dopamine from dark adapted bovine retina; Ca⁺⁺ dependence and effect of TRH. Dark adapted bovine retina, pre-incubated with high specific activity ³H dopamine, was perfused with oxygenated Kreb's bicarbonate buffer pH 7.4 at 37°C until equilibrium release was obtained (about 40 to 45 min). A flashing light stimulus of 2 to 3 Hz frequency and 5 min duration, produced an increase in ³H dopamine release lasting up to 25 min after stimulation. Maximum increase above resting level, 54 ± 17% P < 0.01. Light-evoked release was completely Ca⁺⁺ dependent.*
  TRH, 5 × 10⁻⁴M present in the perfusion fluid, prevented and to some extent reversed the light-evoked release of ³H dopamine. Note that the equilibrium level of release in dark adapted retina, when TRH was present in the perfusion fluid, was higher than when it was absent. Maximum difference in release ± TRH - 31 ± 9% P < 0.01.

●——● *No TRH, Ca⁺⁺2.5mM*   ○——○ *TRH, 5 × 10⁻⁴M., Ca⁺⁺2.5mM*
△——△ *No Ca⁺⁺*

REFERENCES

Ehinger, B. (1976). Biogenic amines as transmitters in the Retina. In "Transmitters in the Visual Process". (Ed. S.L. Bonting), pp. 145-163. Pergamon Press, Oxford.

Kerwin, R.W. and Pycock, C.J. (1979). Thyrotropin-releasing hormone stimulates release of [³H] Dopamine from slices of rat nucleus accumbens *in vitro*. *Brit. J. Pharmac.* **67**, 323-325.

Langer, S.Z., Arbilla S. and Kamal L. (1980). Autoregulation

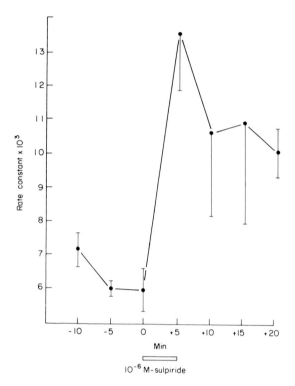

Fig. 3 *L-Sulpiride evoked release of* [3]*H Dopamine from bovine retina. Dark adapted bovine retina, pre-incubated with high specific activity* [3]*H dopamine, was perfused with oxygenated Kreb's bicarbonate buffer pH 7.4 at 37°C until equilibrium release was obtained. L-sulpiride 10⁻⁶M was then introduced for 5 min into the perfusion fluid. This produced a maximum increase in* [3]*H dopamine release of 128 ± 18% P = 0.01, lasting for more than 20 min after introduction of drug.*

of noradrenaline and dopamine release through presynaptic receptors. In "Neurotransmitters and their Receptors" (Eds V.Z. Littauer, Y. Dudai, I. Silman, V.I. Teichberg and Z. Vogel.). pp. 7-21. John Wiley and Sons, New York.

Schaeffer, J.M., Brownstein, M.J. and Axelrod, J. (1977). Thyrotropin-releasing hormone-like material in the rat retina; Changes due to environmental lighting. *Proc. Nat. Acad. Sci., New York.* **74**, 3529-3531.

Stoof, J.C. and Kebabian, J.W. (1981). Opposing roles for D-1 and D-2 dopamine receptors in efflux of cyclic AMP from rat neostriatum. *Nature. Lond.* **294**, 366-368.

IMMUNOLOGY OF RHODOPSIN AND SOME OF ITS PROTEOLYTIC FRAGMENTS

W.J. DE GRIP and R.C.J.F. MARGRY

Department of Biochemistry, University of Nijmegen,
P.O. Box 9101, 6500 HB Nijmegen, The Netherlands

SUMMARY

Anistera are produced by rabbits against various conforma-
tions of bovine rhodopsin. All antisera recognize membrane-
bound antigen irrespective of its conformation ((non)illumin-
ated, denatured). However, when the assay includes detergents,
differences are observed between antisera raised against biochemically intact antigens and denatured antigens respectively.
Then the first type of antiserum only recognizes denatured
antigens, while the second type preferentially reacts with
intact antigens. Suitable conditions therefore enable the
immuno-discrimination between rhodopsin and opsin. Antigenic
sites for the first type of antiserum reside in the N-terminal
half of rhodopsin, probably also involving or close to its
oligosaccharide chains.

INTRODUCTION

Antibodies directed against the visual pigment rhodopsin
evidently present a powerful tool, both for its immuno-
histochemical detection and for the development of ultrasensitive assays. In the latter context, it would be very
exciting if antibodies were to become available which could
discriminate between various intermediate species, e.g. photo-
intermediates. So far, several reports have appeared in the
literature describing the use of antibodies elicited against
rhodopsin (Jan and Revel, 1974; Papermaster *et al.*, 1978;
Godchaux, 1978; Blaustein and Dewey, 1979). In these, the
exact state of the antigen injected is generally not very well
defined, and the antibodies obtained are only partially
characterized. In this paper we will present evidence that

the population of antibodies elicited can be manipulated
by the state in which the antigen is injected and that recognition of antigens by antibodies can be manipulated by
the use of detergents, thereby already enabling discrimination
between rhodopsin and opsin. In addition, some attempts to
locate the antigenic sites in the rhodopsin protein structure
will be described.

METHODS

Preparation of Antigens

In the first place, we wondered whether the state of the
immunogen could influence the antibody population. Consequently, we investigated three conditions: photoreceptor
membranes, handled in darkness (I) in the light (II),
and photoreceptor membranes denatured with SDS (III). It
turned out that the antisera obtained with I and II behaved
comparably but differed from that obtained from III. We will
therefore limit ourselves to a description of the antisera
obtained with immunogens type I and III.
    Bovine rod outer segments (ROS) are isolated as described
by de Grip *et al.* (1980). Photoreceptor membranes are obtained
following hypotonic lysis of ROS and subsequent washing with
aqua dest (3x). Immunogen I is prepared for injection by
dissolving these membranes in isotonic saline containing 2%
Tween 80 and 2% decyldimethylaminoxide, followed by removal
of the aminoxide by dialysis and addition of one volume of
Freund's complete adjuvant. All manipulations with this
immunogen preparation, including the final injection, are
performed in darkness or under dim red light, and it therefore contains spectrally intact rhodopsin. Antigen III is
obtained after treatment of washed photoreceptor membranes
with 0.1% (w/v) SDS at room temperature, and therefore contains thermally denatured rhodopsin. Immunogen III is prepared for injection by mixing it directly with one volume
of Freund's complete adjuvant. For immunization, New Zealand
albino rabbits receive intracutaneous injections at multiple
sites on the back. Booster injections, omitting Freund's
adjuvant, are given over periods of 5 to 20 weeks. Details
of the entire immunization procedure are presented elsewhere
(Margery *et al.*, 1983). For the experiments described here,
the antisera finally obtained are used without further purification. It should be noted, that the antibody titers obtained with antigen III were only in the order of 10 to 30%
of those obtained with antigen I (Margry *et al.*, 1983;
Margry *et al.*, in prep.) as determined by complement fixation
(Levine and Van Vunakis, 1967).

RESULTS AND DISCUSSION

Specificity of the Antisera

Since the rod outer segment membrane contains a small amount
of other proteins in addition to rhodopsin, it is essential
to determine to what extent the antisera are specific for
rhodopsin. Labelling of frozen retina sections by immunofluorescence shows specific label to be confined to the outer
segment region (Magry *et al.*, 1983). Electrophoresis of
rod outer segment proteins, separated in the first dimension
by SDS-polyacrylamide-gradient gel electrophoresis, into a
second dimension of antisera-containing agarose gel, shows
only precipitation rockets derived from the monomers and
oligomers of rhodopsin (Fig. 1). When the protein population
of the entire retina is analysed by the same technique, again
only opsin is recognized by the antisera (not shown, cf.

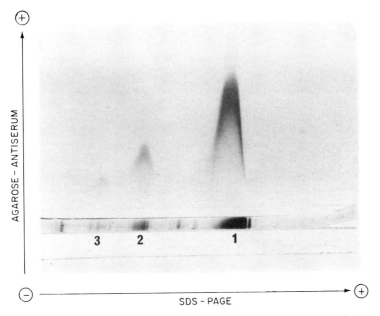

Fig. 1 *Crossed Immuno-electrophoresis of ROS proteins,
adapted from Converse and Papermaster (1975) in the modification of Chua and Blomberg (1969). First dimension: SDS-
PAGE on linear polyacrylamide gradient gels (8–28% w/v acrylamide; ratio bis/monomer = 0.05), run in the Laemmli-system
(Laemmli, 1970). Position of monomer (1), dimer (2) and trimer
(3) of opsin are designated under the gel. Second dimension:
antiserum-containing agarose gel.*

Magry *et al.*, 1982). We may safely conclude therefore that the antisera are monospecific for rhodopsin.

Configurational Specificity of the Antisera

For most immunochemical techniques the antigen has to be soluble in aqueous media. Solubilization of membrane-bound antigens like rhodopsin requires the use of detergents (de Grip *et al.*, 1980). We therefore investigated whether detergents would interfere with the antigen-antibody interaction, using the ouchterlony double-diffusion technique (Ouchterlony and Nilson, 1978). Some intriguing features were observed (Margry *et al.*, 1983) which can be summarized as follows. With antiserum I, both rhodopsin and opsin yield one precipitation line, but only when they are denatured (thermally as well as by acid) or when the detergent used causes thermal denaturation at the ambient temperature (rhodopsin: SDS; opsin: most detergents except mild ones like cholate and dodecylmaltose). Under those conditions all antigens tested (solubilized photoreceptor membranes; purified (rhod) opsin) yield one precipitation line, which fuse with each other, suggesting identical antigenic sites. However, in the presence of detergents which keep the antigens biochemically intact (criteria: rhodopsin: 500 nm absorbance band; opsin: regenerability with 11-cis retinal) no precipitation is observed. Hence, in detergents of intermediate "strength" (like Triton X-100, Emulphogene BC-720, Ammonyx LO), in which rhodopsin remains intact but opsin is denatured, only opsin is recognized by the antibodies. That is, under certain conditions antiserum I is able to discriminate between rhodopsin and opsin.

With antiserum III, comparable, albeit opposite results were obtained. Here, the undenatured species is most reactive, while denatured antigens show little or no precipitation at all. Thus, like antiserum I, antiserum III is able to distinguish rhodopsin from opsin under certain conditions, but its specificity is reversed.

We would like to extend these results to the membrane-bound situation. For this purpose, we have employed the complement fixation test (Levine and Van Vunakis, 1967) which allows both particulate and soluble antigens. Figure 2 shows some major results. When membrane-bound (traingles), all antigens tested (both intact and denatured rhodopsin resp. opsin) are recognized by both antisera. This corroborates the immunofluorescence experiments, where membrane-bound opsin constitutes the antigen. However, in agreement with the double-diffusion test, addition of Emulphogene BC-720 (a detergent which leaves rhodopsin intact but denatures

opsin) leads to differential effects on rhodopsin and opsin
(crosses, circles). With antiserum I, complement fixation
shows for rhodopsin a vertical shift depending on detergent
concentration, being absent in 1% Emulphogene (Fig. 2a).
However, upon solubilization of opsin complement fixation shows
only a slight vertical shift but a fairly large lateral shift
(Fig. 2b), suggesting a considerable increase in available
antigenic sites. With antiserum III, on the contrary, both
opsin and rhodopsin show a comparable vertical shift upon
solubilization and opsin a large lateral shift as well, but
only at relatively low antiserum dilution (Fig. 2c,d). Upon
further dilution of antiserum III, membrane-bound antigens
still show a high degree of complement-fixation (Fig. 2c,d),
but both solubilized rhodopsin and opsin fail to show complement-fixation (not shown). This detail deviates from the
double-diffusion test, where rhodopsin gives much stronger
precipitation lines with antiserum III than does opsin.

The general patterns obtained with the double-diffusion
test and the complement fixation assay are consistent enough
to support the following conclusions:

1. In the membrane, rhodopsin is always recognized by our
antisera, irrespective of its configurational state. This
does not imply that lipids are involved in the antigenic
reaction, since particulate lipid-free rhodopsin is antigenic
as well (Margry *et al.*, in prep.). In any case, for immunochemical assay of (rhod)opsin in the membrane the configurational state of the antigen, both during immunization and in
the final assay, does not appear to be of much importance.

2. Upon solubilization in detergent, profound effects are observed depending on the detergent and the type of antiserum.
With antiserum I, biochemically intact antigens are no longer
recognized and only denaturated samples yield precipitation
lines or induce complement fixation. On the other hand, with
antiserum III, biochemically intact antigens yield stronger
precipitation lines, while the capacity to induce complement
fixation is strongly reduced for all antigens. In view of
the diverse effects obtained with different antisera, the
detergent induced loss in antigenicity is probably not due
to failure of "normal" antigen-antibody complexes to induce
lattice formation or complement fixation, but rather to a
variable decrease in antigen-antibody affinity as a result
of detergent-induced conformational changes around the antigenic sites. Other evidence also supports the latter alternative.

3. In the presence of certain detergents, immuno-discrimination
between rhodopsin and opsin is feasible. Here, the detergent

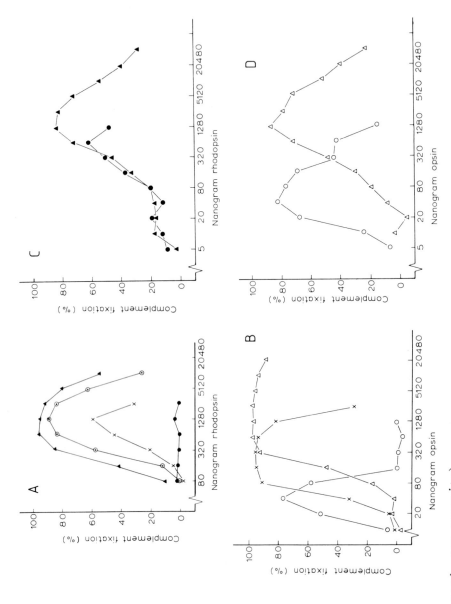

(For legend, see opposite).

appears to intensify subtle conformational differences between rhodopsin and opsin, manifest, for example, in their thermal stabilities. Interestingly, under these conditions anti-serum I, raised against intact rhodopsin, preferentially reacts with denatured samples, while antiserum III, raised against denatured antigens, preferentially appears to recognize biochemically intact antigens.

Location of Antigenic Sites

Both for better interpretation of the results described above, which might permit the design of the promising immunogen-configurations, and for the further use of antibodies in structural and functional studies, it would be very helpful if the location of antigenic sites in the rhodopsin entity could be determined as accurately as possible. Due to the low titer of antiserum III, so far only antiserum I has been investigated in this respect. In the absence of detailed information on the secondary, let alone the tertiary structure of rhodopsin, some first attempts to locate antigenic sites were made using limited proteolysis. With respect to the enzymatic fragmentation pattern of rhodopsin (Mw ~ 36 kD), to date two classes of proleolytic enzymes can be discerned. One class, so far comprising thermolysin, papain, subtilisin and Staphylococcus aureus V8 protease (cf. Hubbell and Bownds, 1979), first releases two small water-soluble C-terminal peptides leaving a membrane bound fragment, which migrates on SDS-polyacrylamide gels with an apparent Mw of about 33 kD. This fragment is subsequently split into two smaller ones: a N-terminal fragment with an apparent Mw of about 23 kD and a C-terminal one of about 12 kD (Fig. 3). Rhodopsin contains two oligo-saccharide chains at residues 2 and 15 (Hargrave, 1977) and N-terminal fragments can thus be identified, for example, by their positive reaction in the periodic acid-Schiff

---

Fig. 2 *Micro-complement fixation curves of rhodopsin preparations obtained with antiserum I (A,B) resp. antiserum III (C,D). The assay is performed in darkness, according to Levine and Van Vunakis, 1979), on spectrally intact rhodopsin (closed symbols; A,C) and illuminated rhodopsin (open symbols; B,D). Triangles represent membrane suspensions; crosses and circles represent antigens solubilized in 0.5% and 1% Emulphogene BC-720 respectively. Antiserum dilution = 1:1700 (A,B), 1:600 (C,D: triangles) and 1:100 (C,D: circles). Immediately before the assay, the detergent concentration was adjusted in all samples to a final value of 0.01%.*

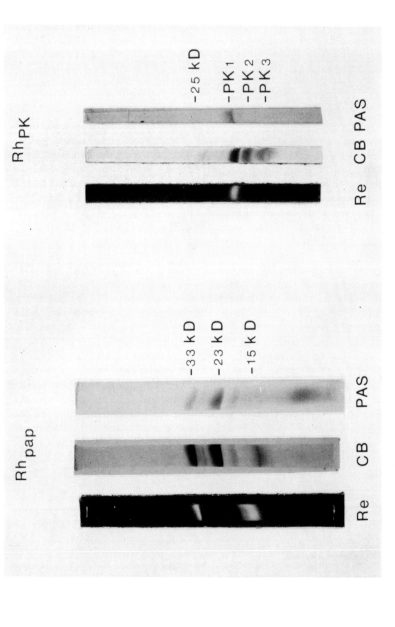

(For legend, see opposite).

(PAS) assay for saccharides. With the first class of enzymes, further splitting of the N-terminal 23 kD fragment is only very limited (Fig. 3). However, a second class of enzymes, so far comprising Chymotrypsin and Proteinase K (de Grip, unpub. results) is able to split this second-largest fragment into two smaller fragments of apparent Mw 18 kD (designed PK_1) and 8 kD (PK_3), of which only PK_1 is PAS-positive, and is therefore located N-terminally in rhodopsin.

The antigenicity of these various fragments is determined by the same crossed immunoelectrophoresis technique, described in Fig. 1, using SDS-polyacrylamide gel electrophoresis in the first dimension. Of the fragments obtained with thermolysin or papain only the N-terminal ones (33 kD, 23 kD) and their oligomers react with antiserum I (Fig. 4). In agreement with this, again only the N-terminal fragment obtained with Chymotrypsin or Proteinase K (PK_1) reacts with antiserum I (Fig. 4). Similar results were obtained using the antibody/^{125}I-Protein A overlay technique of Adair *et al.* (1978). Thus, the antigenic sites for antiserum I reside in the N-terminal half of rhodopsin. Preincubation of rhodopsin with the lectin Concanavalin A, which binds to the N-terminal oligosaccharide chains, strongly reduces the antigenicity of rhodopsin towards antiserum I. This suggests that one or more antigenic sites are located close to and/or include the N-terminal oligosaccharide moieties. Residual activity suggests that (an)other site(s) are present in the N-terminal part of rhodopsin located on the other (*in vivo*: intracellular) side of the membrane, which is not "covered" by Concanavalin A. Clearly, further refinement of this first positioning is required. Another important question requiring further investigation asks how these sites are manipulated by the presence of detergents to produce the effects on antibody affinity described above.

Fig. 3 *Fragmentation pattern of rhodopsin obtained with papain (Rh_{pap}) or proteinase K (Rh_{PK}) analysed by SDS-PAGE on linear polyacrylamide gradient gels (cf. Fig. 1). The same gel is first analysed for retinylfluorescence (Re) by previous reductive fixation of the chromophore (de Grip, unpub.) then assayed for carbohydrate by the PAS-reaction (PAS) and finally stained for protein with Coomassie Blue R-250 (CB) according to Fairbanks et al. (1971). Rh_{pap} shows an intermediate fragmentation pattern with the 33 kD-intermediare still present. Rh_{PK} shows the final pattern of 18 kD (PK_1), 14 kD (PK_2) and 8 kD (PK_2) fragments. PK_2 corresponds to the 14 kD fragment in Rh_{pap}.*

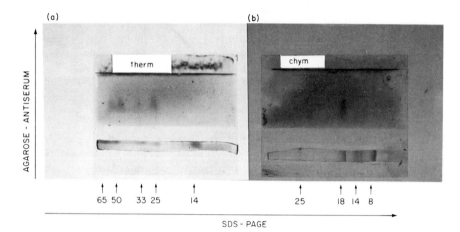

Fig. 4 *Crossed immuno-electrophoresis, performed as in Fig. 1, of proteolytic fragments of rhodopsin obtained with thermolysin (A), or chymotrypsin (B). Figures under the gel denote the apparent molecular weight of the fragments, derived from comparison with calibration proteins.*

ACKNOWLEDGEMENTS

We would like to thank Prof. Dr F.J.M. Daemen for his critical interest and Mr B. Kessels, A. Timmers and C. Jacobs and Mrs P. Bovee-Geurts for technical assistance with several of the described experiments.

REFERENCES

Adair, W.S., Jurivich, D. and Goodenough, U.W. (1978). Localization of cellular antigens in sodium dodecylsulfate-polyacrylamide gels. *J. Cell. Biology* **79**, 281–285.

Blaustein, D.I. and Dewey, M.M. (1979). Localization of rhodopsin in isolated, osmotically intact rod outer segment discs. *J. Histochem. Cytochem.* **27**, 788–793.

Chua N.-H. and Blomberg, F. (1979). Immunochemical studies of Thylakoid membrane polypeptides from Spinach and Chlamydomonas reinhardtii. *J. Biol. Chem.* **254**, 215–223.

Converse, C.A. and Papermaster, D.S. (1975). Membrane protein analysis by two-dimensional immunoelectrophoresis. *Science* **189**, 469–472.

Fairbanks, G., Steck, T.L. and Wallach, D.F.H., (1971) Electrophoretic analysis of the major polypeptides of the human erythrocyte membrane. *Biochem.* **10**, 2606–2617.

Godchaux III, W., (1978). Protein biosynthesis in a cell-free system from bovine retina. *Biochim. Biophys. Acta* **520**, 428–440.

De Grip, W.J., Daemen, F.J.M. and Bonting, S.L. (1980). Isolation and purification of bovine rhodopsin. In "Methods in Enzymology" (Eds D.B. McCormick and L.D. Wright), **67**, pp. 301–320. Academic Press, New York.

Hargrave, P.A. (1977). The amino terminal tryptic peptide of bovine rhodopsin; A glycopeptide containing two sites of oligosaccharide attachment. *Biochim. Biophys. Acta* **492**, 83–94.

Hubbell, W.L. and Bownds, M.D. (1979). Visual transduction in vertebrate photoreceptors. *Ann. Rev. Neurosci.* **2**, 17–34.

Jan, L.Y. and Revel, J.-P. (1974). Ultrastructural localization of rhodopsin in the vertebrate retina. *J. Cell Biol.* **62**, 257–273.

Laemmli, U.K. (1970). Cleavage of structural proteins during assembly of the head of bacteriophage T4. *Nature* **227**, 680–685.

Levine, L. and Van Vunakis, H. (1967). Micro complement fixation. In "Methods in Enzymology 11" (Eds C.H.W. Hirs), pp. 928–936. Academic Press, New York.

Margry, R.J.C.F., Bonting, S.L. and Daemen, F.J.M. (1983). Effects of detergents on the antigenicity of rhodopsin. *Biochim. Biophys. Acta*, (in press).

Ouchterlony, O. and Nilson, L.A. (1978). Immunodiffusion and immunoelectrophoresis. In "Handbook of Experimental Immunology" (Ed. D.M. Weir) (3rd edition) pp. 19.1–19.23. Blackwell, Oxford.

Papermaster, D.S., Schneider, B.G., Zorn, M.A. and Kraehenbuhl, J.P. (1978). Immunocytochemical localization of opsin in outer segments and Golgi zones of frog photoreceptor cells. *J. Cell Biol.* **77**, 196–210.

ROD AND CONE ELECTRORETINOGRAMS IN THE CAT

*SAMUEL G. JACOBSON and HISAKO IKEDA

*Vision Research Unit of the Sherrington School,
Rayne Institute, St. Thomas' Hospital, London, UK*

INTRODUCTION

Isolating the rod and cone components of the electroretinogram
(ERG) with full-field visual stimulation is a commonly used
technique in clinical electroretinography (Gouras, 1970).
The independent evaluation of rod and cone function with such
methods has proven valuable for assessing and classifying
patients with hereditary retinal degenerations (Berson, 1981).
Like man, the cat also has rods and cones and the distribution of the two types of photoreceptors across the cat retina
is similar to that in the human retina, although the absolute
numbers of cells are different (Steinberg *et al.*, 1973). Rod
and cone ERGs in the cat, therefore, might be expected to
show similar features to human ERGs, if methods like those
of clinical testing were used to elicit the responses. This
was shown to be the case in previous ERG studies of cats with
retinal degeneration (Rabin *et al.*, 1973; Bellhorn *et al.*,
1974).
    Preliminary to a study of the cat full-field ERG during
postnatal development (Jacobson and Ikeda, in prep.), we felt
it necessary to establish our own control data. In addition,
we wanted to determine whether some of the characteristic
changes in amplitude and timing occur in the human full-
field ERG with different stimuli and under different states
of adaption occur in an analogous manner in the cat. This

*Dr Jacobson is supported by a Research Career Development
Award of the Retinitis Pigmentosa Foundation (Baltimore,
Maryland, USA).

paper describes some of our results.

METHODS

Cats from a specific pathogen-free colony were anaesthetized
with intravenous alphaxolone-alphadolone acetate (Saffan,
14.5 mg/kg/h). The pupil was dilated and the nictitating
membrane retracted with cyclopentolate 1% and phenylephrine
10%. A double corneo-scleral contact lens electrode, similar
in principle to the Burian-Allen electrode, but with an artificial pupil of 7 mm diameter, was used to record the ERGs.
Amplification (bandpass 0.8 to 320 Hz) and computer averaging
of the signals were performed with a Medelec AA6-DAV6. Heart
rate and body temperature were monitored to be certain of
the physiological condition of the animal during all recordings.

The stimulus was a dome with a matt white inner surface and
two light sources situated at the top. One light source was
a xenon-filled gas discharge tube stroboscope (Devices Photic
Stimulator 3180) with peak luminance in the dome of 3.8 log
cd/m^2 and time to peak of 4 μs with exponential decay to
1/e of peak in 25 μs. The other light source was a tungsten
lamp which provided a steady white background light in the
dome with maximum luminance of 214 cd/m^2.

To isolate the rod ERGs in Fig. 1, the cat was dark
adapted for 2 h. Responses were then elicited with a short
wavelength flash (Wratten 47 and 47B and Cinemoid 18 and 25)
and a long wavelength flash (Wratten 25) matched for the rods
according to the method of Rabin *et al.* (1973). Intensity
of the background light was changed by interposing neutral
density filters between the tungsten source and the dome.

To isolate the cone ERGs shown in Fig. 2 A-D, the cats
were light adapted for at least 20 mins prior to the recordings. The stimulus was the maximum intensity white light
flashed at 3 Hz and superimposed on a steady white background
at the maximum luminance. In Fig. 2E, the cat was dark
adapted for 4 h prior to having cone ERGs elicited with the
same stimulus (but at 10 Hz) and background lights as described above. Recordings were taken immediately at onset of
light adaption and 20 min later. Both stimulus and background lights were kept on during the 20 min of light adaptation.

Amplitude of the b-wave of ERGs was measured between the
cornea-negative trough (a-wave) and the cornea-positive peak.
The implicit time of the b-wave was measured from stimulus
onset to the major cornea-positive peak.

RESULTS

Figure 1 shows ERGs from a normal adult cat elicited with
scotopically balanced short (left column) and long (right
column) wavelength stimuli. Each recording in Fig. 1A is
the sum of 2 consecutive responses. In the top row are
records obtained after 2 h of dark adaptation. ERGs in the
next three rows were elicited with stimuli of the same intensity but in the presence of increasing levels of full-field

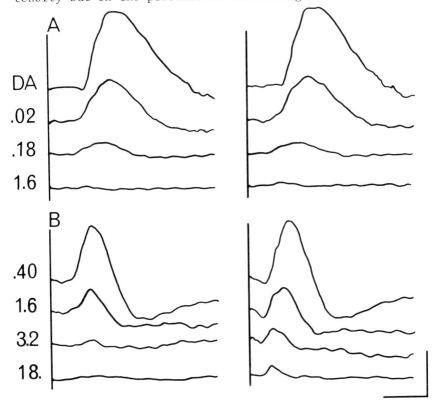

Fig. 1 *Full-field ERGs to scotopically balanced short (left
column) and long (right column) wavelength stimuli. A. ERGs,
representing the sum of 2 consecutive responses, in the dark
adapted state (DA) and with increasing levels of steady white
adapting light. B. ERGs, representing the computer summation
of 50 or 100 responses, with increasing levels of steady
white adapting light. Numbers on left signify full-field
background luminance in cd/m². Calibration (lower right)
represents 100 μv vertically for A and 8 μv vertically for B;
horizontal bar is 50 msec.*

background light. The b-wave amplitude and implicit time
decrease with the increase in intensity of adapting lights
until the responses can no longer easily be distinguished
from the baseline noise. In the recordings shown in Fig.
1A, there is no apparent difference in the behaviour of the
responses elicited with short and long wavelength stimuli
during increasing light adaptation.

Figure 1B is the continuation of the experiment of Fig.
1A but with the use of computer averaging techniques; each
record represents the sum of 50 or 100 responses. A difference between the responses to short and long wavelength
stimuli can now be noted. With increasing intensity of
adapting light, the monophasic response to the short wavelength stimulus decreases in amplitude and timing until it
becomes indistinguishable from noise. In contrast to this
sequence, the response to long wavelength stimulation becomes
biphasic with increasing background light. The component
with a longer implicit time eventually disappears leaving a
single peaked response with relatively short implicit time.
This latter response is that of the cones.

Figure 2 shows examples of light-adapted full-field cone
ERGs from two normal adult cats (A and B), a cat with a unilateral chorioretinal scar produced by intense xenon photo-
coagulation (C), a kitten at two different ages (D), and an
adult cat during the course of light adaptation (E). All
ERGs represent the computer summation of 200 responses. The
reproducibility of cone ERGs elicited in such a manner is
demonstrated in Fig. 2A. The two ERGs are from the right eye
of the same adult cat recorded at testing sessions separated
by about three months. The responses differ very little in
b-wave amplitude or implicit time. An interocular comparison
of cone ERGs from another adult cat is shown in Fig. 2B.
Again there is little difference in the two records. In
contrast, Fig. 2C displays ERGs from the left and right eyes
of an adult cat with a 5 disc diameter healed chorioretinal
scar in the posterior pole of the right eye. Whereas b-wave
amplitude in the eye with a lesion is much reduced compared
to that of the fellow eye without a lesion, the b-wave implicit
times of both responses are similar and within the adult
range (derived from 60 recordings at different sessions on
left and right eyes of 5 adult cats). Figure 2D shows responses recorded from the right eye of a kitten at age 4
weeks and again at 12 weeks of age. In this example, the
b-wave amplitudes of the two responses are similar but the
implicit times are quite different. A very prolonged b-wave
implicit time, 30.1 ms, is found at age 4 weeks while the
response at 12 weeks has an implicit time of 20.0 ms, which

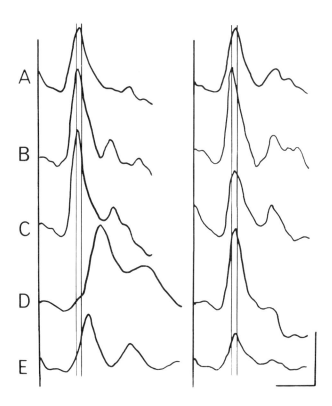

Fig. 2 *Full-field light adapted cone ERGs from 5 cats. A. Right eye responses from 2 sessions separated by nearly 3 months in an adult cat; B and C. Left eye (left column) and right eye (right column) responses from a normal adult cat (B) and from a cat with a chorioretinal scar in the right eye (C); D. Right eye responses at 4 weeks (left column) and 12 weeks of age (right column) in a kitten; E. Right eye responses from an adult cat at the onset of light adaptation (left column) and after 20 min of light adaptation (right column). Cone b-wave implicit time of adult cats ranged from 18.0 to 20.2 ms (vertical lines through responses), while amplitude ranged from 4.2 to 7.4 µv. Calibration (lower right) signifies vertically 4 µv for A–C and 8 µv for D and E; horizontally, it represents 20 ms.*

is within the adult range. Finally, Fig. 2E displays ERGs recorded immediately after light onset in a dark adapted cat and 20 min later. Both b-wave amplitude and implicit time decrease during the course of light adaptation.

DISCUSSION

The full-field rod and cone ERGs of the cat that we elicited
with methods similar to those used in clinical electroretinography provide interesting comparisons to analogous
records from humans. The dark-adapted human ERG obtained
with a long wavelength stimulus is readily distinguished
from its rod-matched short wavelength counterpart by the presence of prominent early oscillations attributable to the
cone system (Gouras, 1970). In contrast, a pair of ERGs
evoked with similar stimuli in the dark-adapted cat are not
easily distinguished from one another. Our demonstration of
how the cat cone ERG can be isolated with progressive light
adaptation of the dark-adapted long wavelength (but not the
short wavelength) response is reminiscent of demonstrations
of the same phenomenon in man (Gouras, 1970; Berson, 1981).
However, our recordings of the cat cone signal required
computer averaging (also found by Rabin, unpubl. results)
while this is not necessary for human recordings. The smaller
number of cones in the cat retina relative to the human
retina (Steinberg et al., 1973) is the likely explanation for
the slightly greater difficulty in obtaining the cone ERG
in the cat than in man.

The importance of examining the temporal aspects of the
ERG has been stressed for clinical recordings (Berson, 1981).
The waveform of the light adapted cone ERG of the cat
especially lends itself to accurate measurements of b-wave
implicit time. Full-field cone ERGs recorded from the same
cat on different days, from both eyes of a normal cat, or
from the two eyes of a cat with a large unilateral chorioretinal scar all had similar b-wave implicit times. Results
from the last-mentioned cat, however, showed a reduced cone
b-wave amplitude in the eye with the delimited area of
retinal destruction when compared with the response from
the normal fellow eye. This example of normal implicit time
in the presence of reduced amplitude is very similar to the
type of cone ERG found in patients with large chorioretinal
scars (Berson, 1981). In contrast, the cone ERG of a 4 week
old kitten had a large amplitude but markedly prolonged
implicit time. There was no prolongation of timing when
the same cat was tested at 12 weeks of age; amplitude, on
the other hand, was almost unchanged. A further demonstration
of an increase in cone implicit time without a decrease in
amplitude was provided by the adult cat at onset of light
adaptation. After a period of time in the light, implicit
time decreased to within the expected adult range. This
particular effect on the timing of the cone ERG of the cat

is analogous to the demonstration in man of a slower cone
b-wave in the dark adapted state than under light adaptation
(Berson, 1981). The only other reported timing delays in the
full-field cone ERG of the cat are in nutritionally-induced
or sporadic retinal degeneration; those ERGs had reduced
amplitudes (Rabin *et al.*, 1973; Bellhorn *et al.*, 1974). In
patients with inherited retinal degenerations, characteristic
delays in the cone b-wave implicit time can occur with normal
or reduced amplitude (Berson, 1981). In the presence of
retinal disease, abnormalities in cone timing are thought to
reflect widespread photoreceptor dysfunction and are in
contrast to examples of localized photoreceptor loss (e.g.
chorioretinal scars) wherein cone b-wave implicit time is
preserved (Berson, 1981).

In conclusion, when the full-field techniques of clinical
electroretinography are applied to the cat, the resulting rod
and cone ERGs can provide interesting analogies to the well-
known patterns of ERG amplitude and timing found in human
recordings.

ACKNOWLEDGEMENTS

We are grateful to Professor R. Fletcher for his generous
help in designing and making the contact lens electrodes
and to Dr A.R. Rabin for helpful discussion. We thank the
Retinitis Pigmentosa Foundation (USA) and the Special Trustees
of St Thomas' Hospital for financial support.

REFERENCES

Bellhorn, R.W., Aguirre, G.D. and Bellhorn, M.B. (1974).
   Feline central retinal degeneration. *Invest. Ophthalmol.*
   13, 608–616.
Berson, E.L. (1981). Electrical phenomena in the retina.
   In "Adler's Physiology of the Eye". (Ed. R.A. Moses) 7th
   edition. pp. 466–529. Mosby, St. Louis, USA.
Gouras, P. (1970). Electroretinography: some basic principles.
   Invest. Ophthalmol. **9**, 557-569.
Rabin, A.R., Hayes, K.C. and Berson, E.L. (1973). Cone and
   rod responses in nutritionally induced retinal degenera-
   tion in the cat. *Invest. Ophthalmol.* **12**, 694–704.
Steinberg, R.H., Reid, M. and Lacey, P.L. (1973). The dis-
   tribution of rods and cones in the retina of the cat.
   J. Comp. Neurol. **148**, 229–248.

LAVAIL asked if there was any evidence that only one type of peptide was associated with any one specific amacrine cell, or did some contain more than one peptide? OSBORNE replied that, unlike the brain, in the case of the retina it was not possible to demonstrate more than one peptide per cell in the retina. IKEDA said that Neal showed acetylcholine in amacrine cells of rabbit retina which could be released. OSBORNE criticized the release experiments on the grounds that they did not show acetylcholine release from presynaptic membranes on physiological stimulation. VOADEN then commented on species differences in retinal transmitters. She said that in mammalian retina, for example, there is no GABA so that it is dangerous to argue that a transmitter in one species will be found to be so in another. She also pointed out that it was possible to load a rat retina with GABA and to cause its release with potassium ions, but that this did not define GABA as a transmitter in that retina. OSBORNE said that he thought that if a substance was established as a true neurotransmitter, it was likely that it would have the same function in all retinas.

VOADEN, commenting on Anderson's data, described her experiments on light-induced retinal damage in the rat and its relation to loss of taurine. She said that damage was seen definitely after 30 to 40h. She had looked at malonyl dialdehyde levels and at ATPase activities in whole retinas, but no changes were found. The reduction in taurine levels were interpreted as being consequent on damage but indicative of permeability changes. ANDERSON pointed out that it was easier to see changes in isolated photoreceptor outer segments, since in whole retina any changes would be diluted by other retinal tissue. He said that they had not yet determined peroxide levels in albino retinas but intended to do so. He also said that one of the difficulties in determining malonyl dialdehyde levels was that vitamin A took part in the reaction, and so the thiobarbituric acid complex must be isolated to demonstrate unequivocally that malonyl dialdehyde was produced. He was intending to use HPLC for

this purpose. **VOADEN** admitted that there was a high background in the malonyl dialdehyde reaction, but the spectrum
they obtained for the thiobarbituric acid-retinaldehyde complex was different from that of the malonyl dialdehyde complex. She also pointed out that Russian workers had found
that when free radicals were formed in retina, then a concomitant and drastic reduction in $Na^+K^+ATPase$ was recorded,
and she would have expected similar reductions in $Na^+K^+ATPase$
in her light-damaged rats. **ANDERSON** stated that they had not
done early determinations in the ferrous sulphate-treated or
albino rats to see whether peroxide formation was a cause or
a consequence of the cellular damage.

BIOCHEMISTRY AND NEUROPHARMACOLOGY: SUMMING UP

H.W. READING

MRC Brain Metabolism Unit, Department of Pharmacology,
1 George Square,
Edinburgh, EH8 9JZ, Scotland.

The session on Biochemistry and Neuropharmacology of the
retina, although covering a wide range of pertinent topics,
unavoidably omitted some important aspects under this heading.

However, both Dr Chader's and Dr Osborne's entertaining
overviews rectified this to some extent by enumerating the
"present state of the art". Many of the advances made in
recent times have been made possible only by the development
of ultrasensitive microanalytical methods combined with the
characterization of specific substances by immunohistochemistry.
Dr Osborne reminded us of the advantages of using the retina
for research in its own right and also as a model for investigations on the C.N.S. His cautionary observations on
the difficulties inherent in positive validification of
chemical transmitters in the retina cannot be overemphasized.

Dr Chader's classification of retinal biochemists was
amusing but not without its serious implications. Too often
researchers forget that the retina works as a miniature
brain, not only transmitting a particular external signal,
but carrying out a great deal of local integration as well.
Some of Dr Chader's remarks, especially those concerning
the controversy between Hagin's (1972) concept of Ca^{++} as
a second messenger in the photoreceptor and that of Liebman's
group (Liebman and Pugh, 1979), that cyclic nucleotides are
involved in the alterations of membrane permeability associated
with light/dark adaptation, are being resolved by the discovery of specific cyclic nucleotide phosphodiesterases
(PDE) and their activation through the mobilization of the
Ca^{++}-binding protein regulator, calmodulin. It still remains
to be seen how the last-named event is brought about when
light is absorbed by the visual pigment. The process may be
coupled to membrane phosphorylation and it is a great pity
that owing to his untimely and sad death, Malcolm Weller,

one of the leaders in this field, was not with us to give his
views. The further elucidation of these processes may have
far-reaching implications in elucidating the processes underlying retinal degenerative diseases such as Retinitis Pigmentosa. The work of Drs Lolley, Farber and Chader (Lolley and
Farber, 1980; Chader *et al*., 1980) and others has shown that
a basic biochemical defect in the metabolism of cyclic
nucleotides involving calmodulin is a common feature of these
conditions.

Dr Chader very rightly paid tribute to the pioneering work
of Oliver Lowry and his group at St Louis (Lowry *et al*.,
1956) which gave us a firm basis for the diverse biochemical
organization of the retina and its relation to morphological
structure.

Dr Anderson's suggestion of lipid peroxidation as a basis
for light-induced retinal degeneration is part of a continuing area of controversy amongst retinal biochemists.
Both Dr Anderson and Dr Voaden's recent work which was
mentioned in discussion, can be looked upon as developments
of much earlier work by both Sorsby (Sorsby and Harding,
1962) and Noell (1965) who were interested in the use of
specific retinotoxic substances to mimic hereditary degeneration. A feature of such substances was the wide variety of
different pharmacological properties possessed by the compounds which prompted many different explanations for the
one common property, that of retinotoxicity. However, the
retinotoxic action of sodium iodate, a powerful oxidant,
could be blocked *in vivo*, by the administration of reduced
glutathione (GSH), a reducing agent. In addition, it was
shown (Reading and Sorsby, 1966) that iodate, in common
with some other retinotoxic agents, had marked effects on
thiol (-SH) groups in the retina. Iodate and the phenothiazines such as thioridazine, are good candidates for the
production of free radicals to produce peroxidation reactions.
It is also worthy of mention in this respect, that in both
drug-induced retinotoxocity and in retinal dystrophy, an
elevation in hexose monophosphate shunt (HMP) activity has
been found   (Reading, 1964, 1965). This metabolic pathway
is normally coupled to the visual cycle and is involved in
the reduction of retinaldehyde to retinol. Activity is
controlled by the levels of specific pyridine nucleotide
cofactors $NADPH^+/NADP$. Normally this ratio is greater than
unity, the reduced form ($NADPH^+$) being in excess. High
HMP activity indicates that the ratio is much less than
unity with the oxidized nucleotide, NADP being in excess.
This will favour conditions in which oxidizing free radicals
are not removed from the photoreceptors. It should not be
assumed that such mechanisms are a primary cause of photo-

receptor degeneration but that all these findings, in some
measure, support the concept that alterations in redox state
are damaging to the retina.

The mode of retinotoxic action of chloroquine and thioridazine is still the subject of discussion but, as Dr Converse
herself pointed out, the drugs are highly lipid-soluble,
therefore toxicity is probably associated with interference
in membrane function. It is possible as outlined above, that
these compounds might offer a useful approach to the problem
of lipid peroxidation and free radical formation in retina.
However, the approach to studying progressive retinal degeneration by the use of toxic drugs has been followed for
more than 30 years and Dr Converse's work follows in the
tradition of giants like Graymore, Sorsby, Noell, Meier-Ruge
and others. Only if some agent producing retinal degeneration
is found, for which there is a specific pharmacological
antagonist, may retinotoxic drug studies help in arresting
the relentless progress of the natural lesion.

Inherited pigmentary degeneration of the retina is a
heterogenetic defect and the aetiology of the lesion is likely
to involve many biochemical anomalies. We have heard throughout this Symposium about the complexities of characterizing
the different forms of retinal degeneration and Dr Lolley's
brilliant suggestion of development and maintenance classes
of the animal condition is based on different types of biochemical anomaly. We have known for many years that the
natural lesion in the rat involves a defect in protein
synthesis in the photoreceptors (Reading and Sorsby, 1964).
This early report was the first observation of a primary
metabolic anomaly in the lesion and LaVail *et al*. (1972)
confirmed and extended this by showing that the defect in
protein synthesis was associated with photoreceptor disc
renewal.

Dr Ikeda's contribution was an elegant example of the
contributions made by electrophysiologists to the study and
characterization of neurotransmitters in the retina. As
Dr Osborne pointed out, a great deal of information is
available on this subject, but even now, much controversy
exists concerning the identity between specific transmitter
and neurone. One of the difficulties lies in the complexity
of retinal neuronal circuitry; there are excitatory and
inhibitory systems as well as those modulating and integrat-
ing information before passing it to the brain. This neces-
sitates an intricate and plastic synaptic system with the
inherent complexities of identification which is further
complicated by the modern physiologist's questioning of
the so-called Dale's principle of one neurone, one transmitter. Different disciplines must therefore be involved

in producing evidence for functional transmitter identity,
with electrophysiology occupying a very major role.

Dr Osborne provided beautiful evidence for the existence
of serotonin and neuroactive peptide containing amacrine
cells in the frog retina and it would appear that he favours
the view that in this species and relevant neuronal population, Dale's principle still holds. Dr Osborne was able
to demonstrate neuroactive peptide containing amacrine cells
and in his overview, to enumerate the different peptides which
have been identified in retina, albeit in the main by immunofluorescence. Since this particular technique is fraught
with difficulties of non-specificity of antibody and cross-
reactivity, Dr Osborne was correct in implying caution in
interpretation of such data. He suggested that the peptides
may have a modulatory function, a term which is difficult to
define physiologically. In fact, the role of neuroactive
peptides in brain, as distinct from the hypothalamic-pituitary
axis and spinal cord, is largely unknown. The short contribution on the interactions between TRH and dopamine
systems in the retina, may in a small way, provide some information on this problem.

The last contribution in this session was given by Dr de
Grip who described work done in Nijmegen on the production
of specific antisera to different comformations of rhodopsin.
This technique should offer a remarkably sensitive tool for
structural studies of different visual pigment derivatives
and may solve some problems associated with recognition of
active sites in the molecule.

REFERENCES

Chader, G., Lin, Y., O'Brien, P., Fletcher, R., Krishna, G.,
    Aguirre, G., Farber, D. and Lolley, R.N. (1980). Cyclic
    GMP phosphodiesterase activator; involvement in a here-
    ditary retinal degeneration. *Neurochemistry* 1, 441-458.
Hagins, W.A. (1972). The visual process. Excitatory mech-
    anism in the primary receptor cells. *An. Rev. Biophys.*
    Bioeng. 1, 131-158.
LaVail, M.M., Sidman, R.L. and O'Neil, D. (1972). Photoreceptor-
    pigment epithelial cell relationships in rats with in-
    herited retinal degeneration: Radiographic and electron
    microscope evidence for a dual source of extralamellar
    material. *J. Cell Biol.* 53, 185-209.
Liebman, P.A. and Pugh, E.N. (1979). The control of phos-
    phodiesterase in rod disc membranes: Kinetics, possible
    mechanisms and significance for vision. *Vision Res.*
    19, 385-380.

Lolley, R.N. and Farber, D.B. (1980). Cyclic GMP metabolic defects in inherited disorders of rd mice and RCS rats. *Neurochemistry* 1, 427–440.

Lowry, O.H., Roberts, N.R. and Lewis, C. (1956). The quantitative histochemistry of the retina. *J. Cell. Biol.* 220, 829–892.

Noell, W.K. (1965). In "Biochemistry of the Eye" (Ed. C.N. Graymore) p. 51, Academic Press, New York.

Reading, H.W. (1964). Activity of the hexose monophosphate shunt in the normal and dystrophic retina. *Nature, Lond.* 203, 491–492.

Reading, H.W. (1965). Protein synthesis and the hexose monophosphate shunt in the developing normal and dystrophic retina. In "Biochemistry of the Retina" (Ed. C.N. Graymore) pp. 51–72. Academic Press, New York.

Reading, H.W. and Sorsby, A. (1964). Metabolism of the dystrophic retina II. Amino acid transport and protein synthesis in the developing rat retina; normal and dystrophic. *Vision Res.* 4, 209–220.

Reading, H.W. and Sorsby, A. (1966). Retinal toxicity and tissue –SH Levels. *Biochem. Pharmacol.* 15, 1389–1393.

Sorsby, A. and Harding, R. (1962). Experimental degeneration of the retina VII — the protective action of thiol donors against the retinotoxic effect of sodium iodate. *Vision Res.* 2, 139–148.

GENETICS AND DEVELOPMENT: AN OVERVIEW

RICHARD N. LOLLEY

*Developmental Neurology Laboratory, V.A. Medical Centre,
Sepulveda, California 91343, and Department of Anatomy,
UCLA School of Medicine, Los Angeles, California 90024, USA.*

Investigations of inherited blindness are passing into a phase
from which an attack may be launched upon the causes of
Retinitis Pigmentosa. Naturally, today's research builds on
that of the past, and vision research has a history that
reaches back for over a century to the discovery of the
visual pigment, rhodopsin. Each decade has offered insight
into the morphology, biochemistry and physiology of rods
and cones, and each new discovery enhances the possibility
that inherited blindness will be understood and cured.

The history of vision research has been influenced by the
concepts and attitudes that prevailed over the past decades.
It is hard to envision now the nature of scientific investigation before the advent of cellular and molecular biology.
Still, vision researchers spent several decades in characterizing the cellular nature of rods and cones and demonstrating
that they metabolized glucose and manufactured ATP like other
cells of the body.

This phase of research blended some four decades ago with
an interest in inherited animal disorders that cause blindness. Blind animals were identified and bred for research.
Their genetic mode of inheritance was identified and the
histopathology of several disorders was characterized. Such
studies were carried out with the stated hope that they might
help explain human diseases like Retinitis Pigmentosa. These
investigators, however, were working at a tremendous disadvantage because little was known about the histopathology
and biochemistry of inherited disease that cause blindness
in humans.

Today, it is widely appreciated that investigations of
human retinas must be carried out. This realization has
prompted a change in attitude among lay persons, vision
researchers and clinicians. The study of human retina must

be pursued actively. Care must be taken with each individual
case in order to clarify the mode of inheritance of the
disease and the clinical manifestations of the disease process. In addition to this, investigators must be prepared
at short notice to study the histopathology and biochemical
abnormalities of the affected photoreceptors if perchance
the eye is offered to research upon the early demise of an
individual. With patience and perseverance a catalogue of
pathologies can be compiled both for the animal disorders
and for human disease. Only then will animal disorders be
identified which are truly models of specific human diseases.

The life of a normal photoreceptor cell begins with cell
division in the embryo or early postnatal life, and it continues through several stages of specialization before it is
established as a mature, functioning visual cell (Fig. 1).
Little is known about the genetics or environmental factors
that induce the newly formed cells to become rods or cones.
It has been shown, however, in normal retina, that some
putative visual cells do not successfully achieve this transformation because about 20% of the newly formed cells degenerate following photoreceptor cell differentiation (Lolley,
1973). Those that do differentiate grow to adult dimensions
and, barring disease or physical injury, they continue to
function throughout the life of the individual.

In the last decade, a surge of information has appeared
which defines in some detail the genetics, histopathology and
biochemistry of several animal disorders. The mode of genetic
transmission of these disorders is uniformly autosomal recessive. Nonetheless, the disorders neither exhibit a uni-
formity of histopathology nor a coincidence in age at which
the animals become blind. I propose that this information
may be helpful in understanding the various animal disorders and, hopefully, it may point out the relevant systems
for investigation in animal and human blindness.

We can ask: "Are there periods in the lifeline of a photoreceptor cell in which the cell is particularly vulnerable
to genetic or environment insults?" Two genetic mutations
which are expressed in the photoreceptor cells of mice suggest that the answer to this question may be yes. Photoreceptors of the *rd* (retinal degeneration) retina are formed
in normal numbers and become transformed into rods and cones,
but all of the rods die in the post-differentiation period
(LaVail and Sidman, 1974). As is seen in most animal and
human diseases, the degeneration of rods precedes that of
cones. The critical event that triggers this disorder appears
to be the process of photoreceptor differentiation.

In contrast to the photoreceptors of *rd* retinas, visual
cells of Purkinje cell-deficient or *pcd* mice survive a perhaps

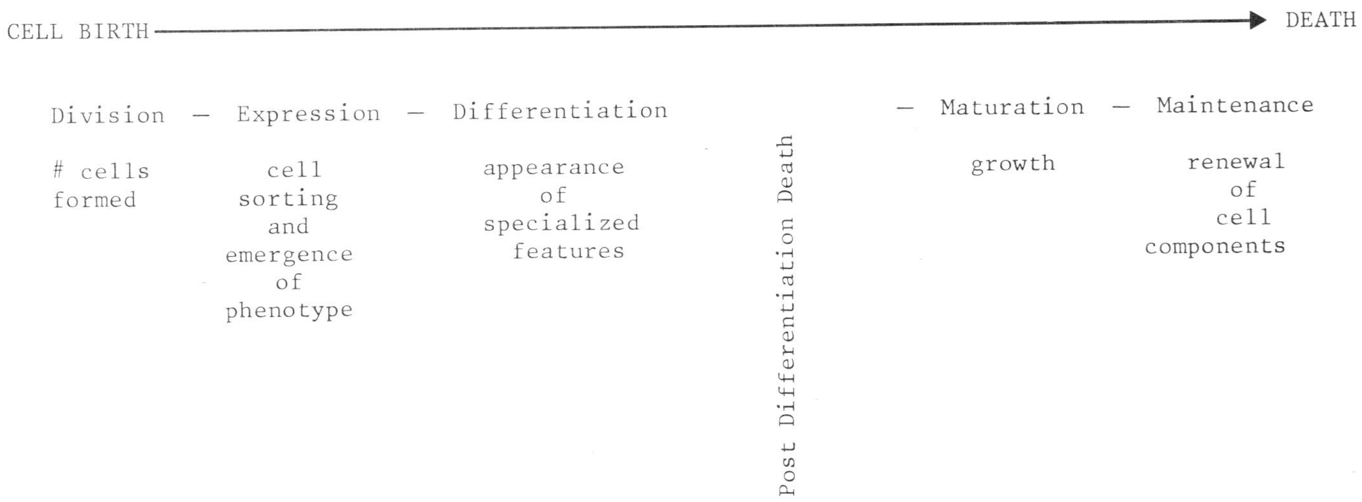

CELL BIRTH ──────────────────────────────────► DEATH

Division — Expression — Differentiation — Maturation — Maintenance

| # cells formed | cell sorting and emergence of phenotype | appearance of specialized features | growth | renewal of cell components |

Post Differentiation Death

Fig. 1 *Lifeline of normal photoreceptor cell.*

atypical differentiation to develop into mature, functional photoreceptors (Blanks *et al.*, 1978). An atypical differentiation is indicated by the transient development of villus-like processes that sprout from the inner segment of the differentiating photoreceptor cells. However, having reached adult dimensions, the rod photoreceptors begin to degenerate slowly over the course of a year. Therefore, the autosomal recessive characteristic of *pcd* mice appears to impact on photoreceptor cells that are attempting to maintain their state of functional differentiation. At present, it is impossible to identify what aspect of photoreceptor renewal is affected by the mutation. In the *pcd*, also, rods are more vulnerable than cones.

One additional difference has been noted between the *rd* and *pcd* disorders. The *rd* photoreceptors characteristically accumulate cyclic GMP before they degenerate (Farber and Lolley, 1976), whereas the photoreceptors of *pcd* mice do not.

Photoreceptor cell development is not an independent process since it can be influenced by environmental factors, some of which may be under the control of the pigment epithelium. The inherited disorder of Royal College of Surgeons or RCS rats is useful to illustrate this point. The RCS disorder has been characterized as one in which the mutant gene is expressed in the pigment epithelium cells, and it renders the pigment epithelium cells incapable of phagocytizing rod outer segment membranes at the rate they are shed by the photoreceptors (Bok and Hall, 1971). The disorder becomes manifest at an age when the photoreceptors have differentiated and have just begun to shed the tips of their rod outer segments. The sheddings accumulate in the subretinal space and, with the build-up of this debris, photoreceptor cells begin to degenerate. Within a month, the rod photoreceptors are lost and only the cones survive. The RCS photoreceptors do not accumulate cyclic GMP before they degenerate. This disorder represents a clear example wherein a faulty renewal system initiates photoreceptor degeneration.

We ask further whether the rodent disorders are special cases or whether they are representative of inherited disorders in other animals. Several inherited disorders that affect the vision of dogs are included in Fig. 2 for comparison with the rodent disorders. It is clear from inspection of the figure that photoreceptor degeneration may occur preferentially at two stages along the lifeline of visual cells. It occurs either at the age when photoreceptor cells are differentiating or later in life when the photoreceptor cells are maintaining a state of functional differentiation. The listing of animal disorders included in Fig. 2 is representative rather than exhaustive, but it

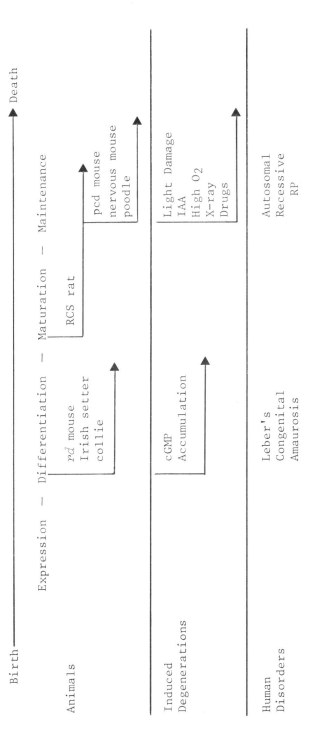

Fig. 2 *Onset of photoreceptor degeneration in inherited or induced blindness.*

illustrates that the disorders of *rd* mice, Irish setter dogs
(Aguirre *et al.*, 1978) and collie dogs (Woodford *et al.*, 1980)
fall into the category of differentiation defects, whereas *pcd*
mice, nervous mice (Mullen and LaVail, 1975), poodle dogs
(Aguirre and Rubin, 1972) and RCS rats are maintenance defects.
    The biochemical mechanisms that cause differentiating
visual cells to degenerate may differ from those that initiate
degeneration in a maintenance defect. From the small sampling
of animal disorders that have been studied biochemically, it
appears that an abnormal metabolism of cyclic GMP may be
characteristic of those disorders that arise from a defect
in differentiation.
    The cause or causes for a maintenance defect are still un-
known. Our findings with the RCS and *pcd* disorders suggest
that a lethal defect need not involve an abnormality in cyclic
GMP metabolism. What does cause rods or cones to degenerate
after they reach maturity is open for speculation.
    It is perhaps enlightening to consider what treatments
are particularly unhealthy for rods and cones. Ulshafer
and Hollyfield (1981) have demonstrated *in vitro* that normal
photoreceptors of animal or humans are vulnerable to incubation conditions that cause cyclic GMP to accumulate.
This means that any chemical or environmental conditions that
stimulate the accumulation of cyclic GMP *in vivo* would most
likely cause visual cell degeneration. However, there is no
reason to postulate that every condition that causes photoreceptor degeneration will do so by involving cyclic GMP.
    Noell (1958) has investigated many conditions that cause
mature photoreceptors to degenerate, and he has pointed out
the similarity between certain induced degenerations and
human Retinitis Pigmentosa. Some of the conditions that he
studied are listed in Fig. 2. All of these conditions share
the capability of creating free radicals, and all agents
affect rods before cones. The common feature between free
radicals and mutant genes may be their ability to disrupt
the normal renewal mechanisms in visual cells. Without the
capacity for continuous rejuvenation, the photoreceptors have
no option but to degenerate.
    Of the autosomal recessive diseases that cause blindness
in man, some may impact upon the differentiation of photoreceptor cells whereas others may disrupt the renewal of rods
and cones. It is too early to know whether the above scheme
for classifying animal disorders has any predictive value
for human diseases. Still, it is worth speculating that
early onset diseases like Leber's congenital amaurosis may
represent a differentiation defect which would exhibit an
elevated level of cyclic GMP in the photoreceptors prior to
their degeneration. Accordingly, Retinitis Pigmentosa that

is transmitted in an autosomal recessive mode might represent
a maintenance defect with an as yet unknown lesion in the
process of photoreceptor renewal. Time will tell whether
this scheme is useful for pinpointing the relevant system
for study in human disorders that cause blindness.

REFERENCES

Aguirre, G.D. and Rubin, L.F. (1972). Progressive retinal
    atrophy in the miniature poodle: An electrophysiologic
    study. *J.A.V.M.A.* **160**, 191—201.
Aguirre, G., Farber, D., Lolley, R., Fletcher, R.T. and
    Chader, G.J. (1978). Rod-cone dysplasia in Irish Setters:
    A defect in cyclic GMP metabolism in visual cells.
    Science **201**, 1133—1134.
Blanks, J.C., Mullen, R.J. and LaVail, M.M. (1978). Ultra-
    structural study of slow photoreceptor degeneration in
    PCD, a cerebellar mutant mouse. *Invest. Ophthalmol. Vis.
    Sci.* **17** (Suppl), 158.
Bok, D. and Hall, M.O. (1971). The role of the pigment epi-
    thelium in the etiology of inherited retinal dystrophy
    in the rat. *J. Cell Biol.* **49**, 664—682.
Farber, D.B. and Lolley, R.N. (1974). Cyclic guanosine
    monophosphate: elevation in degenerating photoreceptor
    cells of the C3H mouse retina. *Science* **186**, 449—451.
LaVail, M.M. and Sidman, R.L. (1974). C57BL/6 mice with
    inherited retinal degeneration. *Arch. Ophthalmol.* **91**,
    394—400.
Lolley, R.N. (1973). RNA and DNA in developing retinae:
    Comparison of a normal with the degenerating retinae of
    C3H mice. *J. Neurochem.* **20**, 175—182.
Mullen, R.J. and LaVail, M.M. (1975). Two new types of
    retinal degeneration in cerebellar mutant mice. *Nature*
    258, 528—530.
Noell, W.K. (1958). Differentiation, metabolic organization
    and viability of the visual cells. *A.M.A. Arch. Ophthal-
    mol.* **60**, 702—731.
Ulshafer, R.J. and Hollyfield, J.G. (1981). The effects of
    PDE inhibitors and ouabain on cultured human retina.
    Invest. Ophthalmol. Vis. Sci. **20** (Suppl), 40.
Woodford, B.J., Chader, G.J., Farber, D.B., Liu, L., Fletcher,
    R.T., Santos-Anderson, R. and Tso, M.O.M. (1980). Cyclic
    nucleotides in inherited retinal degeneration in collies.
    Invest. Ophthalmol. Vis. Sci. **19** (Suppl), 249.

CYCLIC NUCLEOTIDES AND EARLY ONSET RETINAL DYSPLASIA

GERALD J. CHADER

Laboratory of Vision Research, National Eye Institute, National Institutes of Health, Bethesda, MD 20205, USA.

ABSTRACT

Cyclic nucleotides mediate many aspects of normal cellular metabolism. Cyclic GMP and its enzyme of degradation, phosphodiesterase (PDE), seem to be particularly important in retinal photoreceptor function and may actually provide the chemical "signal" in the visual process. Derangement in cyclic GMP metabolism could thus lead to abnormal retinal development (dysplasia) and/or degeneration.

The Irish Setter and Collie both exhibit hereditary retinal abnormalities characterized by early onset photoreceptor degeneration during the postnatal period of outer segment elongation. Biochemically, affected retinas are deficient in cyclic GMP-PDE activity and have greatly elevated levels of cyclic GMP, as has been found in retinas of C3H mice with a similar type of disease. This abnormality appears to precede morphological signs of visual cell degeneration and may constitute the basic biochemical lesion in this disease type. In the Setter disease, calmodulin levels in the young affected retinas are also deficient and the normally Ca^{2+}-independent type of PDE demonstrates a Ca^{2+} and calmodulin-dependency. This latter dependency is not observed in affected Collie retinas, underscoring differences in affected retinas even when other morphological and biochemical characteristics are similar. In general however, derangement in cyclic GMP metabolism may be a common feature in early onset retinal degeneration and may be useful as a working model for one or more types of human RP.

REFERENCES

Chader, G.J., Liu, Y.P., Fletcher, R.T., Aguirre, G., Santos-
    Anderson, R. and Tso, M. (1981). Cyclic GMP phosphodies-
    terase and calmodulin in early-onset inherited retinal
    degeneration. In "Current Topics in Membrands and Transport"
    (Ed. W. Miller), Vol. 15, pp. 135-156. Academic Press,
    London.

OUTER SEGMENT RENEWAL IN CANINÉ
RETINAL DEGENERATION

[+]G. AGUIRRE, [*]P. O'BRIEN, [†]J. MARSHALL, [+]N. BUYUKMIOHI

[+]*School of Veterinary Medicine, University of Pennsylvania 19104, USA*

[*]*National Eye Institute, NIH, Bethesda, Maryland 20205, USA*

[†]*Department of Visual Science, Institute of Ophthalmology, Univetsity of London, London, UK.*

ABSTRACT

Generalized inherited retinal degenerations in dogs (Progressive Retinal Atrophies) are developmental or degenerative. In the developmental form (e.g. rod-cone dysplasia in Irish Setters) photoreceptor development is arrested in the early stages of postnatal retinal differentiation. In the degenerative form (e.g. progressive rod-cone degeneration in miniature poodles), photoreceptors degenerate following normal retinal differentiation.

To determine if these canine retinal degenerations are similar in pathogenetic mechanisms to the RCS strain of retinal dystrophic rats, the renewal of photoreceptor outer segment was investigated. Affected and age-match controls were injected intravitreally with ^{3}H-leucine and eyes enucleated at different post-injection intervals and prepared for standard autoradiographic examination.

In Irish Setters with rod-cone dysplasia, photoreceptor inner segments accumulated ^{3}H-label. Although low density label was present at all levels of the outer segment layer, a distinct band of ^{3}H-label was not present at any post-injection interval. At the time the normal developing photoreceptor outer segments were elongating by the addition of newly formed discs, the affected photoreceptors remained short with disoriented lamellar discs. This suggested a failure in the orderly and continuous addition of newly formed discs during retinal differentiation.

In miniature poodles with progressive rod-cone degeneration,

there was a distinct band of ^{3}H-label present in the outer
segment layer following the intravitreal injection. However,
the rate of displacement of the band of ^{3}H-label (renewal
rate) was significantly slower in affected than in control
animals (1.3 ± 0.25 microns/24 h and 2.3 ± 0.28 microns/24 h,
respectively). This abnormally slow renewal rate in affected
animals was present both in photoreceptors that were still
structurally normal as well as in those showing the early
stage of the disease. Our results suggest that there was a
slower assembly rate of rod outer segment discs in affected
animals.

These studies indicate that the pathogenesis of these two
canine retinal degenerations differ from the RPE phagocytic
defect present in RCS retinal dystrophic rats.

REFERENCES

Aguirre, G. and Rubin, L. (1972). Progressive retinal atrophy
    in the miniature poodle: an electrophysiologic study.
    J. Am. Vet. Assoc. **160**, 190–201.
Aguirre, G. and Rubin, L. (1975). Rod-cone dysplasia (pro-
    gressive retinal atrophy in Irish setters). *J. Am. Vet.
    Assoc.* **166**, 157–164.
Chader, G., Liu, Y., O'Brien, P., Fletcher, R., Krishna, G.,
    Farber, D. and Lolley, R. (1980). Cyclic GMP phosphodies-
    terase activator: involvement in a hereditary retinal de-
    generation. *Neurochem. Int.* **1**, 441–458.

CYCLIC GMP SYNTHESIS AND HYDROLYSIS IN VISUAL CELLS OF *rd* MOUSE RETINA

RICHARD N. LOLLEY

Developmental Neurology Laboratory, V.A. Medical Centre,
Sepulveda, California 91343,
and Department of Anatomy,
UCLA School of Medicine, Los Angeles, California 90024, USA

Inherited blindness in *rd* (retinal degeneration) mice is transmitted as an autosomal recessive characteristic, and it is expressed in retinal visual cells when they differentiate during postnatal life (Wegmann *et al.*, 1971). The differentiating photoreceptor cells of *rd* retina form rudimentary outer segments, and they start to develop their characteristic ribbon synapses (Blanks *et al.*, 1974). However, neither the synaptic complex nor the rod outer segments develops to full maturity. Nonetheless, *rd* photoreceptors are responsive to light in the brief interval between their differentiation and degeneration (Noell, 1965).

The earliest pathological changes occur in the *rd* photoreceptors on about the eighth postnatal day when rod outer segments are beginning to bud. The developing rod outer segment membranes are thrown into disarray, and the structure of the rod outer segments is disorganized (Lasansky and DeRobertis, 1960). Within the inner segment, some mitochondria become swollen. By day ten, pycnotic nuclei are evident in the outer nuclear layer and, by day 20, all of the rod visual cells have degenerated. The cone photoreceptors of the mouse retina survive longer than the rods (Carter-Dawson *et al.*, 1978), but they too degenerate in the following weeks.

Affected *rd* photoreceptors begin to accumulate cGMP between the 6th and 8th postnatal days (Farber and Lolley, 1974) due apparently to a deficiency in phosphodiesterase activity (Schmidt and Lolley, 1973). This reduced capacity to hydrolyse cGMP is the earliest known abnormality that has been found in the developing *rd* visual cells. A de-

ficiency in phosphodiesterase activity may result from the
expression of the *rd* gene but this has not been verified.

In the *rd* mouse disorder, the accumulation of cGMP may
trigger the degenerative process because it has been shown
experimentally that drugs can cause cGMP to accumulate and
thereby initiate degeneration of normal photoreceptor cells
(Lolley *et al.*, 1977). If we understand the apparent cause
of this disorder, it is possible perhaps to rectify the
abnormality by preventing the accumulation of cGMP.

The concentration of cGMP in rod visual cells is controlled by the relative rate of its synthesis and hydrolysis.
One approach to reducing the concentration of cGMP in *rd*
photoreceptors is to enhance the rate of cGMP hydrolysis via
the enzyme, phosphodiesterase. Another approach is to
diminish the rate of cGMP synthesis by inhibiting the enzyme,
guanylate cyclase.

The phosphodiesterase of rod photoreceptors has been investigated extensively, and it has been shown to be activated
by light in the presence of GTP (Bitensky *et al.*, 1978).
Several steps may be involved in the activation process,
with the bleaching of rhodopsin triggering the activation
of a GTPase which in turn activates the phosphodiesterase
(Fung *et al.*, 1981). This activation process is at least
partially intact in *rd* visual cells because cGMP levels in
dark-adapted retinas are reduced slightly by illumination
(Farber and Lolley, 1977). However, the light-activated
phosphodiesterase of *rd* visual cells is never able to
reduce the concentration of cGMP to levels that are near or
equivalent to those of normal photoreceptors. This observation is consistent with the observation by other investigators that light does not retard the rate of degeneration in the *rd* retina. Therefore, light which is the
most potent activator of visual cell phosphodiesterase
currently known cannot effectively lower the cGMP levels
of *rd* photoreceptors.

Controlling the rate of cGMP synthesis still remains a
viable option for reducing the concentration of cGMP in *rd*
visual cells. The guanylate cyclase which catalyses this
reaction has now been partially characterized. This cyclase
appears to be regulated by calcium ion rather than by light
or GTP. For this enzyme, calcium acts as an inhibitory
effector with activation of the enzyme occurring only at
concentrations of free calcium below about 5×10^{-6} M (Lolley
and Racz, 1981). It is generally assumed that the concentration of free calcium within a cell is about 10^{-7} to 10^{-8}
(Kretsinger, 1979). This would suggest that fluctuation in
the concentration of intracellular calcium could be capable
of regulating the rate of cGMP synthesis.

Adoph Cohen (Cohen *et al.*, 1978) has shown that the calcium chelator, EGTA, can cause normal, dark-adapted retinas
to accumulate cGMP to levels that are comparable to those
found in *rd* mice. We have used this approach to measure the
ability of developing normal retinas to respond to EGTA
treatment. A response to EGTA is noted only after visual
cells differentiate, and the magnitude of the response increases during the period when photoreceptors grow and mature.
The developmental sequence in which the retina becomes responsive to EGTA treatment verifies that only the guanylate
cyclase of visual cells is activated by low levels of free
calcium.

Developing visual cells of *rd* retina respond to EGTA
treatment as they differentiate, indicating that perhaps a
normal guanylate cyclase is produced by these cells. However, a response to EGTA treatment is observed about 1 to
2 days earlier in development than that of normal retinas.
The response to EGTA is consistently less than that of
normal retinas of comparable maturity. However, the
developmental and response characteristics of *rd* guanylate
cyclase are comparable in two strains of mice (C3H/HeJ and
C57BL/6 *rdle*) both of which carry the *rd* gene.

One interpretation of the *rd* findings suggests that the
diminished response of *rd* guanylate cyclase to EGTA treatment occurs because the enzyme is already partially activated
in vivo. It follows from this interpretation that the concentration of free calcium is higher in normal visual cells
than in *rd* photoreceptors and, therefore, the guanylate
cyclase of normal photoreceptors is more inhibited than that
of *rd* visual cells. Little is known about the factors that
regulate the concentration of ionized calcium in rod visual
cells, but it has been shown that *rd* retinas contain lower
than normal levels of total calcium during the postnatal
period when the visual cells are differentiating (Farber and
Lolley, 1976).

To test whether the guanylate cyclase of *rd* visual cells
might be partially active *in vivo*, immature *rd* retinas were
incubated in the dark with increasing concentrations (0.01
to 15.0 mM) of exogenous calcium. Over this range of
calcium, normal retinas do not increase or decrease their
concentration of cGMP, whereas, in *rd* retinas, the concentration of cGMP decreases progressively with increasing
calcium concentration. At these concentrations of calcium,
the normal retina either was able to rigorously control the
intracellular concentration of calcium in visual cells or
an elevation in free calcium did not significantly alter the,
perhaps already, inhibited guanylate cyclase. The fall in
cGMP levels in *rd* retinas may occur from the inhibition of

guanylate cyclase by intracellular calcium and by the continued hydrolysis of cGMP by phosphodiesterase.

In order to verify that cGMP can be hydrolysed in normal,
dark-adapted retina *in situ*, retinas were incubated with
EGTA so as to elevate the concentration of cGMP in the visual
cells. Subsequently, they were incubated with 2.5 mM calcium. Within one minute after transfer to calcium, the concentration of cGMP returned to near normal levels, most likely
by cGMP hydrolysis occurring in the near absence of cGMP
synthesis. Immature *rd* retinas incubated with calcium without prior treatment with EGTA lose their cGMP about eight
times more slowly than the EGTA-treated normal retinas.
These experiments again confirm that the activity of phosphodiesterase in *rd* visual cells is considerably lower than
that of normal photoreceptor cells.

We have been able for the first time to reduce the high
levels of cGMP in immature *rd* visual cells. We have done so
by inhibiting *in vitro* the rate of cGMP synthesis and allowing the endogenous phosphodiesterase of *rd* photoreceptors
to hydrolyse cGMP. As we learn more about the characteristics of the visual cell guanylate cyclase and its regulation by calcium or calcium-agonists, this strategy might be
extended from the incubation flask to the living animal.
Then, we can determine whether the affected visual cells of
rd mice will live and function when cGMP is maintained at
or near normal concentrations.

REFERENCES

Bitensky, M.W., Wheeler, G.L., Aloni, B., Vetury, S. and
    Matuo, Y. (1978). Light and GTP-activated photoreceptor
    phosphodiesterase: Regulation by a light-activated GTPase
    and identification of rhodopsin as the phosphodiesterase
    binding site. *Adv. Cyclic Nucleotide Res*. **9**, 553–572.
Blanks, J.C., Aldinolfi, A.M. and Lolley, R.N. (1974).
    Photoreceptor degeneration and synaptogenesis in retinal-
    degenerative (*rd*) mice. *J. Comp. Neurol*. **156**, 95–106.
Carter-Dawson, L.D., LaVail, M.M. and Sidman, R.L. (1978).
    Differential effect of the *rd* mutation on rods and
    cones in the mouse retina. *Invest. Ophthalmol. Vis.
    Sci*. **17**, 489–498.
Cohen, A.I., Hall, I.A. and Ferrendelli, J.A. (1978). Calcium
    and cyclic nucleotide regulation in incubated mouse
    retinas. *J. Gen. Physiol*. **71**, 595–612.
Farber, D.B. and Lolley, R.N. (1974). Cyclic guanosine
    monophosphate: elevation in degenerating photoreceptor
    cells of the C3H mouse retina. *Science* **186**, 449–451.

Farber, D.B. and Lolley, R.H. (1976). Calcium and magnesium content of rodent photoreceptor cells as inferred from studies of retinal degeneration. *Exp. Eye Res.* **22**, 219–228.

Farber, D.B. and Lolley, R.N. (1977). Light–induced reduction in cyclic GMP of retinal photoreceptor cells *in vivo*: Abnormalities in the degenerative diseases of RCS rats and *rd* mice. *J. Neurochem.* **28**, 1089–1095.

Fung, B. K–K., Hurley, H.B. and Stryer, L. (1981). Flow of information in the light-triggered cyclic nucleotide cascade of vision. *Proc. Nat. Acad. Sci. USA.* **78**, 152–156.

Kretsinger, R.H. (1979). The informational role of calcium in the cytosol. *Adv. Cyclic Nucleotide Res.* **11**, 1–26.

Lasansky, A. and DeRobertis, E. (1960). Submicroscopic analysis of the genetic dystrophy of visual cells in C3H mice. *J. Biophys. Biochem. Cytol.* **7**, 679–684.

Lolley, R.N. and Racz, E. (1981). Calcium regulation of receptor guanylate cyclase activity. *Invest. Ophthalmol. Vis. Sci.* **20** (Suppl), 210.

Lolley, R.N., Farber, D.B., Rayborn, M.E. and Hollyfield, J.G. (1977). Cyclic GMP accumulation causes degeneration of photoreceptor cells: Simulation of an inherited disease. *Science* **196**, 664–666.

Noell, W.K. (1965). In "Biochemistry of the Retina" (Ed. C.N. Graymore), pp. 51–72. Academic Press, London and New York.

Schmidt, S.Y. and Lolley, R.N. (1973). Cyclic-nucleotide phosphodiesterase. An early defect in inherited retinal degeneration of C3H mice. *J. Cell Biol.* **57**, 117–123.

Wegmann, T.G., LaVail, M.M. and Sidman, R.L. (1971). Patchy retinal degeneration in tetraparental mice. *Nature* **230**, 333–334.

DRUG INDUCED PHOTORECEPTOR DEGENERATION: SIMULATION OF INHERITED DEGENERATIVE DISORDERS IN NORMAL RETINAS

JOE G. HOLLYFIELD

*Cullen Eye Institute, Baylor College of Medicine
Houston, Texas 77006, USA*

SUMMARY

Phosphodiesterase inhibitors and cyclic-GMP analogues, when applied to normal retinas maintained in organ culture, cause specific changes in the photoreceptor layer. In developing retinas of the toad, (*Xenopus laevis*) both rods and cones undergo degenerative changes, whereas in adult human retinas only rod photoreceptors are affected. This model may be exploited as a means of evaluating the mechanism of cyclic-GMP toxicity.

Early studies using animal models to describe and analyse the metabolic causes of photoreceptor degeneration which result from inherited diseases pointed toward the possible involvement of altered cyclic nucleotide metabolism. The pioneering studies of Farber and Lolley (1974) indicated that in the C3H mouse homozygous for the *rd* (retinal degeneration) gene, photoreceptor degeneration during the second to third post natal week was associated with an altered cyclic GMP phosphodiesterase. As a consequence of this *rd* defect, the content of cyclic GMP in the outer retina increased, reaching a level 4 to 5 times above normal (Farber and Lolley, 1976). The observation of elevated cyclic GMP levels prior to any visible morphological changes in this mutant suggested that the high cyclic GMP levels may be somehow toxic to rod photoreceptors. In order to test this hypothesis, we began a series of studies utilizing normal retinas maintained *in vitro* in the presence of phosphodiestrase inhibitors or analogues of cyclic nucleotides.

We first demonstrated that the developing retinas of the
toad, *Xenopus laevis* were particularly labile to changes
caused by phosphodiesterase inhibitors. When isobutyl-
methylxanthine (IBMX) or the Squibb inhibitor, Sq 65442,
were present in the culture medium at concentration around
$10^{-3} - 10^{-4}$ M, the differentiating photoreceptors in these
retinas undergo specific degenerative changes. In the drug
treated retinas, the photoreceptors round-up and are extruded into the space between the retina and pigment epithelium. With increasing periods following drug exposure,
many of these extruded photoreceptors become pyknotic. The
degenerative changes were restricted to the photoreceptor
layer and did not affect neurons or glial cells in deeper
retinal lamina. (Figs 1 and 2). In companion biochemical

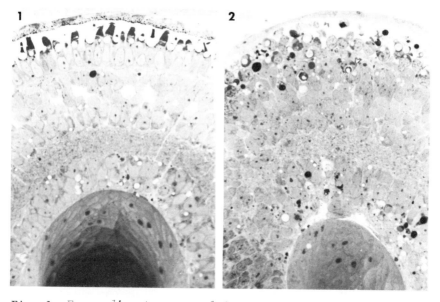

Fig. 1 *Eye rudiments removed from* Xenopus laevis *embryo at
stage 31 of development and grown for three days in hanging
drop cultures. In the presence of 9 × 10⁻⁶ M IBMX, retinal
morphology is normal and well developed photoreceptors are
present with outer segments projecting toward the adjacent
pigment epithelium. This low concentration of IMBX causes
no photoreceptor degeneration and retinas are virtually
identical to retinas cultured in the absence of IBMX
(X2500).*

experiments, elevated cyclic GMP levels were observed after drug treatment which were co-incident with the degenerative changes in the photoreceptors, again suggesting a causal relationship between high cyclic-GMP levels and photoreceptor degeneration (Lolley *et al.*, 1977).

To follow directly the vulnerability of photoreceptor cells in the developing *Xenopus* retina to specific cyclic nucleotides we added either 8-bromo or dibutyryl-derivatives of cyclic GMP and cyclic AMP. Our general observations were that whereas both cyclic AMP and cyclic GMP are toxic to the developing retina in this animal, morphological changes caused by cyclic AMP derivatives occurred throughout all retinal layers whereas the changes caused by the cyclic GMP derivatives were restricted to the photoreceptor layer (Hollyfield *et al.*, 1981).

Additional findings from these studies indicated a stage dependent vulnerability of photoreceptors to high cyclic GMP levels. When retinas were removed to culture at the neuroepithelial cell stage prior to photoreceptor differentiation, in the presence of dibutyryl-cyclic-GMP, retinal histogenesis was blocked as evidenced by the failure of stratification of the nuclear layers and the absence of the appearance of cytological differentiation (Fig. 3). However, if retinas were removed to culture at the time when photoreceptor outer segment differentiation was just commencing (Stage 37–38) and placed in the presence of the same concentration of dibutyryl cyclic GMP, specific photoreceptor degeneration resulted which was virtually identical to changes caused by the phosphodiesterase inhibitors described above (Fig. 4). These findings indicate that photoreceptors in early stages of differentiation are not altered by high levels of cyclic-GMP but that as photoreceptors differentiate they become susceptible to cyclic-GMP toxicity. We concluded from these experiments that high exogenous levels of cyclic-GMP, when aplied at the appropriate stage of retinal differentiation, resulted in a lesion in the outer retina which was comparable to the degeneration obtained when endogenous cyclic-GMP levels increased through the action of phosphodiesterase inhibitors.

The findings suggest that vulnerability to high levels of cyclic-GMP is a consequence of photoreceptor differentiation. To extend these observations on the developing

---

Fig. 2 *Retina cultured for three days in the presence of $9 \times 10^{-4}M$ IBMX. Degeneration is extensive in the photoreceptor cells with cellular debris present between the retina and pigment epithelium. For additional details of this experiment see Lolley* et al., *1977. (X2700).*

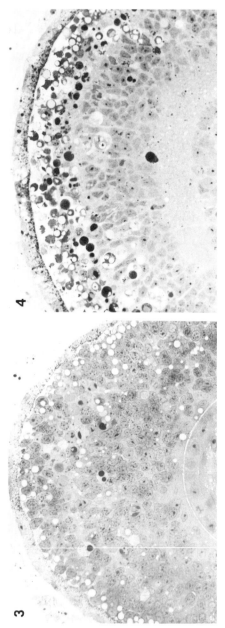

Fig. 3 *Retina removed from stage 31* Xenopus laevis *embryo and maintained for 3 days in culture in the presence of 16 × 10⁻³M dibutyryl cGMP. The cyclic nucleotide analogue causes no degenerative changes but blocks retinal differentiation. Note the absence of the inner and outer plexiform layers in photoreceptor differentiation.*

Fig. 4 *Retinal rudiments from Stage 36/37* Xenopus laevis *embryo maintained for two days in the presence of 16 × 10⁻³M dibutyryl cGMP. Note the extensive degeneration of the photoreceptor cell layer as evidenced by the debris accumulated between the retina and pigment epithelium. For additional details see Hollyfield et al. 1981. (X2700)*

retina to a fully differentiated system, we began to assess
the effects of these drugs on the human retina. Through
the cooperation of the Lions' Eyes of Texas Eye Bank we were
able to obtain eyes enucleated shortly after death of the
donor. Small 3 mm retinal discs were trephined from the
retinas and were cultured in the presence of cyclic nucleotide analogues or phosphodiesterase inhibitors at concentrations similar to those used in the animal studies. Our
initial observations were that both cyclic nucleotide
analogues and phosphodiesterase inhibitors were capable of
producing specific lesions in the photoreceptor layer of
the human retina. When the retinas are cultured for 8 h
in the presence of either dibutyryl cyclic-GMP or IBMX, rod
photoreceptors show profound degenerative changes whereas
cone photoreceptors and other layers of the retina do not
show these alterations (Fig. 5 and 6). We have begun a
series of studies to probe the possible alteration of specific metabolic pathways by elevated cyclic nucleotide levels.
In studies of the effects of these agents on protein synthesis, Dr Robert Ulshafer in my laboratory has observed
that IBMX, as well as several other phosphodiesterase inhibitors, cause inhibition of protein synthesis in the
human retina (Ulshafer and Hollyfield, 1981). When parallel
autoradiographic studies are conducted on human retinal
material cultured in the presence of phosphodiesterase inhibitors using ^{3}H-leucine as a probe for protein synthesis,
a specific inhibition of incorporation of ^{3}H-leucine by rod
photoreceptors was observed prior to the time when degenerative changes take place in this cell type. This suggests
that elevated cyclic-GMP levels may first alter renewal
processes within the rod photoreceptors and that this change
may be followed later by degeneration and cell death.

    At the present time only the studies on the rd mouse
(Farber and Lolley, 1974) and the Irish setter dog (Aquirre
et al., 1978) implicate altered cyclic nucleotide levels as
causally involved in inherited photoreceptor cell degeneration. Although we do not know whether any of the forms of
Retinitis Pigmentosa in man are associated with altered
cyclic nucleotide metabolism, our studies with the normal
human retina provide direct evidence that rod photoreceptors
in man are sensitive to elevated levels of cyclic nucleotides.
We hope that this model system will provide a useful tool
for evaluating the specific mechanisms of cyclic-GMP toxicity.

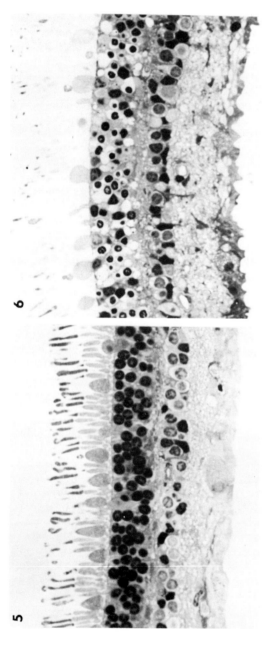

Fig. 5 *Adult human retina maintained in organ culture in control media for 8h. Retinal morphology is normal and no degenerative changes have occurred during this period of time in vitro. (X4000)*

Fig. 6 *Adult human retina maintained in culture for 8h in the presence of 4 mM IBMX. Note extensive degenerative changes in the rod photoreceptors as evidenced by the pyknotic rod nuclei and degenerative changes in rod inner and outer segments. Cone inner segments, though somewhat rounded, show only minor alterations from the normal morphology. For additional details of these studies see Ulshafer et al.,1980. (X4000)*

REFERENCES

Aquirre, G., Farber, D.B., Lolley, R.N., Fletcher, R. and Chader, G. (1978). Rod-cone dysplasia in Irish setters; a defect in cyclic GMP metabolism in visual cells. *Science* **201**, 1133–1134.

Farber, D.B. and Lolley, R.N. (1974). Cyclic guanosine monophosphate: elevation in degenerating photoreceptors cells of the C3H mouse retina. *Science* **186**, 449–451.

Farber, D.B. and Lolley, R.N. (1976). Enzymatic basis for cyclic-GMP accumulation in degenerative photoreceptor cells of mouse retina. *J. Cyclic Nucleotide Res*. **2**, 139–148.

Hollyfield, J.G., Rayborn, M.E., Farber, D.B. and Lolley, R.N. (1981). Selective photoreceptor degeneration during retinal development: the role of altered phosphodiesterase activity and increased levels of cyclic nucleotides. In "Structure of the Eye" (Ed. J. G. Hollyfield), Elsevier-North Holland, pp. 97-114.

Lolley, R.N., Farber, D.B., Rayborn, M.E. and Hollyfield, J.G. (1977). Cyclic GMP accumulation causes degeneration of photoreceptor cells: simulation of an inherited disease. *Science* **196**, 664–666.

Ulshafer, R.J., Garcia, C.A. and Hollyfield, J.G. (1980). Sensitivity of photoreceptors to elevated levels of cGMP in the human retina. *Invest. Ophthalmol. Vis. Sci*. **19**, 1236–1241.

Ulshafer, R.J. and Hollyfield, J.G. (1981). Cyclic nucleotides alter protein synthesis in human and baboon retinas. In "Structure of the Eye" (Ed. J.G. Hollyfield), Elsevier-North Holland, pp. 115-121.

THE INTERPHOTORECEPTOR MATRIX IN RCS RATS: POSSIBLE ROLE IN PHOTORECEPTOR CELL DEATH

MATTHEW M. LAVAIL, DOUGLAS YASUMURA, GREGG GORRIN
and LAWRENCE H. PINTO

*Department of Anatomy, University of California,
San Francisco, School of Medicine,
San Francisco, CA 94143, USA*

SUMMARY

The retinas both of RCS rats with inherited retinal dystrophy and normal control rats have been examined histochemically. Abnormalities in the distribution of the
stainable interphotoreceptor matrix precede photoreceptor
cell loss by 6 to 8 days and may be, at least in part,
responsible for the death of the photoreceptor cells.

Photoreceptor outer segments are surrounded by a complex
mixture of proteoglycans and glycoproteins (Berman and Bach,
1968; Bach and Berman, 1970, 1971a, 1971b) known as the
interphotoreceptor matrix (IPM) (Rohlich, 1970). Several
roles for the IPM have been suggested, including optical
refraction, retinal adhesion to the pigment epithelium (PE),
cell (or outer segment) recognition for phagocytosis, and
facilitation of diffusion of metabolites and vitamin A
between the PE and photoreceptor cells. (Sidman, 1958;
Zimmerman and Eastham, 1959; Zimmerman, 1961; Zauberman and
Berman, 1969; Hall and Heller, 1969; Feeney, 1973a, 1973b).
This wide range of functions implicates the IPM in the
maintenance of the normal physiological state of photoreceptor cells and their interactions with the PE.

If the IPM plays a key role in normal photoreceptor physiology, it seems important to examine the IPM in those
disease states in which photoreceptors degenerate. In the
case of inherited retinal degenerations, remarkably little
is known about the IPM. Despite the occurrence of inherited

retinal degenerations in many laboratory animal populations
and man, the IPM has been examined in only two mutants.
In the mouse with retinal degeneration, gene symbol *rd*,
Zimmerman and Eastham (1959) found histochemically that the
prominently staining IPM adjacent to the apical surface of
the PE appears normal in the developing mutant and remains
unaltered even after photoreceptor degeneration is well
underway. Therefore, in the *rd* mouse the IPM probably does
not play a role in photoreceptor degneration. In the rat
with inherited retinal dystrophy, *rdy*, however, we (LaVail,
Pinto and Yasumura, 1981) have recently found that the IPM
is evident 6 to 8 days before photoreceptor cell death.
Thus, in this mutant the IPM may well play a role in the
loss of photoreceptors. In this symposium report, we will
briefly review our histochemical findings on the IPM of the
rdy rat retina and will indicate further studies undertakn in
this area.

Retinal dystrophy in the rat is characterized by a grossly
reduced level of outer segment phagocytosis by the PE (Bok
and Hall, 1971; Goldman and O'Brien, 1978), resulting in an
accumulation of outer segment "debris" membranes at the
surface of the PE. During development the build up of
whorls of membrane debris is evident by about postnatal day
12 (P12), when outer segments begin to be synthesized
rapidly. By about P25, the outer segment zone consists of
a relatively normal region of outer segments with a layer
of membrane debris between it and the PE. At older ages,
the outer segment zone becomes almost totally a zone of
debris which remains for several months. Photoreceptor cells
are progressively lost beginning about P20 and continuing
until about P60, when most have degenerated and disappeared.

Using three histochemical stains for mucosubstances in
the IPM, Alcian blue, metachromatic staining with toluidine
blue and the colloidal iron reaction, we found consistent
differences in the distribution of stainable IPM in mutant
(RCS strain) and normal (RCS-*rdy*+ strain) retinas as early
as P12 in the posterior regions of the retinas. (For details
of procedure and specificity of histochemical stains, see
LaVail, Pinto and Yasumura, 1981). In normal retinas
beginning on P12 and at all ages thereafter, an intense
band of IPM staining occurs at the apical surface of the
PE, with less intense staining between the outer segments
throughout the outer segment zone (Figs 1A, 2A and 3A).

By contrast, in the dystrophic retinas the intense band
of IPM staining is incompletely formed at the apical surface
of the PE at P12. As whorls of debris accumulate, IPM staining almost disappears along the PE cell surface and in the
debris zone (Figs 1B, 2B and 3B). In addition, the basal

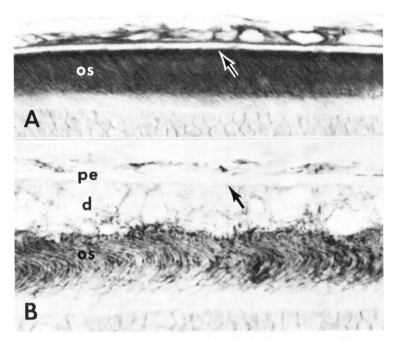

Fig. 1 *Light micrographs of colloidal iron-stained retinas*
from normal RCS-rdy+ (A) and dystrophic RCS (B) rats at P24.
In the normal retina (A), the highest concentration of
stained IPM is at the apical surface of the PE (arrow), but
stained IPM is present throughout the outer segment (os)
zone. In the dystrophic retina (B), the colloidal iron
reaction product surrounds the relatively intact outer
segments (os), but it appears to be mostly excluded from
the debris zone (d), and little is present at the apical
surface of the PE (arrow). pe: pigment epithelium. 10 um
polyester wax. Uncounterstrained. X965. (From Lavail et al.,
1981, with permission from Mosby Press).

outer segment region stains much more heavily in dystrophic
retinas than in normal retinas (Fig. 2B and 3B), a feature
which presumably represents an abnormal accumulation of IPM
in this region of mutant retinas.

An interpretation of our histochemical findings with
respect to the role of the IPM in the photoreceptor degeneration is that the abnormal IPM distribution alters
normal diffusional processes, which then results in photoreceptor cell death. Proteoglycans such as those present
in the IPM may influence the diffusional properties of

ionic and possibly non-ionic species (Preston and Snowden, 1972). Therefore, the exclusion of the IPM from the debris zone might act as a physiological diffusion barrier to metabolites originally destined to reach the photoreceptor cells from the choriocapillaris. Alternatively or additionally, the abnormal accumulation of IPM in the basal

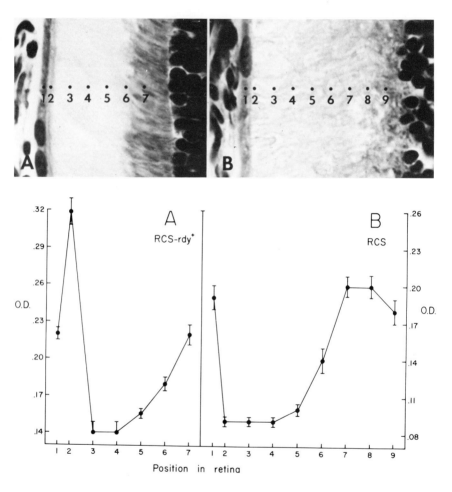

(For legends, see opposite).

outer segment region may affect metabolite diffusion.

A potentially important correlation exists between the development of PE function and temporal sequence of IPM changes. The intense band of IPM staining at the apical surface of the PE appears about P12 in the normal retina. This is the same age when outer segment disc shedding and phagocytosis by the PE begin in the developing rat retina (Tamai and Chader, 1979). If the IPM in this region is necessary for phagocytosis, then the diminished concentration of IPM in this region of the mutant retina might explain the grossly reduced level of phagocytosis in the rat.

Several questions remained unanswered in our initial histochemical study. One was the issue of subcellular localization of the staining. What is represented by the band of intense IPM staining at the apical PE surface in the normal and its absence in the mutant retinas? What is the subcellular localizaton of the intense IPM staining in the basal outer segment region in the mutant retina? We have begun to answer these questions by ultrastructural cytochemistry and stereological analysis. Although our

Fig. 2 *Light micrographs of toluidine blue-stained sections of RCS-rdy[+] (A) and RCS (B) rat retinas at P26. The numbered points correspond to the positions indicated in the microphotometric readings shown in Fig. 3. The magnifiction has been set so that the points show not only the positions measured, but also the area covered by the aperture in the microscope photometer. In the normal retina (A), an intense band of metachromatic staining is present at the apical surface of the PE (position number 2), whereas the band of staining is absent from the mutant retina (B, position number 2).*

Fig. 3 *Microphotometric readings of absorbance (exressed in standard optical density OD units) at 485 nm taken from single retinal sections similar to those in Fig. 2. In the normal retina (A), the highest absorbance is that of the band of pink metachromatic staining (position 2); the outer segment zone (position 3-5) shows the lowest absorbance. In the dystrophic retina (B), the position corresponding to the apical band at the surface of the PE (position 2) has the lowest absorbance and equals that of the outer half of the outer segment zone (positions 3-5); the absorbance is highest in the basal half of the outer segment zone (positions 6-8), suggesting an accumulation of IPM there. For further details see Fig. 16 in LaVail et al., 1981. (From LaVail et al., 1981, with permission from Mosby Press.)*

findings are only preliminary, we have observed one here-
tofore unrecognized feature of the dystrophic rat retina
that may, at least in part, explain the intense IPM staining in the basal outer segment region. In this zone, including the inner segment-outer segment junctional region,
the extracellular space is much more abundant in the mutant
than in the normal retina (Figs 4A and 4B), and this space
presumably is filled with IPM. Consistent with the visual
impression in Figs 4A and 4B, our preliminary stereological
data indicate that in the normal P23 retina the extracellular space in this basal zone only occupies about 4 to
6% of the total cross-sectional area (areal density), with
inner and outer segments making up the remainder. In the
rdy retina at P23, however, the areal density of the extracellular space is about 14 to 18%.

   Another issue is the cause of the greatly diminished
band of IPM staining at the apical PE cell surface in the
mutant. Since the IPM is synthesized, at least in part, by
the PE (Berman, 1964; Rohlich, 1970; Feeney, 1973*a*), could
the weak staining be due to a decreased rate of IPM synthesis by the PE? We have begun to explore this problem
by autoradiographic analysis following *in vitro* incubation
of the PE in tissue culture medium containing ^{35}S-sulphate.
Preliminary data based on silver grain counts in autoradiograms show that both the mutant and normal PE in-
corporate the isotope. Moreover, the mutant PE appears

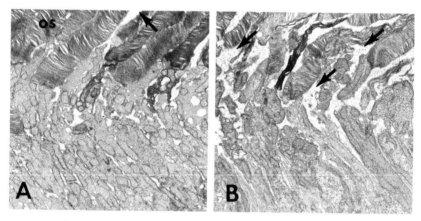

Fig. 4 *Electron micrographs of retinas from normal RCS-rdy^{+}*
(A) and dystrophic RCS (B) rats at P23. The extracellular
space (arrows) near the base of the outer segments (os) is
greater in the mutant (B) than in the normal (A) retina.
(X4975)

less heavily labelled than the normal PE, but these data are
derived from only a single incorporation (incubation) time
and, therefore, should be taken only as an indication of a
promising approach to the problem.

We presently are also perfecting histochemical stains
for tissues previously embedded in epoxy resins. When
these are available, they will provide a means of examining
many important and valuable tissues, such as retinas from
rat chimeras (Mullen and LaVail, 1976), other retinal
degenerations in laboratory animals and from patients with
Retinitis Pigmentosa. Our goals are to provide further insight into the cellular mechanisms in retinal dystrophy, in
the case of the rat chimeras, and to determine whether any
other forms of inherited retinal degeneration show abnormalities of the IPM similar to that seen in the *rdy* rat.

ACKNOWLEDGEMENTS

We thank Nancy Lawson for maintenance of the animal colony,
Jack Essig for secretarial assistance, and Carson Optical
Co. for the use of a Zeiss microscope photometer. This in-
vestigation was supported in part by USPHS Research Grants
EY-01919 (MML) and EY-02536 (LHP) and by Core Grant EY-
02162 from the National Eye Institute.

REFERENCES

Bach, G. and Berman, E.R. (1970). Characterization of a
    sialoglycan isolated from cattle retina. *Ophthal. Res.*
    1, 257–272.
Bach, G. and Berman, E.R. (1971*a*). Amino sugar-containing
    compounds of the retina. I. Isolation and identification.
    Biochim. Biophys. Acta **252**, 453–461.
Bach, G. and Berman, E.R. (1971*b*). Amino sugar-containing
    compounds of the retina. II. Structural studies.
    Biochim. Biophys. Acta **252**, 461–471.
Berman, E.R. (1964). The biosynthesis of mucopolysaccharides
    and glycoproteins in pigment epithelial cells of bovine
    retina. *Biochim. Biophys. Acta* **83**, 371–373.
Berman, E.R. and Bach, G. (1968). The acid mucopolysac-
    charides of cattle retina. *Biochem. J.* **108**, 75–88.
Bok, D. and Hall, M.O. (1971). The role of the pigment
    epithelium in the etiology of inherited retinal dystrophy
    in the rat. *J. Cell Biol.* **49**, 664–682.
Feeney, L. (1973*a*). Synthesis of interphotoreceptor matrix.
    I. Autoradiography of H-fucose incorporation. *Invest.
    Ophthalmol.* **12**, 739–751.

Feeney, L. (1973*b*). The interphotoreceptor space. II. Histochemistry of the matrix. *Devel. Biol.* **32**, 115-128.

Goldman, A.I. and O'Brien, P.J. (1978). Phagocytosis in the retinal pigment epithelium of the RCS rat. *Science* **201**, 1023–1025.

Hall, M.O. and Heller, J. (1969). Mucopolysaccharides of the retina. In "The Retina" (Eds. B.R. Straatsma, M.O. Hall, R.A. Allen and F. Crescitelli), pp. 211-224, University of California Press, Los Angeles, California.

LaVail, M. (1981). Analysis of neurological mutants with inherited retinal degeneration. *Invest. Ophthalmol. Vis. Sci.* **21**, 638-657.

LaVail, M., Pinto, L. and Yasumura, D. (1981). The interphotoreceptor matrix in rats with inherited retinal dystrophy. *Invest. Ophthalmol. Vis. Sci.* **21**, 658-668.

Mullen, R.J. and LaVail, M.M. (1976). Inherited retinal dystrophy: primary defect in pigment epithelium determined with experimental rat chimeras. *Science* **192**, 799–801.

Preston, B.N. and Snowden, J.M. (1972). Model connective tissue systems: the effect of proteoglycans on the diffusional behavior of small non-electrolyes and microions. *Biopolymers* **11**, 1627–1643.

Rohlich, P. (1970). The interphotoreceptor matrix: electron microscopic and histochemical observations on the vertebrate retina. *Exp. Eye Res.* **10**, 80–96.

Sidman, R.L. (1958). Histochemical studies on photoreceptor cells. *Ann. New York Acad. Sci.* **74**, 182–195.

Tamai, M. and Chader, G.J. (1979). The early appearance of disc shedding in the rat retina. *Invest. Ophthalmol. Vis. Sci.* **18**, 913–917.

Zauberman, H. and Berman, E.R. (1969). Measurement of adhesive forces between the sensory retina and the pigment epithelium. *Exp. Eye Res.* **8**, 276–283.

Zimmerman, L.E. (1961). Acid mucopolysaccharides in ocular histology and pathology. *Proc. Inst. Med. Chicago*, **23**, 267-277.

Zimmerman, L.E. and Eastham, A.B. (1959). Acid mucopolysaccharide in the retinal pigment epithelium and visual cell layer of the developing mouse eye. *Am. J. Ophthal.* *47 (Part II)*, 488–499.

A SURVEY OF CYTOMORPHOLOGICAL CHANGES DURING EXPRESSION OF THE RETINAL DEGENERATION (rd) GENE IN THE MOUSE

SOMES SANYAL

Department of Anatomy, Erasmus University, Medical Faculty, Postbox 1738, 3000 DR Rotterdam, The Netherlands

SUMMARY

A review of the developmental anomalies in the retina of the rd mutant mice suggests that the gene acts within the visual cells starting from the time when the presumptive visual cells are still proliferating. Early effects are seen in slow in- crease of visual cells, retarded differentiation at the receptor and the synaptic ends, and delayed segretation of the perikarya. Lytic changes start with the Golgi vesicles, soon affect the entire cell, and result in nuclear pycnosis. This is followed by invasion of macrophages which phagocytose the dying nuclei and rapidly reduce the outer nuclear layer. Factors which retard or inhibit growth of the outer segments slow down the rate of degeneration. It is speculated that the genetic defect is such that the cells can undergo retarded development till the initiation of functional dif- ferentiation when the factor becomes lethal for the whole visual cell.

INTRODUCTION

Brückner (1951) reported a trait in mice causing anomalous vision which was histologically identified as due to selective loss of visual cells following their initial development (Tansley, 1951; Karli, 1952; Sorsby *et al.*, 1954). The gene, since called retinal degeneration, symbol rd, is an auto- somal recessive gene located in chromosome 5, and has been shown to be present in many inbred strains (Sidman and Green, 1965). A wealth of information on structural changes during the development and degeneration of retina of rd mutant mice

has now accumulated. This short survey will relate the structural changes within the visual cells to the sequence of their
appearance during the time course of development and degeneration of the mutant retina with the aim of reviwing the morphological basis of the phaenogenesis of the *rd* gene.

RESULTS

*Early Embryogenesis and Proliferation of Presumptive
Visual Cells*

Since the retina in the newborn mutant mouse is indistinguishable from the normal, it is generally inferred that early
embryogenesis of the eye in these mutants also follows the
normal pattern. Occasional mention is made in the literature
that fewer mitoses are observed in the mutant retina. The
autoradiographic data of Blanks and Bok (1977) have revealed
no differences in the mitotic rate of bipolar and Müller
cell precursors between mutant and normal after birth.
Similar data about visual cell precursors are not available.
The observed preponderance of normal cells in the visual cell
layer of $rdrd \leftrightarrow ++$ chimaeras (Mintz and Sanyal, 1970; LaVail
and Mullen, 1976; Sanyal and Zeilmaker, 1976) could result
from a difference in growth rate between cells of the two
genotypes. This question has been examined by Sanyal and
Zeilmaker (1976) who observed that in a group of chimaeras
animals with chimaeric distribution in the retinal pigment
epithelium with a fully normal neural retina occurred but
that there was no animal showing the reverse pattern of distribution and they suggested that cell selection during the
extended period of mitosis in the neural retina was a likely
cause. Since similar types and proportions of chimaeric
distribution were also observed in a comparable group of
chimaeras derived from congenic mice with reversed allelic
composition at the *rd* locus, differences in background genes
between the strains as a factor could be eliminated, leading
to the conclusion that the *rd* gene specifically affects the
proliferation rate of the visual cell precursors. It will
be interesting to know if this is due to a general slowing
down of cellular activity or to a specific change in any
particular phase of the cell cycle.

Differentiation of Visual Cells

Morphological differentiation of the visual cells is highly
asynchronous; while some cells become post-mitotic (Sidman,
1961) and show signs of development at the receptor end

(Bhattacharjee, 1977) many cells continue to divide. In the retina of the newborn, rudiments of receptor inner segments have developed and appear identical in both normal and mutant mice. As the inner segments grow in length a clear difference between the normal and the mutant could be detected as early as 4 days after birth (Sanyal and Bal, 1973). From this stage on, retarded growth of the inner segments (Figs 1 and 2), and reduced and disorganized outer segment production remain a consistent feature of the visual cells in the retina (Karli *et al.*, 1965; Caley *et al.*, 1972; Sanyal and Bal, 1973). At the same time, segregation of the visual cell perikarya into the outer nuclear layer by outward migration (Figs 4, 5 and 6) is also delayed in the mutant retina (Sanyal and Bal, 1973). At the synaptic end of the cell, Blanks *et al.* (1974) have shown that while dyad con- figurations resulting from contacts between horizontal and receptor cell terminals occur in the normal way, triad con- figurations resulting from further contact with bipolar cell dendrites fail to develop in the mutant retina. Therefore, in the 3 different aspects of differentiation in which effective comparison can be made between the mutant and the normal, that is, receptor growth, perikaryal migration and synapto- genesis, the visual cells in the *rd* mutant show clearly discern- ible deviation prior to the appearance of the degenerative changes. Since most of the above differences could be ob- served between congenic littermate individuals the effects must be ascribed to the specific activity of the *rd* gene.

Degeneration of Visual Cells

The first indication of degeneration has been observed in the appearance of vesicular structures and mitochondrial lysis within the developing inner segments (Lasansky and de Robertis, 1960). Such inner segments occur sporadically from the age of 7 days (Fig. 3) and as their frequency increases lytic changes appear throughout the visual cells. An early indication of such changes has been observed in the appearance of perinuclear activity of the lysosomal enzyme acid phosphatase (Sanyal, 1970) as early as 8 days and frequently at 10 days (Fig. 7) preceding the appearance of pycnotic nuclei. At about the same time lytic changes are also recorded in the synaptic terminal (Lasansky and de Robertis, 1960; Blanks *et al.*, 1974). The appearance of pycnotic nuclei in the outer nuclear layer is followed by migration of macrophages into this layer (Fig. 8) which actively ingest the dying visual cell nuclei and digest them *in situ* (Fig. 9). The origin and transformation of the macrophages have been described in detail (Sanyal, 1972)

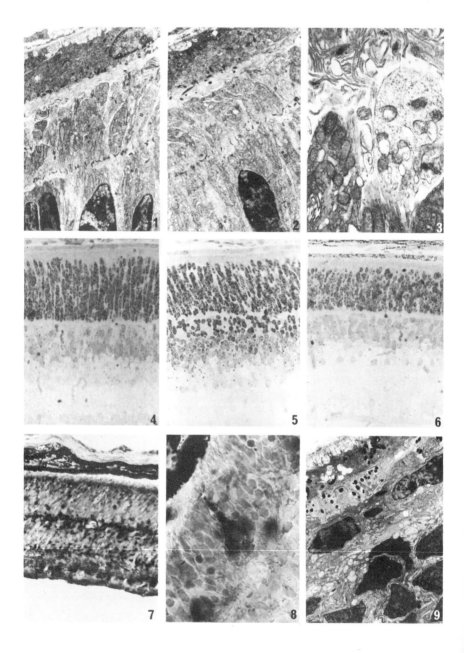

(For legends, see opposite).

Fig. 1 *Electron micrograph of the developing receptor layer from the retina of 8 day old normal Balb/c mouse. The inner segments are well developed with accumulation of mitochondria, Golgi elements and ciliary structures. Outer segments have also started to appear.*

Fig. 2 *Similar picture as in Fig. 1 from a congenic littermate mouse which is homozygous for* rd *gene. Inner segments are retarded in length.*

Fig. 3 *Electron micrograph from 7 day old mutant retina of C3H mouse showing a degenerating inner segment with vacuoles and mitochondrial lysis next to a normal appearing inner segment.*

Fig. 4 *Light micrograph of retina from 8 day old normal Balb/c mouse. Note complete separation of outer and inner nuclear layer.*

Fig. 5 *Light micrograph from a congenic littermate homozygous* rd *mouse showing presence of visual cell perikarya at the inner side of the outer plexiform layer due to slower perikaryal migration.*

Fig. 6 *Mutant retina from C3H mouse at 10 days showing progress of development.*

Fig. 7 *Cryostat section of mutant retina from C3H mouse at 10 days stained for (α-naphthyl) acid phosphatase activity. Note enzyme positive granules near the outer limiting membrane and scattered nuclei showing perinuclear enzyme activity.*

Fig. 8 *Cryostat section of retina from 12 day old C3H mouse stained for N-Acetyl-β-glucosaminidase activity showing a large macrophage cell which has ingested several visual cell perikarya.*

Fig. 9 *Electron micrograph of mutant retina from C3H mouse at 26 days. Outer nuclear layer is reduced to a single row. Note extensive growth of pigment epithelial villous processes and accumulation of Müller cell fibres.*

and appear to be an important factor in the rapid reduction
of the outer nuclear layer. In the absence of any focal
lesion the degenerated cells appear singly and scattered.
This has been taken to imply that the immediate cause of death
resides within individual visual cells. A central to peripheral progression of cell loss has been observed (Noell,
1958) and considered to be the result of a similar direction
in the progression of differentiation of the visual cells,
as well as of general retinal development. Recent observations of Carter-Dawson *et al.* (1978) show that the *rd* gene
has a differential effect on rod cells which, as a result,
degenerate rapidly in comparison to the cone cells which
survive much longer in the central, and even more so in the
peripheral, retina. This also illustrates strikingly how the
initiation and rate of degeneration may be related to factors
within the visual cells.

Changes at Other Retinal Sites

In *rd* mutant mice actual loss of cells is restricted to the
visual cell layer. The possibility that some cells of the
inner nuclear layer, particularly some of the bipolar cells,
also degenerate has been considered and discounted (Blanks
and Bok, 1977). However, distinct structural changes have
been reported at several retinal sites. As with changes
within the visual cells, changes at other sites have been
observed before, during and after the beginning of the degenerative events. Changes which appear early, such as
delayed transformation from rough to smooth endoplasmic
reticulum in the pigment epithelium (Caley *et al.*, 1972) and
structural changes within the Müller cell fibres (Shiose and
Sonohara, 1968), have not been observed in studies using congenic littermate animals of other strains (Sanyal and Bal,
1973; Robb, 1974). The appearance of phagosomes in the pigment epithelium (Sanyal and Bal, 1973) and the observed in-
clusion of cell debris in the cytoplasmic processes of Müller
cells (Blanks *et al.*, 1974) coincide with the period of cell
loss and indicate some additional role of these elements, together with the macrophages, in the scavenging operation.
These, as well as other changes at various retinal sites at
still later stages, reported in several studies, can be considered as secondary, and presumably consequential, to the
loss of visual cells.

Factors Affecting Rate of Degeneration

DiPaolo and Noell (1962) observed that visual cell degeneration was "very rigidly determined, and little modified by

other genetic factors". Very similar rates of degeneration
have indeed been observed in different studies using albino
and pigmented strains of mice with varying genetic backgrounds.
(Caley *et al*., 1972; Sanyal and Bal, 1973; LaVail and Sidman,
1974). It is known that nutritional and growth factors,
especially the ones which retard or accelerate receptor cell
differentiation, likewise affect the rate of degeneration
(Lucas and Newhouse, 1957). Recently it has been reported
(Sanyal and Hawkins, 1981) that a new gene called retinal
degeneration slow (*rds*), which completely prevents development of rod outer segments and causes very slow degeneration
of visual cells, if combined with *rd* (i.e., in animals which
are homozygous for both *rd* and *rds*), significantly retards
the progression of degeneration due to the *rd* gene. Thus
it appears that, though degeneration is rigidly determined,
the rate of cell loss is somehow related to acquisition of
functional differentiation.

CONCLUSIONS

While the degenerative changes in the visual cells of the *rd*
mutant mice and their immediate cause have been the subject
of many studies, changes observed during the differentiation
of the visual cells and preceding the actual process of
degeneration have remained largely unnoticed or ignored.
However, if one looks at the visual cells in the *rd* mutant
mice through their entire developmental course it becomes
clear that manifestation of the gene is detectable in
retarded growth and differentiation before the appearance of
the lytic changes leading to cell death. These findings are
compatible with the view that the *rd* gene is expressed very
early in development but that the cells can survive and
develop in a defective way to a certain stage of differentiation at which time the genetic factor becomes lethal for the
whole visual cell. Attempts to identify the nature of action
of the *rd* gene at the subcellular level will have to take
both of these aspects of cytomorphological changes into
consideration.

REFERENCES

Bhattacharjee, J. (1977). Sequential differentiation of retinal
    cells in the mouse studied by diaphorase staining. *J.
    Anat*. **123**, 273-282.
Blanks, J.C., Adinolfi, A.M. and Lolley, R.N. (1974). Photo-
    receptor degeneration and synaptogenesis in retinal-

degenerative (*rd*) mice. *J. Comp. Neur*. **174**, 95–106.

Blanks, J.C. and Bok, D. (1977). An autoradiographic analysis of postnatal cell proliferation in the normal and degenerative mouse retina. *J. Comp. Neur*. **156**, 317–328.

Bruckner, R. (1951). Spaltlampenmikroskopie und Ophthalmoskopie am Auge von Ratte und *Maus*. *Doc. Ophthalmol*. **5-6**, 452.

Caley, D.W., Johnson, C. and Liebelt, R.A. (1972). The postnatal development of the retina in the normal and rodless CBA mouse: a light and electron microscopic study. *Am. J. Anat*. **133**, 179–212.

Carter-Dawson, L.D., LaVail, M.M. and Sidman, R.L. (1978). Differential effect of the *rd* mutation on rods and cones in the mouse retina. *Invest. Ophthalmol. Vis. Sci*. **17**, 489–498.

Dipaolo, J.A. and Noell, W.K. (1962). Some genetic aspects of visual cell degeneration in mice. *Exp. Eye Res*. **1**, 215–220.

Karli, P. (1952). Rétines sans cellules visuelles. Recherches morphologiques, psychologiques et physio-pathologiques chez les rongeurs. *Arch. Anat. Hist. Embry*. **35**, 1–76.

Karli, P., Stoeckel, M.D. and Porte, A. (1965). Dégénérescence des cellules visuelles photo-réceptrices et persistence d'un sensibilité de la rétine à la stimulation photique. Observations au microscopie electronique. *Z. Zellforsch. Mikrosk. Anat*. **65**, 238–252.

Lasansky, A. and de Robertis, E. (1960). Submicroscopic analysis of the genetic dystrophy of visual cells in C3H mice. *J. Biophys. Biochem. Cytol*. **7**, 679–83.

LaVail, M.M. and Mullen, R.J. (1976). Role of the pigment epithelium in inherited retinal degeneration analyzed with experimental mouse chimeras. *Exp. Eye Res*. **23**, 227–45.

LaVail, M.M. and Sidman, R.L. (1974). C57BL/6J mice with inherited retinal degeneration. *Arch. Ophthalmol*. **91**, 394–400.

Lucas, D.R. and Newhouse, J.P. (1957). The effects of nutritional and endocrine factors on an inherited retinal degeneration in the mouse. *Arch. Ophthalmol*. **57**, 224–35.

Mintz, B. and Sanyal, S. (1970). Clonal origin of the mouse visual retina mapped from genetically mosaic eyes. *Genetics 64 (Suppl.)* 43–44.

Noell, W.K. (1958). Studies on visual cell viability and differentiation. *Ann. N.Y. Acad. Sci*. **74**, 337–61.

Robb, R.M. (1974). Electron microscopic histochemical studies of cyclic 3', 5'-nucleotide phosphodiesterase in the developing retina of normal mice and mice with hereditary retinal degeneration. *Tr. Am. Ophth. Soc*. **72**, 650–69.

Sanyal, S. (1970). Changes of lysomal enzymes during hereditary degeneration and histogenesis of retina in mice. I. Acid phosphatase visualized by azo-dye and lead nitrate methods. *Histochemie* **23**, 207-19.

Sanyal, S. (1972). Changes of lysosomal enzymes during hereditary degeneration and histogenesis of retina in mice. II. Localization of N-Acetyl-β-glucosaminidase in macrophages. *Histochemie*, **29**, 28-36.

Sanyal, S. and Bal, A.K. (1973). Comparative light and electron microscopic study of retinal histogenesis in normal and *rd* mutant mice. *Z. Anat. Entwickl.-Gesch.* **142**, 219-38.

Sanyal, S. and Hawkins, R.K. (1981). Genetic interaction in the retinal degeneration of mice. *Exp. Eye Res.* **33**, 213-22.

Sanyal, S. and Zeilmaker, G.H. (1976). Comparative analysis of cell distribution in the pigment epithelium and the visual cell layer of chimaeric mice. *J. Embryol. Exp. Morph.* **36**, 425-30.

Shiose, Y. and Sonohara, O. (1968). Studies on retinitis pigmentosa. XXVI. Electron microscopic aspects of early retinal changes in inherited dystrophic mice. *Acta Soc. Ophthalmol. Jap.* **72**, 1127.

Sidman, R.L. (1961). Histogenesis of mouse retina studied with thymidine-H . In "The Structure of the Eye" (Ed. G.K. Smelser) pp. 487-505. Academic Press, New York.

Sidman, R.L. and Green, M.C. (1965). Retinal degeneration in the mouse; location of the *rd* locus in linkage group XVII. *J. Heredity* **56**, 23-29.

Sorsby, A., Koller, P.C., Attfield, M., Davey, J.B. and Lucas, D.R. (1954). Retinal dystrophy in the mouse: histological and genetic aspects. *J. Exp. Zool.* **125**, 171-98.

Tansley, K. (1951). Hereditary degeneration of the mouse retina. *Br. J. Ophthalmol.* **35**, 573-82.

EARLY DEVELOPMENT OF A NEW RP-LIKE MUTANT IN THE CHICK

M.A. WILSON, B.J. POLLOCK, R.M. CLAYTON and [+]C.J. RANDALL

*Department of Genetics, West Mains Road
Edinburgh EH9 3JN, UK*

[+]*Ministry of Agriculture, Veterinary Laboratory,
Eskgrove, Lasswade, Midlothian, UK.*

Blindness in a strain of commercial laying fowl was described by Randall and McLachlan (1979). At hatching the affected chicks are generally less active than normally sighted birds, but quickly adapt to their surroundings. The affected birds appeared to have some vision initially, but the majority made no response to visual stimuli by 6 months of age. The condition behaves like a single recessive mutant (Pollock and Randall, unpubl.). We propose that the mutant be referred to as *rdd*: partial retina dysplasia and degeneration. Preliminary observations of histological sections from older embryos and hatched chicks revealed abnormalities in the retina extending from the pigment epithelium (PE) to the inner nuclear layer. A more extensive examination of histological sections has now been undertaken including earlier embryological stages.

Eyes from embryos and hatched chicks were processed for plastic embedding by immersion in Karnovsky's fixative at pH 7.3 (Karnovsky 1965). After a buffer wash the eyes were postfixed in 1% osmium tetroxide, dehydrated in a graded series of alcohols and embedded in araldite. Sections were cut at 1μm on a Porter Blum MtI ultramicrotome and stained with toluidine blue.

Abnormalities in the PE layer were observed as early as 8 days of incubation. Holes in this layer occurred on either side of the chloroid fissure and were just visible to the naked eye and clearly seen in the dissecting microscope (Figs 1a and 1b). In sections of 11 day embryos, discontinuities were observed in the PE layer. Gaps due to a lack of pigment cells were of varying size. EM shows

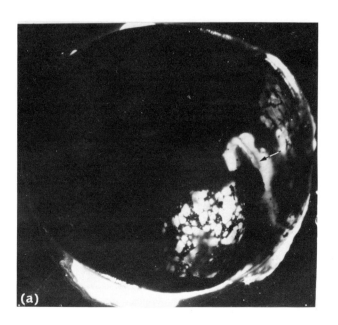

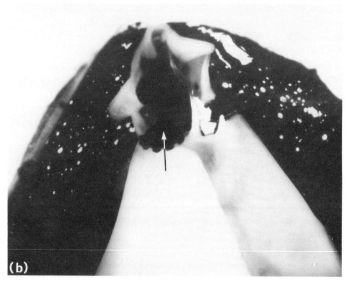

Fig. 1 *Posterior portion of the* rdd *globe with vitreous removed. Note holes on either side of the pecten region. (a) 1 day chick, neural retina removed. Arrow denotes site of the removed pecten. (b) 18 day embryo, neural retina deflected. Arrow denotes pecten.*

that the external basement membrane of the PE remains intact
(Wilson, unpubl. obsv.). In these regions the outer limiting
membrane (LM) generally deviated up to make contact with
the basal regions of the PE cells adjacent to the holes.
The holes were filled with closely packed precursor receptor cells (Fig. 2b). Undulations in the outer plexiform
layer and upper half of the inner nuclear layer were very
obvious in the regions under the holes. Degenerating cells
were seen in the lower half of the inner nuclear layer and
occasionally in the ganglion cell layer (Fig. 2b). The
internal plexiform layer appeared to be normal at the light
microscope level.

In histological sections of 16 day embryos, the holes
in the PE were more obvious macroscopically than in 11 day
embryos. The holes, measuring up to 1mm in diameter, were
evenly distributed on each side of the developing pecten.
The area immediately beneath the holes contained fewer
cells than were apparent at the 11 day embryo stage. These
cells were set in a vacuolated matrix (Fig. 2c). Generally,
the cells immediately in the gap stained more lightly than
the photoreceptor precursors which were found immediately
below the vacuolated area and protruded downwards partly
displacing the inner nuclear layer. The OLM was usually
absent under the gap in the PE (Figs 3a and 3b). In some
areas of continuous PE, there were discontinuities in the
OLM which coincided with a decrease in thickness of the
photoreceptor cells. At these foci there was a slight
protrusion of the outer plexiform layer and a vacuolated
appearance immediately beneath the PE (Fig. 2d). Degenerating
cells were found in the ganglion cell layer and the inner
nuclear layer. The inner plexiform layer appeared to be
normal at this stage.

In 4 day old hatched chicks, very obvious holes were
again seen in some of the chicks. However, in other chicks
there were no obvious holes, and no such holes were seen in
older birds which also showed progressive photoreceptor
degeneration, increasing undulations of the outer plexiform
and inner nuclear layers, and some clumping of pigment
(Randall *et al*., in prep.) In older birds the outer nuclear
layer (ONL) becomes progressively thinner and photoreceptor
degeneration progresses until it is virtually complete.
The outer plexiform layer (OPL) and OLM become progressively
more buckled. The average depth of the retina was much
reduced compared to normal retinas, owing to loss of cells
from the inner nuclear layer and the disoriented arrangement
of a reduced number of photoreceptors. (Figs 3c and 3d).
There were few recognizable inner and outer segments. Very

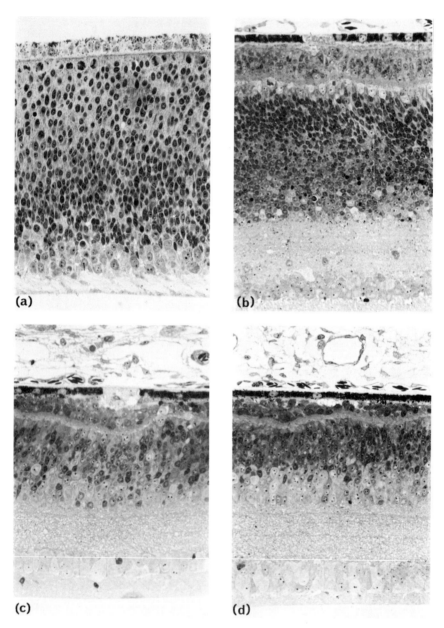

Fig. 2 *Histological sections of the* rdd *mutant retina.*
(a) 8 day embryo. (b) 11 day embryo. (c) and (d) 16 day
embryos.

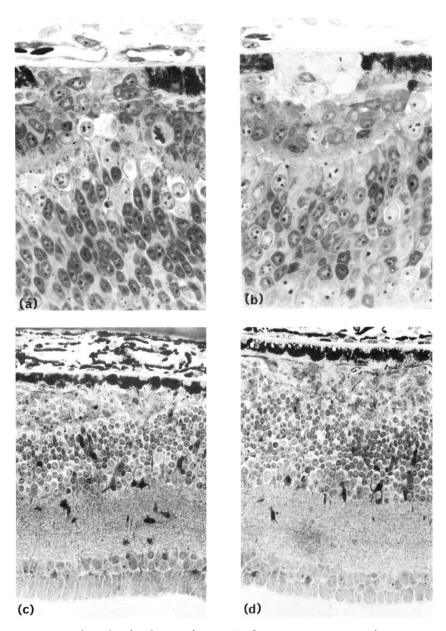

Fig. 3 *Histological sections of the* rdd *mutant retina.*
(a) and (b) 16 day embryos. (c) and (d) 4 day chick.

occasionally, pigment granules were found in the inner nuclear layer. This layer had a "lacy" appearance due to loss of cells and the diffuse appearance of the cytoplasm in the remaining cells.

The aetiology of these histological abnormalities is as yet unknown. Cell culture experiments using neural retina from mutant embryos revealed that retinal degeneration is programmed in the NR cells (Kondoh *et al*., 1980). Death of a proportion of NR cells was found to occur on the 13th day of culture from 3.5 day embryos, on the 10th day from 6 day embryo cultures and after 5 to 6 days in cultures for 8 day embryos, suggesting that some cell death is programmed and tends to follow the same course *in vitro* as *in vivo*. We have observed that in NR cultures of 7 day mutant embryos, the growth rate falls by about 30% after approximately 30 days in culture, compared to controls (Pollock, unpubl. obsv.). Dying cells are apparent in the cultures and many are localized in regions of PE foci which arose from the trans-differentiation of NR cells, suggesting a relationship between pigmented and neuronal cells possibly related to the correspondence between them seen *in vivo*. The appearance of holes in the PE in embryonic life and in the hatched chick and the later disappearance of such obvious features requires explanation. The PE cell population appears to be heterogeneous *in vivo*: clearly some PE cells in particular locations degenerate and the holes might represent either local areas of degeneration, or represent areas normally filled by the progeny of such cells. The disappearance of holes post-hatch suggests that PE cells on their margins are able to divide and colonize these areas. These changes are now being examined further.

Results of electroretinograms performed on week old mutant chicks when vision is poor but not yet lost indicate that the degeneration of the retina is well advanced at this stage. The sensitivity of the rods and cones is greatly diminished compared to control chicks, (G. Arden, unpubl.). The visual acuity of the birds has been measured using low and high frequency grids in standard visual acuity tests. The activity of the mutant birds at this age was lower compared to controls and fell sharply in the high frequency grid tests using decreasing light intensity. (T. Bower, unpubl.).

Blindness in strains of chickens has been reported previously (Hutt, 1935; Smyth *et al*., 1977; Cheng *et al*., 1978; Pollock *et al*., this volume). As far as we can ascertain this is the first chick mutant to undergo a progressive loss of vision similar to the human Retinitis Pigmentosa diseases. Electron microscopy and further cell culture studies are in progress.

ACKNOWLEDGEMENTS

We thank J. Nicol and E. Leitch for their technical assistance, F. Johnston for photography, and J. Bard and A. Ross for making available their facilities at the Western General Hospital, Edinburgh. This work was supported by the Medical Research Council.

REFERENCES

Cheng, K.M., Shoffner, R.N., Gum, G.G., and Gelatt, K.N. (1978). An induced retinal mutation (*rc*) in the chicken. (Abstract). *Poultry Sci.* **57**, 1127.

Hutt, F.B. (1935). Hereditary blindness in the fowl. *Poultry Sci.* **14**, 297.

Karnovsky, M.J. (1965). A formaldehyde-glutaraldehyde fixative of high osmolarity for use in electron microscopy. *J. Cell Biol.* **27**, 137A-138A.

Kondoh, H., Okada, T.S., Randall, C., Brodie, J., Zehir, A. and Clayton, R.M. (1980). Intrinsic programming of neural retina degeneration in a mutant chick. Abstracts of the annual meeting of the Japanese Society of Developmental Biologists.

Pollock, B.J., Wilson, M.A., Randall, C.J. and Clayton, R.M. (1982). Preliminary observations of a new blind chick mutant (beg). (this volume.)

Randall, C.J. and McLachlan, I. (1979). Retinopathy in commercial layers. *Vet. Rec.* **105**, 41-42.

Smyth, J.R., Jr., Boissey, R.E. and Gawron, M.F. (1977). An inherited delayed amelanosis with associated blindness in the domestic fowl. (Abstract). *Poultry Sci.* **56**, 1758.

PRELIMINARY OBSERVATIONS OF A NEW BLIND
CHICK MUTANT *(beg)*

B.J. POLLOCK, WILSON, M.A., +C.J. RANDALL and R.M. CLAYTON

*Department of Genetics, University of Edinburgh,
West Mains Road, Edinburgh EH9 3JN, UK*

*+Ministry of Agriculture, Veterinary Laboratory,
Lasswade, Midlothian, UK*

Preliminary studies have been made of a gene causing blindness found in a commercial strain of white feathered, brown
egg-laying chickens. The affected birds are blind at hatch
and the condition as first observed by P. Hunton (pers. comm.)
is inherited as an autosomal recessive. The newly hatched
chicks have some difficulty at first in finding food and
water, but soon adapt moderately well to their environment.
As the birds mature, turning and circling motions of the
head become pronounced. At times individual birds can be
seen to spin in circles with no particular preference for a
clockwise or anticlockwise direction. This may indicate
some type of vestibular abnormality. Although hearing
seems unaffected, blind and control birds respond similarly
to both loud and soft noises. Egg and semen production
is normal.

The overall size of the eyes of the mutant birds is larger
when compared to sighted control birds. The birds have
some degree of exophthalmus, and the inner canthus region
of both eyes is exposed, (Fig. 1a). In meridional sections
of fixed eyes the enlarged globe and the large volume of
vitreous is obvious compared to a normal chick eye of the
same age (Fig. 1b). We propose that this mutant be referred
to as "*beg*" for "blindness, enlarged globe". The nomenclature follows the format proposed by the genetics symposium
entitled "Mutant Nomenclature and Gene Symbolism" held
during the 66th Annual Meeting of the Poultry Science Association (1977) as outlined by Somes (1980).

Histological sections of the mutant eyes and controls were
examined by light microscopy using the methods described by
Wilson *et al.* (this volume). In retinas of 8 day embryos,

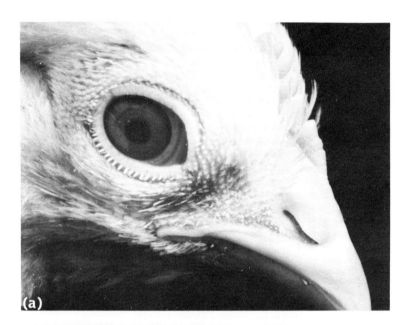

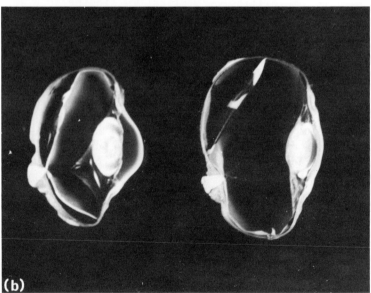

Fig. 1 *Enlarged globe of the* beg *mutant.* (a) *Chick eye with an enlarged and distorted inner canthus region.* (b) *Meridonal section of fixed chick eyes showing examples of the normal (left) and mutant (right).*

a large number of small holes were observed in the mutant
compared to control embryos (Figs 2a and 2b). By the 16
day embryo stage, many more intercellular spaces were
present in the affected embryos. In addition, lightly
stained tracks were visible between nuclei in the upper
half of the inner nuclear layer (Figs 2c and 2d). The
photoreceptor precursor cells appeared normal. In sections
from 4 day post-hatch chicks, obvious holes, 1 to 4 μm in
diameter, were seen in the region extending from the pigment
epithelium (PE) to the external limiting membrane (ELM),
the majority appearing immediately below the PE layer (Fig.
3b). The control retina did not possess such large holes
(Fig. 3a). Some of the holes may be attributed to displacement of the cone oil droplets during sectioning. However,
in the mutant, oil droplets were frequently present beneath
some of the holes. In the adult, the photoreceptors degenerate, and the PE forms irregular clumps (not shown).

Cells from neural retina (NR) and pigment epithelium
(PE) of both normal controls and homozygous *beg* embryos
were grown according to Okada *et al.* (1975) and de Pomerai
et al. (1977). Cells were grown in 6 × 1.5 cm plastic culture
dishes (Flow) and plated at 20 × 10^6 NR cells/plate or
12 × 10^6 PE cells/plate with Eagles MEM containing 10%
Foetal Calf Serum (GIBCO).

No abnormal cell types were observed and plating effi-
ciency was similar in normal and mutant cultures. Taking
an average of 3 separate experiments, the growth rate of
7 day *beg* NR cultures was found to be 1.4 times that of
normal between 16 and 39 days of primary culture. Transdifferentiation of NR cells into melanin-producing PE cells,
and cells producing lens cell-type products (lentoids)
occurred an average of 1 week before control cultures grown
under identical conditions. Similarly, transdifferentiation
of PE cells into lentoids in cultures of PE occurred
approximately 1 week before that in control cultures.

There are a number of factors which affect the likelihood
and the rate of transdifferentiation of neural retina (reviewed Clayton, 1982). These include the age of the embryo,
factors affecting the mitotic rate of the cells in culture,
cell-cell contacts, and medium composition. A high rate
of mitosis is associated with more rapid transdifferentiation,
whether brought about by insulin treatment, (de Pomerai
and Clayton, 1978), the Hy1 genotype (Clayton *et al.*, 1977),
associated with earlier stages of development in the embryo,
(Araki and Okada, 1977; Nomura and Okada, 1979; de Pomerai and
Clayton, 1978). It is not known whether this acceleration
of transdifferentiation is associated with a higher level
of crystallin mRNA in the retina, (Clayton *et al.*, 1979),

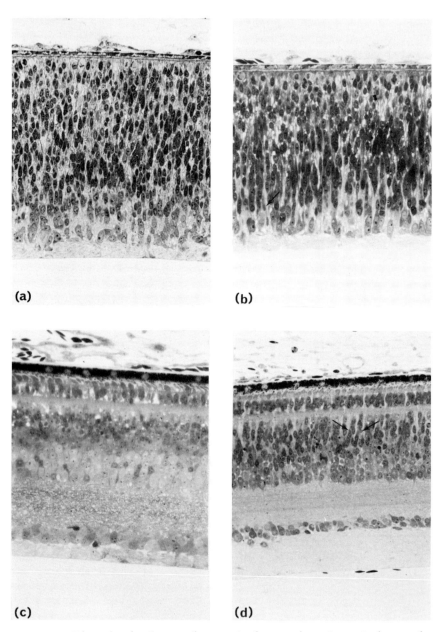

Fig. 2 *Histological sections of the retina from 8 day and 16 day chick embryos. (a) Normal 8 day embryo retina. (b) Mutant 8 day embryo retina. (c) Normal 16 day embryo retina. (d) Mutant 16 day embryo retina.*

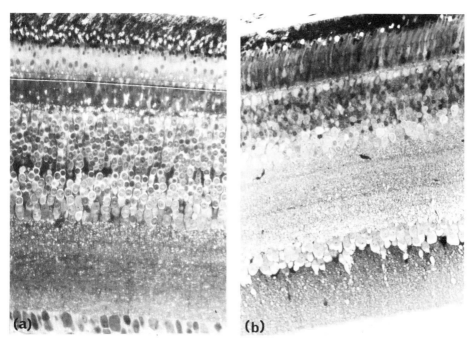

Fig. 3 *Histological sections of the retina from 4 day old hatched chicks. (a) Normal 4 day chick retina. (b) Mutant 4 day chick retina.*

which is age related, or with the cell-cell contacts (Clayton, *et al.*, 1977; Moscona and Degenstein, 1981) which increase as cell number and therefore density increases. In the case of *beg*, the precocious transdifferentiation and the high rate of mitosis in culture may be related either through a requirement for a fixed number of mitoses or to the increased cell contacts associated with a higher cell density. These possibilities will be experimentally assessed. Normal chick retina loses the capacity for transdifferentiation to lens in monolayer culture by 16 to 17 days of incubation (Nomura and Okada, 1979; de Pomerai and Clayton, 1978). However, an unpublished pilot experiment in collaboration with D. de Pomerai indicated that neural retina from post-hatching (*beg*) birds may still be able to transdifferentiate after a prolonged period in culture. Transdifferentiation potential is not expressed unless initial cell-cell contacts are disrupted (reviewed Clayton, 1982); and the possibility that the duration of transdifferentiation potential may be prolonged by the modified cell contacts suggested by the lightly stained material seen in the *beg* retina (Fig. 1d) will also require investigation.

Several blind chick mutants have been reported in the past, none of them dominant. Hutt (1935) described a semilethal autosomal recessive condition in White Leghorns in which chicks were blind at hatching, with bulging of one or both eyes. Smyth *et al.* (1977) reported a type of inherited amelanosis associated with blindness in chicken, which was probably recessive. The *rc* mutant (Cheng *et al.*, 1980; Wolf, this volume) and the *rdd* mutant (Randall and McLachlan, 1979; Wilson *et al.*, this volume) show serious retinal dysplasia affecting the photoreceptor and inner nuclear layers in the embryonic states. The *beg* mutant appears to have features distinguishing it from these other conditions. Further studies of cell behaviour *in vitro*, and the relationship between the growth rate *in vitro*, the excessive volume of vitreous and the size of the globe *in vivo* remains to be ascertained. A more extensive histological examination of the *beg* mutant is under way at both the light and electron microscope level.

ACKNOWLEDGEMENTS

We are grateful to E. Leitch and J. Nicol for their technical assistance, to F. Johnston for photography, and to J. Bard and A. Ross for the use of their facilities at Western General Hospital. This work was supported by the Medical Research Council.

REFERENCES

Araki, M. and Okada, T.S. (1977). Differentiation of lens and pigment cells in cultures of neural retinal cells of early chick embryos. *Devl. Biol.* **60**, 278-286.

Cheng, K.M., Shoffner, R.N., Gelatt, K.N., Gum, G.G., Otis, J.S. and Bitgood, J.J. (1980). An autosomal recessive blind mutant in the chicken. *Poultry Sci.* **59**, 2179-2182.

Clayton, R.M. (1982). Cellular and molecular aspects of differentiation and transdifferentiation of ocular tissues *in vitro* In "Differentiation *In Vitro*" British Society for Cell Biology, Symposium 4. (Eds. M.M. Yeoman and D.E.S. Truman) pp. 83-120. Cambridge University Press.

Clayton, R.M., de Pomerai, D.I. and Pritchard, D.J. (1977). Experimental manipulation of alternative pathways of

differentiation in cultures of embryonic chick neural
retina. *Dev. Growth Diff*. **19**, 319-328.

Clayton, R.M., Thompson, I., and de Pomerai, D.I. (1979).
Relationship between crystallin mRNA expression in retina
cells and their capacity to redifferentiate into lens
cells. *Nature* **282**, 628-629.

Hutt, F.B. (1935). Hereditary blindness in the fowl.
Poultry Sci. **14**, 297.

Moscona, A.A. and Degenstein, L. (1981). Lentoids in
aggregates of embryonic neural retinal cells. *Cell Diff*.
10, 39-46.

Nomura, K. and Okada, T.S. (1979). Age-dependent change in
the transdifferentiation ability of chick neural retina
in cell culture. *Dev. Growth Diff*. **21**, 161-168.

Okada, T.S., Itoh, Y., Watanabe, K. and Eguchi, G. (1975).
Differentiation of lens in cultures of neural retinal
cells of chick embryos. *Devl. Biol*. **45**, 318-329.

de Pomerai, D.I. and Clayton, R.M. (1978). Influence of
embryonic age on the transdifferentiation of chick neural
retina cells in culture. *J. Emb. Exp. Morphol*. **47**,
179-193.

de Pomerai, D.I., Pritchard, D.J. and Clayton, R.M. (1977).
Biochemical and immunological studies of lentoid formation in cultures of embryonic chick neural retina and
day-old chick lens epithelium. *Devl. Biol*. **60**, 416-427.

Randall, C.J. and McLachlan, I. (1979). Retinopathy in
commercial layers. *Vet. Rec*. **105**, 41-42.

Smyth, J.R. Jr., Boissey, R.E. and Gawron, M.F. (1977).
An inherited delayed amelanosis with associated blindness in the domestic fowl. (Abstract). *Poultry Sci*.
56, 1758.

Somes, R.G. Jr. (1980). Alphabetical list of the genes
of domestic fowl. *J. Hered*. **71**, 168-174.

Wilson, M.A., Pollock, B.J., Clayton, R.M. and Randall, C.J.
(1982). Early development of a new RP-like mutant in
the chick (this volume.)

Wolf, E.D. (1982). An inherited retinal abnormality in
Rhode Island Red chickens. (this volume.)

AN INHERITED RETINAL ABNORMALITY IN RHODE ISLAND RED CHICKENS

E. DAN WOLF

*Dept. of Comparative Ophthalmology,
College of Veterinary Medicine, University of Florida,
Gainesville, Florida, USA*

An inbred strain of Rhode Island Red chickens possessing a recessively inherited retinal abnormality, associated with blindness, was initially reported by Cheng and Shoffner (1978). Clinically, the chickens manifest complete blindness from the time of hatching onward. This is demonstrated by random head bobbing, difficulty in finding food, and a lack of participation in the social "pecking" system. A high mortality rate, slow growth rate and nearly zero reproductive rate may result directly from the blindness or be independently determined and merely accentuated by the lack of vision. In our study, artificial insemination, controlled incubation, tube feeding of the hatchlings and segregation from visual chickens were employed to increase reproductive rate and reduce mortality. (Non-carrier age matched chickens obtained at one day of age and raised under similar conditions served as controls.)

Electroretinography was performed at intervals from 1 day to 63 days of age. While the controls demonstrated significant "a" and "b" wave ERG components from 1 day of age onward the affected chickens had no demonstrable electroretinograph response at any age.

Light microscopy of 1 to 2 micron plastic embedded retinal sections was performed periodically from 13 days of embryonic development to 208 days post hatching. All specimens examined were sections from the superior nasal quadrant near the posterior pole. No obvious differences were visible by light microscopy of the embryonic eyes. Lack of development of the complete complement of crystalloid bodies in the inner segments, loss of organization of the components in the photoreceptor space and progressive degeneration (pyknosis,

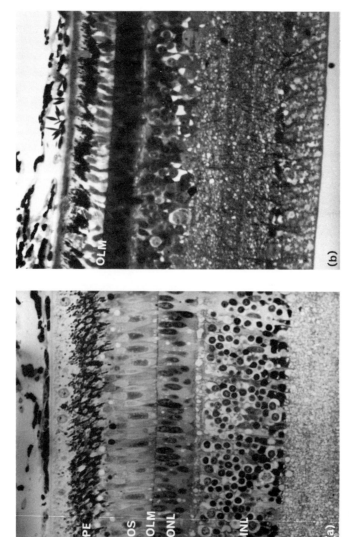

Fig. 1 a) Retina from a normal 43 day old chick, showing organization of the cell layers: pigment epithelium (PE); photoreceptor outer segments (OS); outer limiting membrane (OLM); outer nuclear layer (ONL); inner nuclear layer (INL). b) Retina from a blind, 47 day old chick showing disorganization of photoreceptors.

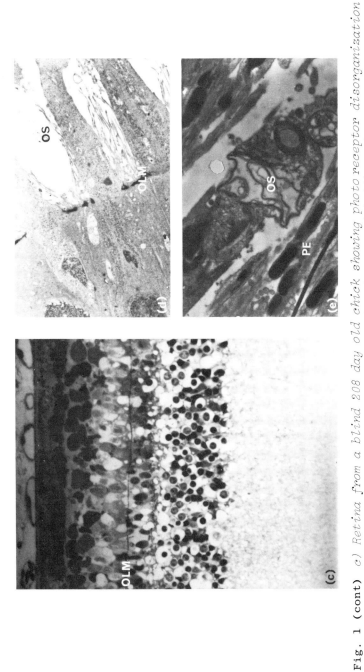

Fig. 1 (cont) c) Retina from a blind 208 day old chick showing photoreceptor disorganization with densely staining globular material against the pigment epithelium. The outer nuclear layer has thinned with degeneration of the nuclei, and the inner nuclear layer is pyknotic.
d) Disorganized photoreceptor outer segments in retina of blind 47 day old chick.
e) Disorganized outer segments in retina of blind 103 day old chick.

then thinning) of the outer nuclear and inner nuclear layers occurred between 1 day and 208 days of age. An accumulation of clumps of darkly staining material within the photoreceptor space was noted from 180 days onward.

Electron microscopy of the 1 day old affected retina demonstrated disorganized outer segment lamellae with vesiculation of the outer segments. Progressive deterioration of the photoreceptor inner and outer segments was noted in successive ages examined. Distinct narrowing of the photoreceptor space with marked reduction of photoreceptor nuclei, as well as inner segments, was noted by 43 days of age. The photoreceptor space contained an abundance of Muller cell processes, degenerating inner segments, occasional photoreceptor nuclei (apparently migrating outside the external limiting membrane) and occasional outer segment material interspersed between pigment epithelial apical processes. By 20 weeks of age only a few inner segments and nuclei remained. Small clusters of grossly degenerate outer segment discs were seen only rarely and the inner nuclear layer was thinned and a proportion of the nuclei were pyknotic.

By 25 and 30 weeks of age a significant proportion of darkly staining clumps of homogeneous material had joined degenerating inner segments, pigment epithelial processes and migrating nuclei in occupying the photoreceptor space. Increasing degeneration of the inner nuclear layer continued. This homogeneous material is compatible in appearance with degenerated nuclear chromatin but this has not yet been confirmed. Also observed clinically but not yet investigated, is the presence of anterior axial cataracts in the majority of the affected birds over 30 to 40 weeks of age.

In conclusion, although much further elucidation is necessary, a form of retinal degeneration exists in chickens which is autosomal recessively inherited, and although present at hatching, progresses relatively slowly. Further studies to evaluate R.P.E. function, differential rates of rod and cone loss and the biochemical characterization of the abnormality are underway.

REFERENCES

Cheng, K.M. and Shoffner, R.N. (1978). An induced retinal mutation (*RC*) in the chicken. *Poultry Science* **57**, 1127.

A SCANNING ELECTRON MICROSCOPY STUDY OF INHERITED RETINAL DEGENERATION IN THE RAT

H.W. READING and D.G. MACINNES

M.R.C. Brain Metabolism Unit, Department of Pharmacology, University of Edinburgh, 1 George Square, Edinburgh EH8 9JZ.

INTRODUCTION

Inherited pigmentary degeneration of the retina occurs in rat, mouse and dog. In these species it is transmitted as an autosomal recessive characteristic. Degeneration in the rat commences after the retina has begun to mature and differentiation has commenced, but before its final stages. Sorsby *et al.* (1954) suggested the term dystrophy rather than abiotrophy to describe the disorder. There are temporal differences in the development of the lesion in different species and Lolley (this volume), has suggested a classification based on development and maintenance diseases. Most of the early experimental studies were carried out on the pink-eyed RCS or Campbell strain of rat, originally described by Bourne *et al.* (1938). Dowling and Sidman (1962) carried out an elegant series of investigations using both light and transmission electron microscopy to study the progress of the lesion in the eyes of dystrophic (RCS) rats. They reported an accumulation of swirling sheets of debris of lamellar form associated with excess rhodopsin lying between the rod outer segments (ROS) and pigment epithelium (PE).

Autoradiographic studies carried out by LaVail and his colleagues (1972 and 1975) in the RCS rat showed anomalies in protein synthesis associated with the production of rod outer segment material. Bok and Hall (1971) had shown that the accumulation of extracellular debris containing rhodopsin consisted of material from shed, effete ROS and discs which had not been phagocytosed in the normal way by the PE. In fact, the rates of shedding and digestion of ROS in the RCS rat are unequal, since the PE loses its capacity to phagocytose (LaVail *et al.*, 1972). After accumulation of

the debris, degenerating nuclei are visible and breakdown
of the photoreceptor neuroepithelium occurs. All the research
described above was carried out on the pink-eyed RCS strain
of rat. In 1974, the breeding of a congenic strain, homozygous for the retinal dystrophic allele was reported (Yates
et al., 1974). This is the so-called Hunter rat. In this
congenic strain, as judged by light microscopy and biochemistry, the lesion follows a slower but similar course
to that in the albino rat. Changes are delayed by about 1
week and it was concluded that the presence of pigment in
the eye retards the degeneration process.

METHODS

Scanning electron micrographs (*sem*) were made of retinas
dissected from (a) normal rats with pigmented eyes (PVG
strain), (b) congenic dystrophic rats, homozygous for the
blind allele (Hunter strain, Yates *et al.*, 1974), (c) normal,
non-pigmented pink-eyed rats, (Wistar strain) and (d) dystrophic, non-pigmented pink-eyed rats, homozygous for the
blind allele, (RCS strain, Bourne *et al.*, 1938)
   Whole retinas were fixed in 2.5% glutaraldehyde in 0.1 M
cacodylate buffer pH 7.3 for 4h at room temperature. The
retinas were then washed in the same buffer, dehydrated in
an ethanol series, transferred to acetone, then critically
point dried using carbon dioxide according to standard procedure. The retinas were then fractured; the fragments
sputter coated with gold in a Polaron E 5100 sputter coater
and then examined in an ISI 60 scanning electron microscope.

RESULTS AND DISCUSSION

The *sem* of Fig. 1 represent a vertical cross sectional
fracture of each retina and show all layers from the photoreceptor outer segments (ROS) to the ganglion cell layer
(GC). The *sem* show quite clearly that degeneration progresses
at a faster rate in the non-pigmented albino eye (Figs 1A
and 1C) so confirming earlier studies using other procedures.
In both normal retinae at this age (24 days), the photoreceptor layers are well developed and show differentiation
into inner (RIS) and outer (ROS) segments. The external
limiting membrane (ELM) between the inner segments and the
photoreceptor nuclear layer (ONL) is well defined (Figs 1B
and 1D.
   The ROS of the dystrophic albino (Fig. 1A), show marked
degenerative changes with foreshortening and coalescence.

Some of the extracellular lamellar debris described by Dowling
and Sidman (1962) and LaVail *et al.* (1972) can be seen clinging
to the outer segment layer, although as Dowling and Sidman
(1962) pointed out, most of this material remains attached to
the pigment epithelium during the dissection and removal of the
retina for examination. It is almost impossible to distinguish the inner from the outer segments and in fact, the photoreceptors present a "melted candle" appearance. The ELM has
virtually disappeared in the albino at this stage and the
ONL appears abnormal.

On the other hand at this age, the pigmented dystrophic
retina (Fig. 1C) does not show such marked degeneration.
The ROS have lost their normal pallisade appearance and show
some changes reminiscent of the albino retina. Remains of
the inner segments still exist but show much less degeneration than the corresponding structure in the albino retina.
The ELM can still be faintly discerned. The ONL appears
normal whereas this layer in the albino (Fig. 1A) is already
showing degenerative changes. The minor breakdown in the
ROS of the pigmented dystrophic retina (Fig. 1C) is seen
earlier than previously recorded by light microscopy (Yates
et al., 1974).

Figures 2 and 3 are high power *sem* of the outer surface of
the retinal neuropithelium (ROS layer) of pigmented rat retina
at 40 days of age; normal retina (Fig. 2, PVG strain) and
dystrophic retina (Fig. 3, Hunter strain) at magnifications
of ×4410 and ×5000 respectively. The normal retina shows
the ROS arranged regularly in columnar form and in some of
them can be seen the outline of the outer segment discs. In
this picture, the outer segment plasma membrane is obviously
in a healthy condition. In contrast, the dystrophic ROS
(Fig. 3) present a random appearance with some coalescing
and appear to lack turgidity. They are swollen and the outer
plasma membrane has a "fluffy" appearance. This may correspond to the interphotoreceptor matrix material described by
Dr LaVail (LaVail, this volume). In addition, some of the
extracellular amorphous debris associated with the condition
can be seen surrounding the outer segments and invading the
inner depths of the photoreceptor layer.

Figures 4, 5 and 6 represent *sem* of retinae from albino
rats of 40 days of age; both normal, Wistar strain (Fig. 4)
and dystrophic, RCS strain (Figs 5 and 6). Figures 4 and
5 were made at the same magnification (×5000) and like the
corresponding *sem* of pigmented retinae (Figs 2 and 3) are
taken looking down on the outer surface of the photoreceptor
layer. Figure 4 shows the normal pallisaded appearance of
ROS, whilst Fig. 5 shows an advanced stage of degeneration
of the photoreceptor layer wherein only debris of the rod

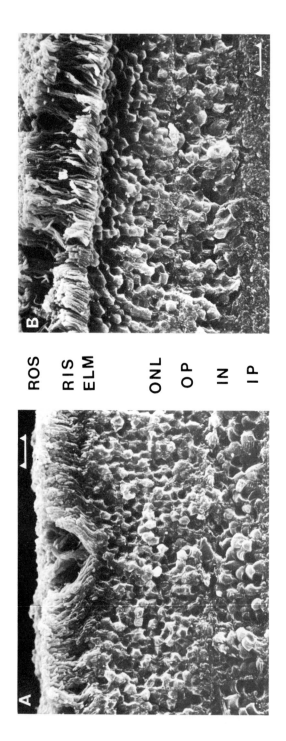

ROS
RIS
ELM

ONL
OP
IN
IP

Fig. 1 *Scanning electron micrographs of rat retinae, dystrophic and normal, albino and pigmented at 24 days of age. A. Albino, dystrophic. B. Albino, normal. C. Pigmented, dystrophic. D. Pigmented, normal. ROS, rod outer segments; RIS, rod inner segments; ELM, external limiting*

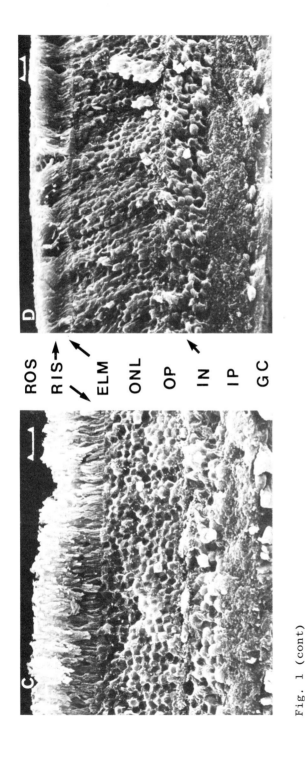

ROS
RIS→
ELM
ONL
OP
IN
IP
GC

Fig. 1 (cont)

membrane, ONL, outer nuclear layer (photoreceotpr nuclei), OP, outer plexiform layer, IN, inner nuclear layer (bipolar cell layer), IP, inner plexiform layer, GC, ganglion cell layer. Bars represent 10 μm. Note severe degeneration in 1A, together with disappearance of external limiting membrane.

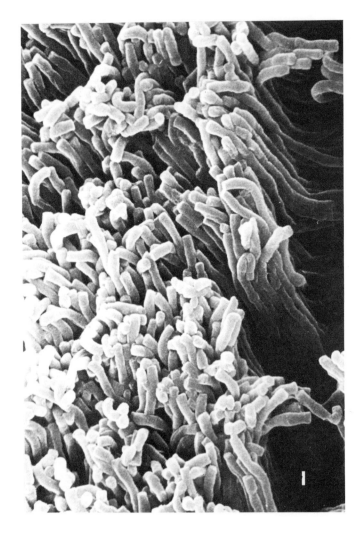

Fig. 2 *Scanning electron micrograph of outer surface of photoreceptor layer in normal pigmented eye of rat at 40 days of age. Bar = 1 μm. The rod outer segments have a normal, regular columnar appearance. The outline of some of the rod discs can be seen in the rod outer segment cylinders.*

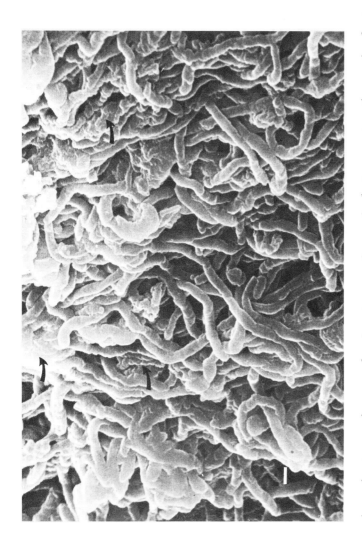

Fig. 3 *Scanning electron micrograph of outer surface of photoreceptor layer in dystrophic pigmented eye of rat at 40 days of age. Bar = 1μm. The rod outer segments are swollen and collapsed and appear to have lost turgidity. They show changes in the plasma membrane which appears to have a "fluffy" coat. Extracellular debris can be seen (arrows), surrounding some of the outer segments and larger masses can be seen within the inner part of the photoreceptor layer.*

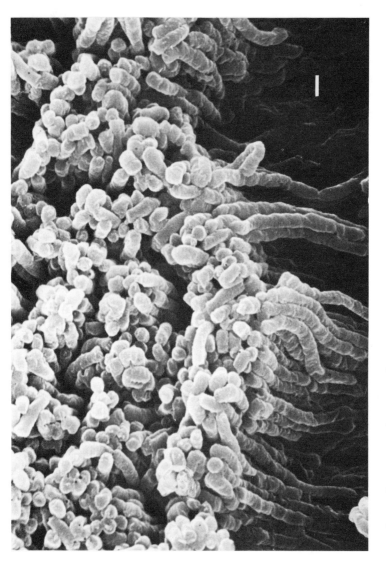

Fig. 4 Scanning electron micrograph of outer surface of retina of 40 day old normal albino rat. Bar = 1 μm. The rod outer segments have a normal regular columnar appearance. The interior of the photoreceptor layer is clear and free of any form of debris.

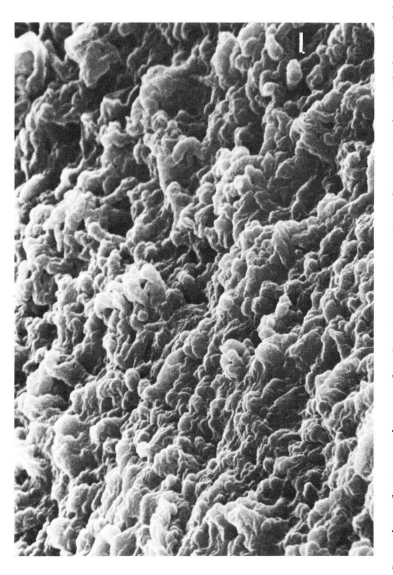

Fig. 5 *Scanning electron micrograph of outer surface of retina of 40 day old dystrophic albino rat. Bar = 1 μm. The photoreceptor layer is in an advanced state of degeneration and is reduced to a carpet of debris covering the outer nuclear layer.*

ANIMAL MODELS AND HUMAN DISEASE : SUMMING UP

M. M. LAVAIL

Except for the papers of Drs Anderson and Converse, this
session has marked the junction between those studies primarily on normal retinas with the remainder of the sessions
in the symposium, which will be on abnormal retinas. At
the outset, Dr Lolley provided us with an intriguing concept or model which groups the retinal degenerations into two
general classes of defects, differentiation and maintenance.
This summing-up attempts to see how Dr Lolley's model fits
the presentations. As I see it, there were 2 examples in
favour of the model. Dr Aguirre described in the miniature
poodle a slowing of the rod renewal rate, that is to half or
a little over half the normal rate, and this mutant falls
into the category of a maintenance defect in Dr Lolley's
classification. There are also two other mutants for which
we have either published or unpublished data that fall
into the maintenance category, and these are the RCS rat and
the *pcd* mouse. In the early 1970s, it was shown that the
RCS rat also had a reduced rate of rod renewal prior to any
overt degeneration of photoreceptor cells, and from some
unpublished work with Drs Blanks and Mullen, we know
that the rate of outer segment renewal in the *pcd* mouse is
also about half the rate in the normal. So it looks as if
this similarity in grouping might hold up, at least at this
level of analysis.
   The other point in favour of this model is Dr Chader's new
data on the collie, which is at the other end of the spectrum;
that is, it is a differentiation mutant. It has an elevated
cyclic GMP level just as do the other differentiation
mutants, the *rd* mouse and the Irish setter. So again, at
this level of analysis, the collie data support the hypothesis that Dr Lolley put forward, that perhaps the differentiation class of mutants will turn out to involve abnormalities
in cyclic nucleotide metabolism.
   On the other side, however, Dr Chader pointed out a
possible problem - that the calmodulin dependence of phos-
phodiesterace in the collie is never calcium dependent,

unlike the situation in the setter, and he suggested that it might be a different type of "early-onset dysplasia", as he called it. If so, it might be that Dr Lolley's classification system is too coarse. Although this may well turn out to be true, it is also likely that *any* classification system is going to be too coarse the more sophisticated the analysis becomes. However, at present the system does at least stand as a useful model to test and does help to provide us with a useful framework and also a goal: to push for the comparative analysis of mutants.

We are very fortunate to have in this one symposium session representatives from all the major laboratories which have contributed to the most well worked-out photoreceptor cell death mechanism, abnormal cyclic nucleotide metabolism. The work with the *rd* mouse and the Irish setter retinas and with the Xenopus and human retinas in culture has developed a story that really offers a challenge: to analyse the other models and human RP eyes in order to determine whether they also have a similar defect. This sort of comparative analysis is very important. When we look at any RP eye we must ask a comparative question: is this form of RP the same or similar to another form of RP? When we look at an animal model we must ask whether this animal model is the same as another animal model or to one of the human conditions or forms of RP. It is exciting to see that at this symposium, these same workers are already pursuing other animal models, as they have told us, both in search of the cyclic nucleotide defect as well as other phenotypic characteristics of these models. It is also exciting to see these investigators pushing their systems and their techniques to an even greater level of sophistication.

Finally, I think that it is worth reflecting for a moment to see how we stand with the animal model research for RP. There are many inherited degenerations of the CNS in man for which there is not a single animal model and yet, in RP research we have a number of models, and we have worked out at least one fairly well defined degeneration mechanism. We have every reason to be proud of these investigators and with their work which has been presented at the last two seesions. However, we do not have reason enough to be satisfied, because it is likely that the closer we get to the actual gene mechanisms of these defects, the harder the questions are going to become and the more difficult it will be to get definitive answers. On the other hand. if we look at the rate at which we are acquiring new data and the enthusiasm that we are seeing in the research efforts that have been presented here, we have cause for optimism in our search for clues to the cure of Retinitis Pigmentosa.

ANIMAL MODELS AND HUMAN DISEASE — AN OVERVIEW

G.B. ARDEN

Department of Visual Science,
Institute of Ophthalmology, Judd Street, London, UK.

As this meeting has continued, it has become more and more difficult to give a coherent account which is not just a repetition of the excellent surveys we have already heard. Our corpus of knowledge is, after all, not so extensive. I shall try to slant this contribution strictly to my title, and ask what we may learn by comparing human degenerations to animal disease. Although such conditions are common in man, in only a few cases is the aetiology known (e.g. Kaiser-Kupfer *et al.*, 1980), and I shall not attempt to cover the subject comprehensively, but instead will single out those slowly progressive human conditions which are lumped together under the title of *Retinitis Pigmentosa* (R.P.). Thus, I shall not be touching upon the various macular degenerations, or the defects of ageing, to which one could devote an entire symposium. Our models of R.P. have in the main been derived by extrapolation from clinical data to what is known about the fundamental anatomy, physiology and biochemistry of the eye, so it is convenient to consider how our clinical ideas have developed.

Retinitis Pigmentosa was named from the post-mortem appearance of the diseased retina, and was recognized as soon as the ophthalmoscope came into common use. The pigmentation and alterations in retinal vascularity were associated with the changes seen in other chronic inflammatory eye diseases (e.g. syphilis) and theories of the R.P. aetiology were developed along these lines. Some professed treatments for R.P. are still based on this early erroneous pathology! However, recently these ideas have been revived in a reputable form (Jay, M. Ph.D. thesis, 1981: see Bird, this volume) since it appears that a proportion of cases which are diagnosed as R.P. may not be due to alterations in the genome.

The modes of inheritance of the human disease were

established at the turn of the century, and Dominant, X-
linked and Recessive forms are known. The total prevalence
in the population is about 0.2%. It is remarkable that no
inherited degenerations have been detected in other primates.
The human X-linked condition would not, I should have thought,
have been bred out by evolutionary pressure, and the dominant
disease, in most cases, is so mild that visual handicap does
not occur until the end of the reproductive age. Nevertheless, the only animal models of which we know are all recessively inherited* and therefore are not completely satis-
factory for making analogies with human conditions.

One of the prominent symptoms of the human condition is
"night-blindness". This has been known for 100 years, in
fact since the establishment of the duplicity theory. The
early proponents must have found it gratifying that a
naturally occurring pathology could so neatly discriminate
between the (still hypothetical) scotopic and photopic
systems. In some of our animal models, e.g. rodents, the
cone systems are so poorly developed that it is difficult
to determine whether such a selectivity exists, while in
others (e.g. dogs) there is no selectivity. It is encouraging
that recent investigations of abnormally treated retinas
(Hollyfield, this volume; Lolley *et al.*, 1977; Ushafer *et
al.*, 1980) show that a chemically-induced retinal degeneration may be rod-selective. Differences in the metabolism of
cyclic nucleotides between cones and rods have been detected
(Farber *et al.*, 1981). The phagocytosis of cones has been
shown to be different from that in rods, for while disc
shedding in rods occurs soon after sunrise (see Young, 1976,
for a review) in cones it occurs after sunset (Young, 1978).
However, it is by no means certain that such selectivity for
rods occurs in all cases of human Retinitis Pigmentosa (see
Arden, this volume). Some reports are certainly due to the
fact that in many cases the peripheral retina is most
affected, and the concentration of rods drops towards the
central retina: thus any condition which restricts the
visual field will incidentally cause night-blindness.

The nature of the visual field changes in human and
animal dystrophies could also help identify which comparisons might be more appropriate. In man, the mid-peripheral
field is often first affected, and this leads to the appearance of annular scotomata. It was fascinating to see Aguirre's
micrographs of dystrophic poodle retina (this volume), where
the mid-periphery was similarly severely affected, but where,

---

*But see Barnett, this volume for central degeneration in
the dog.

histologically, a far peripheral rim of retina preserved
relatively normal morphology. In those few reports of human
disease (e.g. Szamier *et al.*, 1979), similar sharp transitions have been noticed. Another feature of human disease
is the frequent occurrence of altitudinal field defects:
sometimes the lower half of the retina is grossly disturbed
in dominant disease, while the upper half seems almost
normal. In X-linked heterozygotes the thinning and pigment
clumping is frequently confined to the lower retina until
late in life. It is sometimes thought that this distribution indicates damage by light, which commonly comes from
above. However, the time scale is really too great. For
visual processes, the reciprocity law breaks down for times
greater than tens of milliseconds: for thermal damage, the
reciprocity may extend to tens of seconds. It is difficult
to conceive of a reciprocity extending for tens of years!
Such an altitudinal defect occurs in one chicken retinal
degeneration (Clayton, pers. comm.) but as far as I know,
in no other model.*

It is often thought that patients with R.P. are suffering
from night-blindness, but, in fact, a much more severe
complaint is that light causes "white-out" and loss of visual
function for extended periods. Thus chemical models which
concentrate on aspects of retinal function related to transduction are of special interest. No abnormality of rhodopsin
itself has ever been demonstrated in laboratory animals
(Dowling and Sidman, 1962; Chaitin and Williams, 1977) or
in man (Ripps *et al.*, 1978). However, the reduction and transport of retinol from the rods to the pigment epithelium has
long been suspected as a link in the rhodopsin cycle which
could, when modified, lead to retinal degeneration. (Dowling,
1960; Reading, 1970; Berman, this volume). There is a
specialized retinol binding protein (Maraini *et al.*, 1977),
which facilitates such transport. The concentration of
retinal in the Rod outer limb ROL is 3 mM, and such a concentration of Vitamin A will lyse cells (Dingle and Lucy, 1962;
Lucy *et al.*, 1963). Thus, abnormalities in the Vitamin A
cycle could cause damage to receptors or to the Retinal
pigment epithelium (R.P.E.). If such damage was discontinuous,
it could lead to a breach of the blood-retinal barrier, and
the development of anti-retinal antibodies, which, subsequently, with another episode of retinal damage, could result in
an auto-immune reaction (Rahi *et al.*, 1976). In the rat,

---

*La Vail (pers. comm., this volume) tells me that altitudinal
defects occur in pigmented RCS rats, and are independent of
the lighting in which the animal lives.

retinal degeneration is associated with a breach in the blood-
retinal barrier (Essner *et al.*, 1980). This may be the mechanism whereby long continued exposure to relatively dim
light causes retinal degeneration in normal animals' eyes
(Hansson, 1970; Kuwabara and Gorn 1971; Noell and Albrecht,
1971; Organisciak and Noell, 1977). It has usually been
thought that the degeneration affected photoreceptors primarily, but Lai *et al.* (1980) found that in the rat, the
R.P.E. showed the earliest changes. Such mechanisms if
occurring in man, would, explain clinical findings such as
the non-uniform progression of the disease, which may appear
stationary for long periods, and then suddenly progress;
the retinal oedema, which may come and go, and the leakage
of retinal vessels.

Other classes of model of R.P. are based on what is known
of the biochemistry of light excitation. Photoreceptors
have large membrane areas, and small internal volumes. The
ROL is normally permeable to sodium in darkness (Tomita,
1972; Arden and Ernst, 1970) and a radial current flows
along the length of the outer limb (Hagins *et al.*, 1970),
which is so large that the entire ionic contents are ex-
changed (in darkness) in a minute or so. Such activity
requires membrane pumps which are localized in the inner
limb (Baylor *et al.*, 1979) and the metabolic activity of the
receptor is very high, accounting for the large mitochindria.
There is also, of course, very active membrane synthesis, and
the processes involving visual transduction are associated
with the splitting of high energy phosphate bonds. Thus,
there are several reasons for the high energy requirement
of photoreceptors (Graymore, 1970) and since these cells are
in an avascular zone, they depend upon the R.P.E. for a
supply of metabolites. Such factors may account for the
high susceptibility of photoreceptors to damage in retinal
degenerations, even if the primary lesion is elsewhere, for
example in the R.P.E. A more specific biochemistry can now
be invoked. When rhodopsin absorbs light, it activates a
specialized phosphodiesterase, which rapidly cleaves cGMP
to 5'-GMP. In darkness, the level of cGMP is extraordinarily
high, and its reduction by light is swift and considerable
(Pober and Bitensky, 1979; Liebman and Pugh, 1979, 1980;
Kawamura and Bownds, 1981; Woodruff and Bownds, 1979). The
level of cGMP may control the ROL membrane permeability. In
one mutant mouse the development and decay of photoreceptors
is associated with a great rise and later fall of the levels
of cGMP (Farber and Lolley, 1974). The same is true in
some canine retinopathies (Lolley *et al.*, 1977.) Moreover,
in developing retina and in human retina, poisoning the
tissue with agents which cause cGMP to accumulate results in

a retinal degeneration (Lolley *et al.*, 1977; Ulshafer *et al.*,
1980). Possibly, such a mechanism might cause some forms
of blindness in man. It may be noted that in mice heterozygous for the retinal degeneration, there is a biochemical
abnormality of cGMP (Ferandelli and Cohen, 1976) and the
receptor potential kinetics are abnormal (Arden and Low,
1980). In man, the kinetics of the receptor response are
difficult to determine since they are masked by the response
of postsynaptic units in the electroretinogram. Even in the
cones, which are less severely affected, the responses appear
to be slowed. (Arden, this volume).

Rods have an active system for progressive renewal (Young,
1976), and about 1/10th of the 1000 intracellular discs are
formed each day, as the ROL lengthens from its base. At the
apex old discs are shed, engulfed by the R.P.E., and digested
in phagosomes. In one animal model, the RCS rat, this mechanism is disrupted, and early in life the rods elongate
and the shed material partially fuses, and forms a great
mass which causes a retinal detachment. (Dowling and Sidman,
1962; Arden and Ikeda, 1965). RCS rat pigment epithelial
cells in tissue culture fail to phagocytose ROL from normal
rats (Edwards and Szamier, 1977) and by making chimeras,
LaVail showed conclusively that the defect lay in the R.P.E.
(Mullen and LaVail, 1976; LaVail and Mullen, 1976; LaVail,
1981). The mechanisms of phagocytosis have been investigated,
and the surface binding properties of the rods (Bridges,
1981) and the interphotoreceptor matrix (LaVail, this volume)
have been analysed. Phagocytosis apparently occurs in
several stages, and while in the RCS rat cell recognition
may be normal, the subsequent engulfment is not (Hall and
Chaitin, 1980).

Although in some human conditions, there seems to be abnormal material retro-retinally, the accumulations of shed
ROL in the RCS rat seem to be a unique phenomenon.

Discs are not shed continuously (LaVail, 1976; Bassinger
et al., 1976; Beharse *et al.*, 1977*a,b*). Although there is
a circadian element, the shedding is light triggered, and
in some species the rate of growth of the outer limb is also
subject to the same influence (Hollyfield and Bassinger,
1978; Flannery and Fisher, 1979), so that the volume of the
outer limb depends on the light regime (Hollyfield and Rayborn, 1979; Dudley and O'Brien, 1981). Thus slight alterations in the rate of formation or loss of discs could lead
to a slow progressive shortening of outer limbs, and then
possibly to cell death, a picture compatible with the few
reports of the histology of human R.P. in which the condition had not entered its final stage (Kolb and Gouras,
1974; Szamier *et al.*, 1979). Hence in animal models (LaVail,

1981) and particularly in the progressive retinal atrophy of
dogs, (Aguirre *et al.*, 1978; Buyukmichi *et al.*, 1980; Buyukmichi and Aguirre, 1976; Aguirre and O'Brien, 1981; Aguirre,
this volume) the rate of growth of ROL has been measured,
and in some it is slowed. It is of interest to consider
what sensory defects might result: these could be little
more than those due to the loss of light-gathering power in
the photoreceptors. It is interesting that in some cases
of human R.P., this appears to be the case (Ripps *et al.*,
1978: Arden, this volume).

Finally, I should like to point out that another class of
models is now being exploited. Photoreceptors are inacces-
ible, but it is suspected that there may be homologies between
the retina and other tissues (Airaksinen *et al.*, 1979; Arden
and Fox, 1979), so possibly although (with the exception of
cataract and deafness, which are common associations) Retinitis
Pigmentosa appears to be an isolated disease of the retina,
the fundamental defects may be determined by studies on man,
without the use of animal models.

REFERENCES

Aguirre, G., Farber, D.B., Lolley, R.N., Fletcher, T. and
     Chader, G.J. (1978). Rod cone dysplasia in Irish Setters:
     a defect in cyclic GMP metabolism in visual cells.
     Science **201**, 1133—1134.
Aguirre, G. and O'Brien, P. (1981). Rod outer segment renewal
     in miniature poodles with progressive rod cone atrophy.
     ARVO Abstracts. *Supp. to Invest. Ophthal. Vis. Sci.*
     20, p. 42.
Airaksinen, E.M., Airaksinen, M.M., Sihvola, P. and Sihvola,
     M. (1979). Uptake of taurine by platelets in retinitis
     pigmentosa. *The Lancet*, **i**, 474—475.
Arden, G.B. and Ikeda, H. (1965). Electrophysiological find-
     ings in congenital retinal degeneration. Proc. IV. ISCERG.
     Supp. 10. *Jap. J. Ophthal.* 222—230.
Arden, G.B. and Ernst, W.J.K. (1970). The effects of ions on
     the photoresponses of pigeon cones. *J. Physiol. (Lond.)*
     211, 311—339.
Arden, G.B. and Fox, B. (1979). Evidence for increased numbers
     of abnormal nasal cilia in patients with retinitis pig-
     mentosa. *Nature (Lond.)* **279**, 534—536.
Arden, G.B. and Low, J.C. (1980). Altered kinetics of the
     photoresponse from retinas of mice heterozygous for the
     retinal degeneration gene. *J. Physiol. (Lond.)* **308**,
     80—81.
Bassinger, S., Hoffman, R. and Mathes, M. (1976). Photoreceptor

shedding is initiated by light in the frog retina. *Science*
194, 1074.

Baylor, D.A., Lamb, T.P. and Yau, K.W. (1979). The membrane
current of single rod outer segments. *J. Physiol.(Lond.)*
286, 589–612.

Beharse, J.C., Hollyfield, J.G., and Rayborn, M.C. (1977*a*).
Photoreceptor outer segments; accelerated membrane renewal in rods after exposure to light. *Science* **196**, 536.

Beharse, J.C., Hollyfield, J.G. and Rayborn, M.C. (1977*b*).
Turnover of rod photoreceptor outer segments II. Membrane
additions and loss in response to light. *J. Cell. Biol.*
75, 507.

Bridges, C.D.B. (1981). Lectin receptors of rods and cones.
Invest. Ophthalmol. Vis. Sci. **20**, 8–16.

Buyukmichi, N., Aguirre, G. and Marshall, J. (1980). Retinal
degenerations in the dog. II. Development of the retina
in rod-cone dysplasia. *Exp. Eye Res.* **30**, 575–591.

Buyukmichi, N. and Aguirre, G.D. (1976). Rod-disc turnover
in the Dog. *Invest. Ophthalmol. Vis. Sci.* **15**, 579–584.

Chaitin, M.H. and Williams, T.P. (1977). Bleaching characteristics of rhodopsin from normal and dystrophic rats.
Exp. Eye Res. **24**, 553–559.

Dingle, J.T. and Lucy, J.A. (1962). Studies on the mode of
action of excess of Vitamin A. 5. The effects of Vitamin
A on the stability of the erythrocyte membrane. *J.
Biochem.* **84**, 611–620.

Dowling, J.E. (1960). Chemistry of visual adaptation in
the rat. *Nature (Lond.)* **188**, 114–118.

Dowling, J.E. and Sidman, R.L. (1962). Inherited retinal
dystrophy in the rat. *J. Cell. Biol.* **14**, 73–109.

Dudley, P.A. and O'Brien, P.J. (1981). Circadian synthesis
of rat retinal membrane phospholipids. ARVO Abstract
Supp. to Invest. Ophthalmol. Vis. Sci. **20**.

Edwards, R.B. and Szamier, R.B. (1977). Defective phagocytosis of isolated rod outer segments by RCS rat retinal
pigment epithelium in culture. *Science* **197**, 1001.

Essner, R., Pino, R.M. and Griewski, R.A. (1980). Retinal
barrier in RCS rats with inherited retinal degeneration.
Laboratory Investigation **43**, 418–426.

Farber, D.B. and Lolley, R.N. (1974). Cyclic guanosine monophosphate elevation in degenerating photoreceptors of
C3H mouse retina. *Science* **181**, 449.

Farber, D.B., Souza, D.W., Chase, D.G. and Lolley, R.N. (1981).
Cyclic nucleotides of cone-dominant retinas. Reduction
of cyclic AMP levels by light and by cone degeneration.
Invest. Ophthalmol. Vis. Sci. **20**, 24–31.

Ferandelli, J.A. and Cohen, A.I. (1976). The effects of
light and dark adaptation on the levels of cyclic nucleo-

tides in retinas of mice heterozygous for a gene for photoreceptor dystrophy. *Biochem. Biophys. Res. Communication.*
73, 421–427.

Flannery, J.G. and Fisher, S.K. (1979). Light-triggered
rod disc shedding in Xenopus retina in vitro. *Invest.
Ophthalmol. Vis. Sci.* **18,** 638–642.

Graymore, C.N. (Ed.), (1970). "Biochemistry of the Eye".
Academic Press, London.

Hagins, W.A., Penn, R.D. and Yoshikami, S. (1970). Dark
current and photocurrent in retinal rods. *Biophys. J.*
10, 380–412.

Hall, M.O. and Chaitin, M.H. (1980). The engulfment phase
of phagocytosis in the dystrophic rat (RCS) pigment
epithelium. ARVO Abstracts p. 96. *Supp. Invest.
Ophthalmol. Vis. Sci.* **20.**

Hansson, H.A. (1970). Ultrastructural studies on rat retina
dama ed by visible light. *Virchows Arch. Zell. Path.
Abt. B.* **6,** 247–262.

Hollyfield, J.G. and Bassinger, S. (1978). Photoreceptor
shedding can be initiated within the eye. *Nature (Lond.)*
274, 794–796.

Hollyfield, J.G. and Rayborn, M.E. (1979). Photoreceptor
outer segment development: light and dark regulate the
rate of membrane addition and loss. *Invest. Ophthalmol.
Vis. Sci.* **18,** 117–132.

Jay, M.R. (1981). On the heredity of Retinitis Pigmentosa.
Ph.D. Thesis, Univ. of London, UK.

Kaiser-Kupfer, M.I., de Monasterio, F.M., Valle, D., Walser,
M., and Brusilow, S. (1980). Gyrate atrophy of the
choroid and retina: improved visual function following
reduction of plasma ornithine by diet. *Science,* **210,**
1128–1131.

Kawamura, S. and Bownds, M.D. (1981). Light adaptation of
the cyclic GMP phosphodiesterase of frog photoreceptor
membranes mediated by ATP and calcium ions. *J. Gen.
Physiol.* **77,** 571–591.

Kolb, H. and Gouras, P. (1974). Electron microscopic
observations of human retinitis pigmentosa dominantly
inherited. *Invest. Ophthalmol. Vis. Sci.* **13,** 489–498.

Kuwabara, T. and Gorn, A. (1971). Retinal damage by visible
light. *Arch. Ophthal.(Chicago)* **79,** 69–78.

Lai, Y-L., Lug, R., Yao, P., Hayasaka, S. and Hayasaka, I.
(1980). Studies of the pathogenic mechanisms of light on
rat retina. *Acta. Anat.* **107,** 407–417.

LaVail, M.M. (1976). Rod outer segment disc shedding in
relation to cyclic lighting. *Exp. Eye. Res.* **23,** 277–280.

LaVail, M.M. (1981). Photoreceptor characteristics in
congenic strains of RCS rats. *Invest. Ophthalmol. Vis.*

Sci. **20**, 671–675.

LaVail, M.M. and Mullen, R.J. (1976). Role of the pigment epithelium in inherited retinal degeneration analysed with experimental mouse chimeras. *Exp. Eye Res.* **23**, 227–245.

Liebman, P.A. and Pugh, E.N. (1979). The control of phosphodiesterase in rod disk membranes — kinetics, possible mechanisms and significance for vision. *Vision Res.* **19** 375–386.

Liebman, P.A. and Pugh, E.N. (1980). ATP mediates rapid reversal of cyclic GMP phosphodiesterase activation in visual receptor membranes. *Nature (Lond.)* **287**, 734–736.

Lolley, R.N., Farber, D.B., Rayborn, M.E. and Hollyfield, J.G. (1977). Cyclic GMP accommodation causes degeneration of photoreceptor cells: simulation of an inherited disease. *Science* **196**, 664–667.

Lucy, J.A., Liscombe, M. and Dingle, J.T. (1963). Studies on the mode of action of excess of Vitamin A. 8. Mitochondrial swelling. *J. Biochem.* **89**, 419–423.

Maraini, G., Ottonello, S., Gozzoli, F. and Merli, A. (1977). Identification of a membrane protein binding the retinol in retinal pigment epithelium. *Nature (Lond.)* **265**, 68–69.

Mullen, R.J. and LaVail, M.M. (1976). Inherited retinal dystrophy primary defect in pigment epithelium determined with experimental rat chimeras. *Science* **192**, 779–801.

Noell, W.K. and Albrecht, R. (1971). Irreversible effects of visible light on the retina: role of Vitamin A. *Science* **172**, 76–80.

Organisciak, D.T. and Noell, W.K. (1977). The rod outer segment phospholipid/opsin ratio of rats maintained in darkness or cyclic light. *Invest. Ophthalmol. Vis. Sci.* **16**, 188–190.

Pober, J.S., and Bitensky, M.W. (1979). Light regulated enzymes of vertebrate retinal rods. *Adv. Cyclic Nucleotide Res.* **11**, 265–301.

Rahi, A.H.S., Lucas, D.R. and Waghe, M. (1976). Experimental immune retinitis. Induction by isolated photoreceptors. *Mod. Probl. Ophthalmol.* **16**, 30–40.

Ripps, H., Brin, K. and Weale, R.A. (1978). "The aetiology of retinitis pigmentosa". International Congress. XXIII Concilium Ophthalmologicum, Kyoto. Ed. Shimizu, K. and Oosterhuis, J.A., Elsevier, North-Holland.

Szamier, B., Berson, E.L., Klein, R. and Meyers, S. (1979). Sex linked retinitis pigmentosa: ultrastructure of photoreceptors and pigment epithelium. *Invest. Ophthalmol. Vis. Sci.* **18**, 148–160.

Tomita, T. (1972). Light induced potential and resistance

changes in vertebrate photoreceptors. In "Handbook of Sensory Physiology". VII/2 (Ed. M.G.F. Fuortes). Springer Verlag, Berlin, Heidelberg, New York.

Ulshafer, R.J., Garcia, C.A. and Hollyfield, J.G. (1980). Sensitivity of photoreceptors to elevated levels of cGMP in the human retina. *Invest. Ophthalmol. Vis. Sci.* **19**, 1236–1241.

Woodruff, M.L. and Bownds, M.D. (1979). Amplitude, kinetics and reversibility of a light induced decrease in guanosine 3', 5' — cyclic monophosphate in frog photorece-ptor membrane. *J. gen. Physiol.* **73**, 629–653.

Young, R.W. (1976). The Friedenwald Lecture: Visual cells and the concept of renewal. *Invest. Ophthalmol. Vis. Sci.* **15**, 700–725.

Young, R.W. (1978). The daily rhythms of shedding and degradation of rod and cone outer segment membranes in the chick retina. *Invest. Ophthalmol. Vis. Sci.* **17**, 105–116.

RETINAL DISEASES IN DOMESTIC ANIMALS

K. C. BARNETT

Comparative Ophthalmology Unit,
Animal Health Trust Small Animals Centre,
Lanwades Park, Kennett,
Newmarket, Suffolk   CB8 7PN.

INTRODUCTION

Much information is now available on retinal disease in
domestic animals (horse, ox, sheep, dog and cat). The
aetiology is varied; several diseases, particularly in the
dog, are inherited but others are due to infectious agents,
deficiency and toxicity. These comparative retinopathies
have been little used as animal models in the study of human
eye disease, in spite of their similarity and availability.
Much more comparative study has taken place in the laboratory
species such as the mouse, rat and rabbit. However, it would
seem that the dog is now becoming more widely used in the
study of human Retinitis Pigmentosa.

The Dog

"Retinitis Pigmentosa" was first described in the dog by
Magnusson (1911) in the Gordon Setter in Sweden in the early
part of this century, as an hereditary retinal degeneration
similar to the condition in man. Since that time it has
been recorded in several breeds of dog and the veterinary
surgeon now recognizes two principal types of what is commonly called progressive retinal atrophy (PRA) (Barnett, 1976).
These two types differ in their ophthalmoscopic appearance,
their effect on vision, the pathological changes, the modes
of inheritance and the breeds affected. The first type is
usually called "generalized progressive retinal atrophy" and
is more like Retinitis Pigmentosa than the second type,
"central progressive retinal atrophy", which has similarities
to the heredo-macular degenerations.

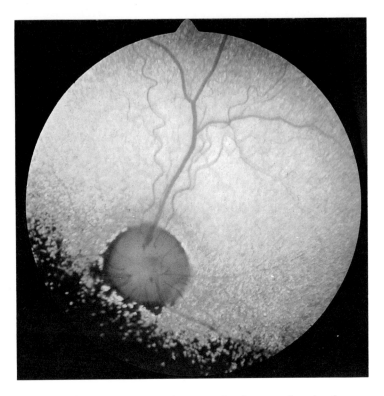

Fig. 1 *Generalized progressive retinal atrophy (rod-cone dysplasia) Irish Setter, female, 6 months of age.*

Generalized PRA commences as a night-blindness, with loss of the rods, occurring some time (months or years) after birth, but with progression, day vision is also lost as the cones degenerate. The condition is undoubtedly hereditary and ophthalmoscopic examination reveals increased tapetal reflectivity indicating thinning of the retina, attenuation of the retinal blood vessels, appearance of the choroidal circulation, pallor and later atrophy of the optic disc and secondary cataract — all similar to Retinitis Pigmentosa. In all cases the retinopathy is bilaterally symmetrical and slowly progressive with ultimate total blindness. Generalized PRA has been described in several breeds of dog with a similar ophthalmoscopic picture but different breeds are affected at different ages. The age of onset of PRA is breed specific, although clinically generalized PRA is similar in all breeds in which it has been recorded. It is interesting that all forms of generalized PRA in the dog which have been studied genetically have been shown to be due to a simple autosomal recessive gene. Histologically, there is a progressive

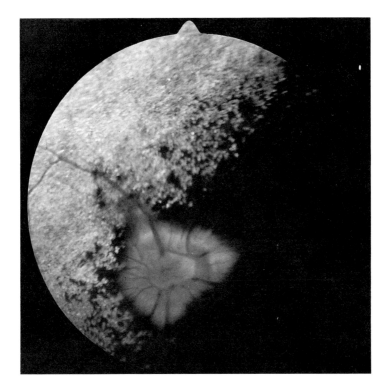

Fig. 2 *Generalized progressive retinal atrophy (progressive rod-cone degeneration) Miniature Poodle, male, 5 years.*

degeneration of the photoreceptors, most severe peripherally, which has no doubt led to the report by the owners of "tunnel vision" in some affected animals, with gradual change to less advanced degeneration in the central region. Diagnosis by the electroretinogram is possible before ophthalmoscopic changes are apparent.

Aguirre (1976) has further classified generalized PRA, by ERG and ultrastructural studies, into different diseases, structurally, functionally and genetically. This subdivision relates to the different ages of onset in the different breeds mentioned above. He names the condition in the Irish Setter "rod-cone dysplasia", as the rods and cones degenerate before reaching maturity; in the Elkhound, "rod dysplasia with cone degeneration", as only the rods do not develop normally, the cones becoming dystrophic later in the course of the disease; in the Miniature Poodle, "progressive rod-cone degeneration", as there is normal development of both rods and cones followed by gradual photoreceptor degeneration. Similar studies in other breeds listed below may reveal other subdivisions. Also, it is possible that more than one form

of generalized PRA may occur in the same breed, in particular
the Irish Setter. Generalized PRA is, therefore, not one
condition but a complex of several different conditions, as
is the case with Retinitis Pigmentosa.

Breeds affected include the following: Gordon Setter,
Irish Setter, Miniature and Toy Poodle, Rough Collie, Tibetan
Terrier, Tibetan Spaniel, Cocker Spaniel, Cardigan Corgi,
Miniature Long-Haired Dachshund, Elkhound and English Springer
Spaniel. Other breeds have been described in other countries
by different authors.

Central PRA does not commence with night-blindness, in
fact, affected dogs have better vision in dull light than in
bright sunlight. The condition is progressive but total
blindness is not invariable and some peripheral vision may
be retained. Ophthalmoscopically, central PRA starts as a
pigmentary disturbance with hyper-reflectivity in the area
centralis, a region of high cone density lateral to the
optic disc. The changes soon affect the whole of the tapetal
fundus but the tapetum nigrum region remains free of obvious
ophthalmoscopic abnormality. Later in the course of the
disease some attenuation of the retinal blood vessels occurs.

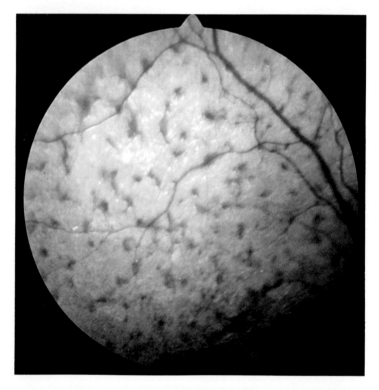

Fig. 3 *Central progressive retinal atrophy Labrador, female,
5 years.*

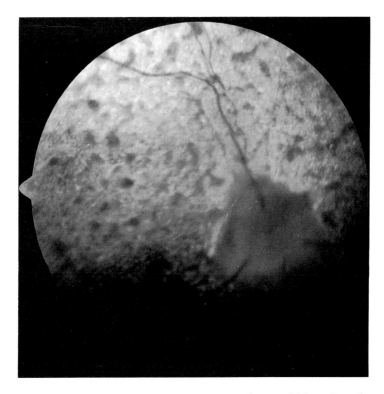

Fig. 4 *Central progressive atrophy Border Collie, female, 6 years.*

The tapetum lucidum is covered with small brown pigment spots of varying size, shape and density and between these there is an increased reflection from the tapetum. Secondary cataract is not as common as with generalized PRA but irregular forms of cataract do occur in some cases. Pathologically, this condition develops as a hyperplasia of the retinal pigment epithelium with migration of these cells to form cell nests on the surface of the retina and with loss of the photo-receptors. There is a clear line of demarcation between affected and non-affected retina.

Central PRA particularly affects the working breeds including the Labrador Retriever, Golden Retriever, Rough Collie, Border Collie and, more recently, the Briard.

The Cat

Hereditary retinal degeneration has been suspected for some time in the Siamese breed due to the number of cases occurring in this breed in comparison to others, but so far it is un-proven. Hereditary retinal degeneration in young Persian kittens due to a recessive gene has been reported in America, but it seems that the condition was self-limiting in some way and no further cases have been reported.   In 1981 an hereditary degeneration (generalized progressive retinal atrophy) was described in Sweden by Narfstrom in the Abyssinian cat (Narfstrom, 1981).   Affected animals are young adults of both sexes and initial genetic studies again indicate a recessive mode of inheritance.   This condition has also been seen in the U.K.

   Another interesting retinopathy in the cat is due to a deficiency of the sulphur-containing amino acid, taurine (Burnett and Burger, 1980).   This condition occurs naturally in cats fed certain diets and can readily be produced experimentally by feeding casein-based taurine deficient diets.   Feline central retinal degeneration (FCRD) commences in the area centralis as a well defined focal and oval area of hyper-reflectivity with a darker border, which later extends just superior to the optic disc to join another, but smaller, oval area developing on the medial side of the disc. The affected area progresses, as long as the cat is kept on

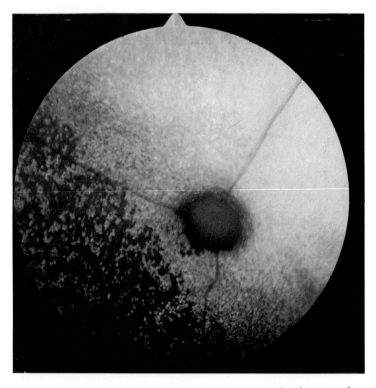

Fig. 5 *The Cat. Hereditary generalized retinal atrophy (Abyssinian, 6 months)*

a deficient diet, and ultimately the whole fundus is involved and attenuation of the retinal blood vessels becomes obvious. Throughout this condition there is a remarkable similarity between the shape of the retinal lesion and cone distribution in the cat's retina. The histopathological changes consist of degeneration of photoreceptors in the area centralis with preservation of photoreceptor nuclei immediately outside this zone. Loss of other layers occurs in advanced cases. The ERG changes show a reduction in amplitude of cone and rod ERGs and delayed implicit times.

The Horse

Retinal degeneration of any cause is not common in the horse in spite of the fact that many horses are allowed to live most of their natural lifespan, as are dogs and cats, (Barnett, 1971) but not the agricultural animals. Retinal degeneration in the horse, when it occurs, is probably post-inflammatory in origin although the aetiology is basically unknown. The majority of cases appear as a pigmentary change in the peripapillary region and appear to have little

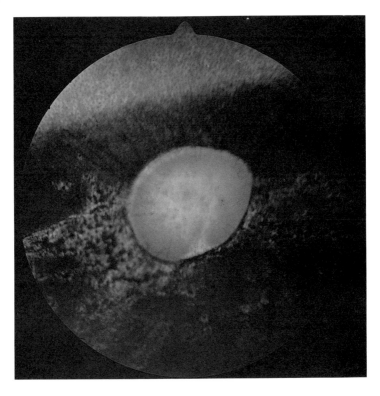

Fig.6 *The Horse. Peripapillary retinopathy.*

effect on vision. They are sometimes bilateral but not
symmetrical. It has been suggested that they may be associated with equine periodic ophthalmia (recurrent uveitis) but
this is not proven and certainly is not always the case.

One interesting case of retinal degeneration in a horse
occurred in an American-bred, yearling, thoroughbred colt.
The condition was bilaterally symmetrical and progressive
with ophthalmoscopic changes of hyper-reflectivity in the
tapetal fundus. Histology showed loss of the photoreceptor
layer. To date there is no evidence that this case was
hereditary but it showed remarkable similarities to generalized PRA in the dog and cat.

The Cow

Vitamin A deficiency as a cause of blindness in animals has
been known since Biblical times. Vitamin A deficiency
retinopathy in cattle still occurs under natural conditions,
particularly in the young rapidly growing beast, and was
very prevalent in recent years during the barley-fed beef

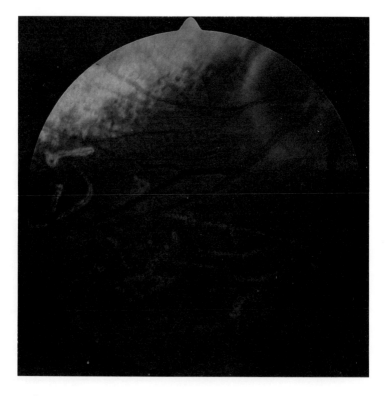

Fig.7 *The Cow. Vitamin A deficiency retinopathy.*

era (Barnett *et al.*, 1970).   The first clinical sign of hypo-
vitaminosis A in cattle is papilloedema due to raised
cerebrospinal fluid pressure and altered bone growth around
the optic nerve.   Papilloedema ultimately develops into optic
atrophy but, prior to this, retinal degeneration occurs,
appearing ophthalmoscopically as irregular focal areas mainly
in the non-tapetal fundus.   Histologically the changes were
confined to the outer retinal layers and choroid.   Retinal
degeneration due to vitamin A deficiency has also been described in the horse, dog, cat, rat and rabbit as an experimental condition.   It is interesting that in cattle no
corneal changes occurred even in field cases in totally
blind animals.

The Sheep

Bright blindness is a toxic retinopathy only occurring in
sheep and due to the ingestion of bracken (pteris aquilina)
(Barnett *et al.*, 1977).   It is a bilaterally symmetrical,
progressive, generalized retinopathy with ophthalmoscopic
changes of hyper-reflectivity in the tapetum lucidum pro-

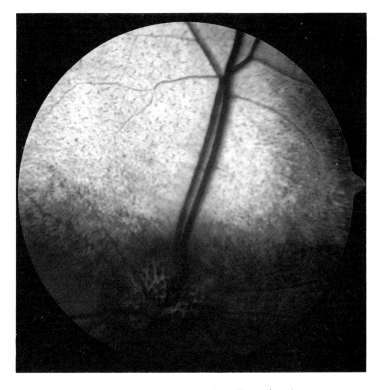

Fig. 8 *The Sheep.   Toxic retinopathy (bracken).*

ducing a mirror-like appearance, pallor of the tapetum
nigrum and visible choroidal vessels in some parts, attenuation of the retinal blood vessels and pupillary dilation.
Histologically, the photoreceptor layer is degenerate
together with portions of the outer nuclear layer. The
changes are most severe in the tapetal region with a gradual
change to less affected retina peripherally. This condition
occurs naturally in bracken infested areas in hill sheep
breeds, in particular Yorkshire, Lancashire, Durham,
Northumberland and Westmoreland, as well as in Scotland and
Wales. It can also be produced experimentally by feeding
bracken nuts to any breed of sheep.

CONCLUSION

Human retinal degenerations are evidently due to a multi-
plicity of causes. The availability of so many animal
conditions leading to retinal disease must offer a valuable
resource to the experimenter.

REFERENCES

Aguirre, G. (1976). Inherited retinal degenerations in the
    dog. *Transactions American Academy Ophthalmology and
    Otolaryngology* **81**, 667-676.
Barnett, K.C. (1972). The ocular fundus of the horse. *Equine
    Veterinary Journal* **4**, No. 1, 17-20.
Barnett, K.C. (1976). Comparative aspects of canine hereditary
    eye disease. *Advances in veterinary science and compara-
    tive medicine* **20**, 54-59.
Barnett, K.C., Palmer, A.C., Abrams, J.T., Bridge, P.S.,
    Spratling, F.R. and Sharman, I.M. (1970). Ocular changes
    associated with hypovitaminosis A in cattle. *The British
    Veterinary Journal* **126**, No. 11, 561-573.
Barnett, K.C., Blakemore, W.F. and Mason, J. (1972). Bracken
    retinopathy in sheep. *Transactions of the ophthalmolo-
    gical societies of the United Kingdom* **XCII**. 741-744.
Barnett, K.C. and Burger, I.H. (1980). Taurine deficiency
    retinopathy in the Cat. *J. Small Anim. Pract.* **21**, 521-534.
Magnusson, H. (1911). Uber retinitis pigmentosa und
    konsanguinitat beim hunde. *Arch. Vergleich Ophtalmol.*
    2, 147-163.
Narfstrom, K. (1981). Progressiv retinal atrofi hos
    abessinierkatt. *Svensk Veterinartidning* **33**, 6.

EFFECT OF ORNITHINE ON MACROMOLECULAR BIOSYNTHESIS IN EMBRYONIC PIGMENT EPITHELIUM

GERALD J. CHADER, SHAY-WHEY M. KOH and EILEEN MASTERSON

Laboratory of Vision Research, National Eye Institute, National Institutes of Health, Bethesda, MD 20205, USA

SUMMARY

The effects of ornithine and putrescine on macromolecular synthesis in embryonic chick retina and pigment epithelium (PE) *in vitro* were investigated. Ornithine (20 mM) greatly inhibited protein synthesis but not incorporation of glucose into macromolecules. Putrescine (20 μM) inhibited protein synthesis in young cultured PE cells but a stimulatory effect was seen in older cells. An abnormally high ornithine or putrescine level could thus adversely affect protein synthesis during embryonic and/or early neonatal development and may contribute to cellular dysfunction in Gyrate Atrophy.

INTRODUCTION

Gyrate atrophy (GA) is a hereditary disease characterized by progressive chorioretinal degeneration (Simell and Takki, 1973). Ocular findings include myopia, cataract, night blindness, constricted visual fields, diminished ERG response, and the appearance of well-defined areas of chorioretinal atrophy in the midperiphery at about the time of puberty. Systemically, histological changes in muscle fibres and liver mitochondria have been reported (McCulloch and Marliss, 1975; Arshinoff *et al.*, 1979) which may involve degeneration of type 2 fibres (Sipila *et al.*, 1979; Kaiser-Kupfer *et al.*, 1981).

Biochemically, affected patients have plasma ornithine levels that are 10- to 20-fold above normal (Simell and Takki, 1973). In 1974, Takki (Takki, 1974) reported a deficiency in the enzyme ornithine: 2-oxoacid aminotransferase in a liver biopsy of a GA patient although no data were

given. Subsequently, definitive evidence for such a deficiency has been given for transformed lymphocytes (Valle
et al., 1977) and cultured fibroblasts (Sengers *et al.*, 1976;
O'Donnell, *et al.*, 1977, 1978; Shih *et al.*, 1978) of GA
patients and heterozygous carriers.

The high ornithine levels may adversely affect a variety
of important metabolic pathways and functions in the body
including creatine biosynthesis (Sipila *et al.*, 1979) and
inhibition of the enzyme arginine-glycine amidinotransferase
(Sipila, 1980). Sipila *et al.* (1979) and Kaiser-Kupfer *et
al.* (1981) have shown marked systemic effects in GA patients
with striking tubular aggregates in muscle tissue. Moreover, exogenous ornithine was found to be toxic to cultured
muscle cells from GA patients in contrast to the lack of
such an effect in muscle cells from control patients (Askan-
sas *et al.*, 1980; Kaiser-Kupfer *et al.*, 1981). In the present communication we report on the acute effect of high
ornithine concentration on macromolecular synthesis in pigment epithelium (PE) and neural retina of the chick embryo.

MATERIALS AND METHODS

Tissue Culture

White leghorn embryonic chick PE cells were dissected and
dissociated as previously described (Redfern *et al.*, 1976).
Cultures were seeded at approximately 200,000 cells/35 mm
culture dish (Falcon Plastics, Los Angeles, CA) and maintained in 1.5 ml of Eagles' No. 2 Minimal Essential Medium
(NIH media unit) containing 5% heat-inactivated fetal calf
serum (GIBCO, Grand Island, NY).

Macromolecular Synthesis

Tissue culture medium from culture dishes was decanted and
2 ml of Glucose-Bicarbonate Ringer's (GBR) solution, pH 7.4,
added. The GBR contained test substances at appropriate concentrations. Cells were incubated for 2 h at 37°C followed
by addition of approximately 2,203,400 dpm of ^{3}H-leucine
(New England Nuclear, sp. act. 5.0 Ci/mmol) or of ^{14}C-
glucose (51.6 mCi/mmol) to each culture dish. Incubation
was continued for an additional 30 min. At the end of this
time, cells were scraped from the plate, homogenized in
2.0 ml of GBR; 0.5 ml of a 5% trichloracetic acid (TCA)
solution was then added and the suspension was sonicated to
disrupt the cells. After a 30 min extraction period at 4°C,
the homogenate was filtered (Watman No. 2) and the filter

washed three times with cold TCA solution and three times
with acetone. Filter papers were treated with 2.0 ml NCS
solubilizer (New England Nuclear Corp.) plus 200 μl of water
overnight and assayed for radioactivity.

In other experiments, pigment epithelial sheets or neural
retinal tissue was cleanly dissected from embryonic eyes for
organ incubation. In general, the tissue equivalent of two
retinas or three pigment epithelia were pooled for each incubation flask. The same experimental procedure as above
was then followed. Results were normalized for protein by
the method of Lowry *et al.* (1951).

RESULTS

PE cells in culture for about two weeks are well-differentiated
and non-dividing in the central portion of each colony but
are still actively dividing at the periphery (Fig. 1). In
cells of this age, ^{3}H-leucine is readily incorporated into

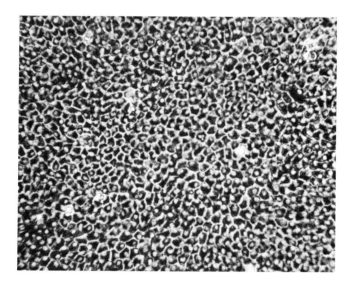

Fig. 1 *Typical pigment epithelial cells in culture for
approximately two weeks.*

protein over the 30 minute incubation period (Table 1). Preincubation of the cells for 2 h with 20 mM ornithine decreased incorporation by about 4-fold. Similarly, 20 μM
putrescine greatly inhibited protein synthesis although
putrescine at a concentration of 2 μM had no significant

TABLE 1

Macromolecular synthesis in cultured pigment epithelial cells

Condition	^{3}H-leucine incorp. (dpm/mg protein)	^{14}C-glucose incorp. (dpm/mg protein)
A) 13 DAY OLD CELLS		
control	114,850 ± 21,160	1350 ± 910
+ 20 mM ornithine	27,010 ± 3,850	1430 ± 160
+ 20 µM putrescine	28,010 ± 1,700	1140 ± 210
+ 2 µM putrescine	130,920 ± 1,730	1030 ± 430
B) 30 DAY OLD CELLS		
control	331,810 ± 63,190	10,109 ± 2,180
+ 20 mM ornithine	71,990 ± 10,030	7,848 ± 2,410
+ 20 µM putrescine	656,750 ± 79,750	–
+ 20 µM putrescine	572,890 ± 71,010	–

For cell cultures, PE cells were dissected from 9 day old embryos and were maintained in culture for 13 or 30 days before use. Subsequently, the tissue culture medium was removed, 2 ml Glucose-Bicarbonate Ringers' solution with or without ornithine or putrescine was added and cells were incubated at 37°C for 2 h. ^{3}H-Leucine or ^{14}C-glucose was then added, cells incubated for an additional 30 min, cells collected and assayed for radioactive precursor incorporation into macromolecules. Values given are $\overline{X}$ ± S.E. of 6 to 8 replicate culture places.

effect. Incorporation of ^{14}C-glucose into macromolecules was not significantly altered by the presence of ornithine or putrescine.

Somewhat surprisingly, basal incorporation of ^{3}H-leucine into protein was almost 3-fold higher in 30 day old cultures than in 13 day old cultures (Table 1B); ^{14}C-glucose incorporation was also higher. Ornithine inhibited protein synthesis by about 4.7-fold but had no significant effect on ^{14}C-glucose incorporation as seen in the 2 week old cultures. In contrast to the 2 week old cultures however, putrescine had a distinct stimulatory effect on protein synthesis both at the 20 and 2 μM concentrations.

Organ incubation of relatively intact sheets of freshly dissected PE cells and neural retina was also conducted (Table 2). In PE cells (Table 2A), the presence of 20 mM ornithine inhibited protein synthesis (2.6 fold) but had a small stimulatory effect on ^{14}C-glucose incorporation. Putrescine appeared to have a small stimulatory effect on

TABLE 2

Macromolecular synthesis in incubated retinal and pigment epithelial tissues

Condition	^{3}H-leucine incorp. (dpm/mg protein)	^{14}C-glucose incorp. (dpm/mg protein)
A) PIGMENT EPITHELIUM		
control	89,650 ± 9,480	11,640 ± 980
+ 20 mM ornithine	34,810 ± 2,900	15,680 ± 1,400
+ 20 μM putrescine	110,440 ± 12,680	16,770 ± 1,140
+ 2 μM putrescine	140,550 ± 16,760	23,130 ± 1,620
B) NEURAL RETINA		
control	52,270 ± 2,560	1,280 ± 430
+ 20 mM ornithine	29,630 ± 1,780	1,820 ± 490
+ 20 μM putrescine	49,020 ± 1,760	1,400 ± 310
+ 2 μM putrescine	64,010 ± 6,580	2,850 ± 810

Tissues were dissected from 7 day old embryos. The equivalent of three pigment epithelia or 2 retinas was pooled for each experimental parameter. Other conditions are given in Table 1. Values given are $\bar{X}$ ± S.E.

protein synthesis (although not statistically significant) and a definite increase in ^{14}C-glucose incorporation. In the neural retina under these conditions (Table 2B), protein synthesis, as well as ^{14}C-glucose incorporation was somewhat lower than in the PE sheets possibly due to differential diffusion of the radiolabeled amino acid into the multilayer retina versus the single cell thick sheets of pigment epithelium. A 1.8 fold inhibition of protein synthesis was observed with 20 mM ornithine with no significant effect on ^{14}C-glucose incorporation. Putrescine at 20 µM had no effect on macromolecular biosynthesis although some stimulation was observed at the 2 µM level.

In a separate series of experiments (Table 3), the specificity of the ornithine effect was examined. Incorporation of ^{3}H-leucine in control cultures and those treated with 20 mM ornithine was 108,750 and 16,910 dpm/mg protein respectively, a 6.4-fold inhibition by ornithine (Table 3A). In

TABLE 3

Comparative effect of ornithine and arginine on protein synthesis in embryonic chick pigment epithelium

Condition	^{3}H-Leucine incorporation (dpm/mg protein)
A) CELL CULTURE	
control	108,750 ± 21,430
+ 20 mM ornithine	16,910 ± 3,900
+ 20 mM arginine	38,530 ± 7,750
B) TISSUE INCUBATION	
control	96,250 ± 6,380
+ 20 mM ornithine	21,110 ± 1,020
+ 20 mM arginine	17,190 ± 2,860

For cell cultures, PE cells were dissected from 9 day old embryos and were maintained in culture for 14 days before use. For tissue incubation, PE sheets were dissected from 10 day old embryos. Incubation conditions were as given in Table 1. Values given are $\bar{X}$ ± S.E.

comparison, incorporation by cells similarly treated with 20 mM arginine exhibited only a 2.8-fold inhibition of incorporation. With incubation of freshly dissected sheets of PE cells (Table 3B), ornithine and arginine have a 4.6- and 5.6-fold inhibitory effect respectively.

DISCUSSION

Ornithine is best known as a component of the urea cycle where it aids in ammonia detoxification. Besides this, it is important in several other, less well-known metabolic pathways (Fig. 2). The missing enzyme in gyrate atrophy, ornithine transaminase (OTA) begins the conversion of orni-thine to glutamic acid under normal circumstances. Sub-sequently, glutathione can be formed or, in another meta-bolic pathway, γ-amino butyric acid (GABA) and ultimately carnitine which is involved in fatty acid oxidation. Orni-thine has also recently been found to be a direct pre-cursor of proline (Mestichelli et al., 1979). Through decarboxylation by ornithine decarboxylase, polyamines such as putrescine are formed which play a pivotal role in DNA synthesis, cell replication and embryonic differentiation. Ornithine is also involved in creatine phosphate biosynthesis since the amino acid is a precursor for creatine through a guanidoacetic acid intermediate. Interestingly, the amidino-transferase enzyme has been shown to be inhibited by orni-thine, thus both low and high ornithine levels can affect cellular energy levels.

The specific cause of the pathology in gyrate atrophy has not been pinpointed. High ornithine itself may directly inhibit an important metabolic process causing the de-generation although a report in the literature (Fell et al., 1974) indicates that hyperornithinemia per se is apparently not always linked with chorioretinal atrophy. Theoretically, a decrease in product subsequent to the OAT enzyme defi-ciency and/or an increase in product from another of the metabolic pathways depicted in Fig. 2 could be involved in the disease. Serum ornithine in GA patients is high but other serum amino acids such as glutamic acid, glutamine and proline are close to normal. Determinations using whole blood (Arshinoff et al., 1979), however, demonstrate a decrease in circulating glutamate and glutamine, leaving open the question of a relatively subtle derangement in general amino acid metabolism, use of amino acids as neuro-transmitters (e.g., GABA, glutamic acid) or in protein syn-thesis (e.g., collagen). The work of Sipila and coworkers (Sipila et al., 1979; Sipila, 1980) offers strong evidence that ornithine can directly impair cellular metabolism by inhibiting the mitochondrial enzyme, ornithine trans-aminidase. This would cause a deficiency in creatine and creatine-P with a subsequent deficit in cellular energy equivalents and may be one mechanism for the pathological changes seen in choroid, pigment epithelium and retina and in the formation of tubular aggregates in type II muscle

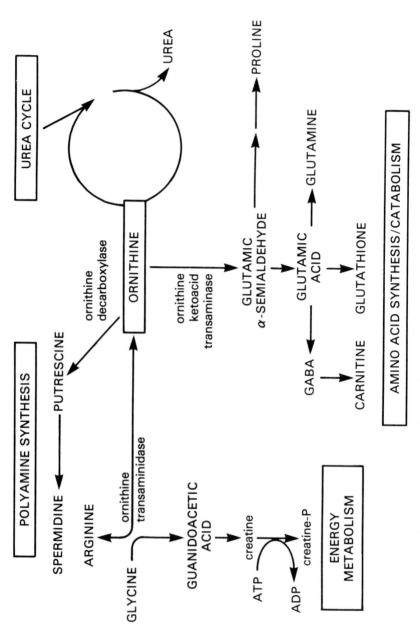

Fig. 2 *Major metabolic pathways involving ornithine.*

fibres (Sipila *et al.*, 1979; Kaiser-Kupfer *et al.*, 1981).
It is interesting that morphologically abnormal mitochondria
have been described in liver biopsy specimens from a GA
patient (Arshinoff *et al.*, 1979).

A recent study of Kuwabara *et al.* (1981) has shown that
intravitreal injection of ornithine *in vivo* leads to rapid
swelling of PE cells (within 4 h) followed by PE cell degeneration and subsequent degeneration of retinal photoreceptor cells. This indicates the rapidity with which a
high ornithine concentration can affect the pigment epithelium of even an adult animal. In our study, high ornithine quickly inhibited protein synthesis in embryonic cultured PE cells and in organ incubations of both embryonic
PE and retina. Even though the concentration of ornithine
used in the present experiments was about 10-fold higher than
the 1-2 mM ornithine levels chronically observed in the
serum of GA patients, it was effective within the acute
2.5 h incubation period and could very well have a similar
inhibitory effect in the embryo *in vivo* at a lower concentration but over a much longer, chronic period of time.
The effect is relatively specific for protein synthesis
since ornithine did not markedly alter ^{14}C-glucose incorporation into macromolecules. The effect on protein synthesis is not specific for ornithine though since a high
level of a similar basic amino acid, arginine, also inhibited ^{3}H-leucine incorporation into protein to approximately the same extent particularly in the tissue incubation
experiments. This is not a troublesome finding however,
since there is no *a priori* reason why substances other than
ornithine (and putrescine) should not interfere with normal
protein synthesis in a cell.

Putrescine is a polyamine product of ornithine decarboxylase that is a well known promoter of cell division and
hyperplasia *in vivo* and in cell culture. We felt that its
concentration may rise in some tissues of GA patients due
to the increased circulating ornithine levels and may cause
selective damage particularly to cells that normally would be
postmitotic by the time of late fetal development (e.g., PE).
Our results show markedly different effects of the polyamine
under the differing conditions of our experiments. In two
week old cultured cells, 20 µM putrescine was as effective
as 20 mM ornithine in inhibiting protein synthesis. In contrast, in 30 day old cells, both 20 and 2 µM putrescine
actually stimulated protein synthesis as it also did to
a lesser extent under the organ culture conditions. Although
complex, these results indicate that increased polyamine
synthesis could play a role in the etiology of the disease
either in inhibiting normal metabolism in early development

or stimulating synthetic machinery at an inappropriate time or to an inappropriate extent. Future studies should include an investigation of the effects of polyamines (putrescine and spermidine) on DNA synthesis.

The present study certainly does not give direct evidence that protein synthesis is actually altered by ornithine or putrescine *in vivo* during embryonic development in patients with GA. It does indicate however that this is a distinct possibility and that such an alteration may at least contribute to the pathogenesis of the disease in the human as a primary factor in the PE or a secondary contributing factor in the retinal photoreceptor cell during the critical stages of embryonic development.

REFERENCES

Arshinoff, S., McCulloch, C., Matuk, Y., Phillips, M., Gordon, B. and Marliss, E. (1979). Amino acid metabolism and liver ultrastructure in hyperornithemia with gyrate atrophy of the choroid and retina. *Metabolism Clin. Exptl*. **28**, 979–988.

Askanas, V., Valle, D. ad Kaiser-Kupfer (1980). Cultured muscle fibres of gyrate atrophy patients: tubules, ornithine toxicity and 1-ornithine-2-oxoacid aminotransferase (OAT). *Neurology* **30**, 368.

Fell, V., Pollitt, R., Sampson, G. and Wright, T. (1974). Ornithinemia, hyperammonemia and homocitrullinuria: A disease associated with mental retardation and possibly caused by defective mitochondrial transport. *Am. J. Dis. Child*. **127**, 752–760.

Kaiser-Kupfer, M., Kuwabara, T., Askanas, V., Brody, L., Takki, K., Dvoretzy, I. and Engel, W. (1981). Systemic manifestations of gyrate atrophy of the choroid and retina. *Ophthalmology* **88**, 302–306.

Kuwabara, T., Ishikawa, Y. and Kaiser-Kupfer, M. (1981). Experimental model of gyrate atrophy in animals. *Ophthalmology* **88**, 331-334.

Lowry, O., Rosebrough, J., Farr, A. and Randall, R. (1951). Protein measurement with Folin phenol reagent. *J. Biol. Chem*. **193**, 265–275.

McCulloch, C. and Marliss, E. (1975). Gyrate atrophy of the choroid and retina with hyperornithinemia. *Am. J. Ophthalmol*. **80**, 1047–1057.

Mestichelli, L., Gupta, R. and Spenser, I. (1979). The biosynthetic route from ornithine to proline. *J. Biol. Chem*. **254**, 640–647.

O'Donnell, J., Sandman, R. and Martin, S. (1977). Deficient

L-ornithine: 2-oxoacid aminotransferase activity in cultured fibroblasts from a patient with gyrate atrophy of
the retina. *Biochem. Biophys. Res. Comm.* **79**, 396–399.

O'Donnell, J., Sandman, R. and Martin, S. (1978). Gyrate
atrophy of the retina: inborn error of L-ornithine: 2-
oxoacid aminotransferase. *Science* **200**, 200–201.

Redfern, N., Israel, P., Bergsma, D., Robison, W., Whike-
hart, D. and Chader, G. (1976). Neural retinal and pigment epithelial cells in culture. Patterns of differentiation and effects of prostaglandins and cyclic
AMP on pigmentation. *Exp. Eye Res*. **22**, 559–568.

Sengers, R., Trijbels, J., Brussaart, J. and Deutman, A.
(1976). Gyrate atrophy of the choroid and retina and
ornithine-ketoacid aminotransferase deficiency. *Pediatr*.
Res. **10**, 894.

Shih, V., Berson, E., Mandell, R. and Schmidt, S. (1978).
Ornithine ketoacid transaminase deficiency in gyrate
atrophy of the choroid and retina. *Am. J. Hum. Genet*.
30, 174–179.

Simell, O. and Takki, K. (1973). Raised plasma-ornithine
and gyrate atrophy of the choroid and retina. *Lancet* **1**,
1030–1033.

Sipila, I. (1980). Inhibition of arginine-glycine amidino-
transferase by ornithine. *Biochim. Biophys. Acta* **613**,
79–84.

Sipila, I., Simell, O., Rapola, J., Sainio, K. and Tuuteri,
L. (1979). Gyrate atrophy of the choroid and retina with
hyperornithinemia: tubular aggregates and type 2 fibre
atrophy in muscle. *Neurology* **29**, 996–1005.

Takki, K. (1974). Gyrate atrophy of the choroid and retina
associated with hyperornithinaemia. *Br. J. Ophthalmol*.
58, 3–23.

Valle, D., Kaiser-Kupfer, M. and Del Valle, L. (1977).
Gyrate atrophy of the choroid and retina: deficiency of
ornithine amino-transferase in transformed lymphocytes.
Proc. Nat. Acad. Sci. (USA) **74**, 5159–5161.

IODOACETATE-INDUCED DEGENERATION OF CONE VISUAL CELLS IN GROUND SQUIRREL RETINA

DEBORA B. FARBER and DAVID G. CHASE

Jules Stein Eye Institute, UCLA School of Medicine,
Los Angeles, California 90024, USA
and the
Developmental Neurology Laboratory
and the
Cell Biology Research Laboratory,
Veterans Administration Medical Center,
Sepulveda, California 91343, USA

During the last few years, extraordinary progress has been made in the understanding of the morphology, chemistry, electro-physiology and cellular biology of the normal retina. A wealth of information has become available from which improvements in clinical eye care are continuously evolving. However, the etiology or treatment of blinding diseases such as Retinitis Pigmentosa has not been established as yet.

In Retinitis Pigmentosa, the basic elements of the visual process, the photoreceptors, malfunction and die. Studies of normal animal retinas, with which planned investigations can be accomplished, have demonstrated that visual cells are char-acterized by their unique metabolic and synthetic properties, by their membrane composition and dynamics as well as by their specific vulnerability to chemical and physical agents. Further-more, work with animal models of retinal degeneration has helped to elucidate not only the localization of some important components of the photoreceptors but also the description and identification of morphological and biochemical changes that occur before, during, and after the process of cell death. For example, it is now known that the rod-dominant retinas of mice, which are homozygous for the rd gene, are affected with an abnormality in cyclic GMP metabolism that precedes the death of the vast population of rod photoreceptors (Farber and Lolley, 1974). The same is true for the rod-cone dysplasia of the duplex retina (containing rods and cones) of Irish setter dogs (Aguire *et al.*, 1978). The accumulation of cyclic

GMP in the visual cells, as a consequence of defective phosphodiesterase (Farber and Lolley, 1976), and uninhibited
guanylate cyclase activities (Lolley *et al.*, 1980) seems
to promote the degeneration of the photoreceptors. A similar
situation was created in normal retinas of toad embryos
maintained *in vitro* which confirmed the toxic effect of cyclic
GMP specifically on visual cells (Lolley *et al.*, 1977) in
the *rd* mouse and Irish setter dog diseases, the degeneration
of rods occurs prior to that of cones. During the progress
of the pathological condition and following the removal of
cone outer segments, cone cell bodies continue for some time
to have synaptic contact with horizontal and bipolar cells.
This survival may account for the residual photoreceptive
capacity of animals with advanced retinal degeneration (Noell
et al., 1971). Cone cell death in these diseases may then
be a secondary event, probably the consequence of lack of
support by rods.

   Cyclic GMP is enriched in normal rod photoreceptors;
its concentration is higher by severalfold than that in cone
visual cells, and it is regulated by light. This suggests
a role for cyclic GMP in the function or metabolism of rod
photoreceptors. Furthermore, rods malfunction and die when
they have an imbalance in cyclic GMP synthesis and degradation which results in abnormal levels of this cyclic nucleotide.

   Comparable genetic models for studying the cause and
development of degeneration of cone photoreceptors are not
available. Yet, it is very important to learn which kind
of metabolic or control mechanisms operate in cones since
these cells are also affected in several human blinding
diseases including Retinitis Pigmentosa.

   We have been able to induce cone degeneration in the
cone-dominant retina of ground squirrel by iodoacetic acid
treatment (Farber *et al.*, 1981). Iodoacetate was injected
intracardially in one or two doses of 20 mg/kg body weight
each, given 24 h apart.

   Iodoacetic acid exposure of less than 24 h had little
effect on retinal morphology. By 24 h, however, altered cone
cells were observed. Ten to 15% of the cone cells were degenerating and had dense cytoplasm and pycnotic nuclei whereas
the remaining photoreceptors showed minor changes in outer
segments and pedicles. Otherwise, retinal morphology was
normal.

   After 3 days of exposure to iodoacetate about one-half
of the photoreceptors were in advanced stages of degeneration,
and outer segments, synaptic ribbons and synaptic vesicles
were significantly reduced in number in the remaining intact
cone cells. Pigment epithelial and other retinal cells were

still relatively unchanged. Small numbers of macrophages
were present at the inner margin of the photoreceptor layer.

The photoreceptor layer contained only dense cone cells
with pycnotic nuclei and occasional macrophages in the 4-day
iodoacetate-treated retina. Pigment epithelial cells were
also markedly altered. Basal infoldings were replaced by flat
surface and apical processes were swollen and fused. Pigment
granules were not confined to apical cytoplasm, as in control
retinas of non-treated ground squirrels, but were scattered
randomly throughout the cells. The outer limiting membrane
was still apparent but pursued an irregular course and was
often interrupted. Macrophages were present in small numbers.
Occasional pycnotic nuclei were seen in the inner nuclear layer.

These same features also characterized the 10-day iodoacetate-treated retina. Greater inward expansion of the
apical surfaces of pigment epithelial cells and disappearance
of the outer limiting membrane were the major differences
noted.

In 4- and 10-day iodoacetate-treated retinas, there
was little evidence to suggest that removal of photoreceptor
cell debris had occurred to any great extent. The layer of
debris was unbroken and contained recognizable synaptic,
nuclear, inner segment and outer segment components still in
their typical inner to outer sequence.

More advanced retinal degeneration was evidenced in the
11-day retina by the presence of a greater number of macrophages, many of which contained photoreceptor and pigment
epithelial cell debris, and by partial removal of photoreceptor debris. The removal of debris was patchy and varied
in degree in different areas of the retina. Thus, alternat-
ing patches of photoreceptor layer were either empty, leaving
pigment epithelium in contact with second order neurons, contained macrophages alone, contained macrophages and inner and
outer segment debris or contained macrophages plus an intact
layer of debris. Macrophages were also seen around blood
vessels in the inner retinal layers and in the inner nuclear
layer. They were always located vitread of cone cell debris
and never appeared in the pigment epithelium. The distribution of macrophages suggests that they entered the neuroretina from the circulation, moved into the photoreceptor
layer and phagocytized cone cell debris and fragments of cast
off pigment epithelial cells in a pedicle to outer segment
sequence, and then departed the area. There was no evidence
to suggest that the pigment epithelium participated in the
removal of dead cone cells.

Another interesting feature of this preparation was that
pigment epithelium was most severely modified, where it con-
tacted photoreceptor debris, and showed a partial return

toward normal morphology in areas of reduced or no contact
with debris. This suggests that the modification of the
pigment epithelium was secondary to that of photoreceptors.
Cells of the inner retinal layers survived the degeneration
of the photoreceptor layer. Occasionally, a few scattered
pycnotic nuclei corresponding to horizontal cells were observed.

We have reported previously that in contrast to rod-
dominant retinas, the normal ground squirrel retina is enriched in cyclic AMP and has considerably lower levels of
cyclic GMP. Furthermore, light reduces selectively the concentration of cyclic AMP with no significant effect on that
of cyclic GMP (Farber *et al.*, 1981).

With iodoacetic acid treatments, the levels of cyclic AMP
in dark-adapted ground squirrel retina were rapidly increased
and had doubled by 24 h after injection. At this time, light
did not reduce any longer the cyclic AMP content of the experimental retina. Between one and three days after iodoacetate injection, when the photoreceptors were actively
degenerating, cyclic AMP levels dropped sharply and stabilized at about 50 to 55% of the dark-adapted level of control
retina.

Changes in cyclic GMP concentration with iodoacetic acid
treatment followed a pattern similar to that observed for
cyclic AMP. Levels increased rapidly and were maximal
(3 to 4 times higher than control) at about 4 to 5 hours
post-injection. Then, they declined gradually, but, by day
1, they were still above the concentration present in untreated retinas. At day 4 and later, cyclic GMP could be
barely detected in the experimental retina.

The biochemical results described above resemble those
observed in the degenerating retinas of *rd* mice during
development. The main difference is that whereas in the *rd*
mice only cyclic GMP becomes elevated prior to the pathological morphology of the cells, in the iodoacetic acid-
treated retina, cyclic AMP and cyclic GMP both reach values
much higher than normal before any sign of degeneration is
detected. This may be related to a non-specific blockage
by iodoacetic acid of all types of phosphodiesterase activity present in the ground squirrel retina (Farber and Souza,
1981). In fact, iodoacetate is a potent inhibitor of sulf-
hydryl enzymes. We have found that, at least in the test
tube, it prevents the hydrolysis of cyclic nucleotides. This
may also explain the loss of sensitivity to light of retinal
cyclic AMP that we observe after iodoacetic acid treatment.

Another point that became clear through this work is the
localization of cyclic nucleotides within the ground squirrel
retina. After the iodoacetic acid-induced degeneration and

removal of the cones, about 50% of cyclic AMP and almost no cyclic GMP were present in the surviving inner layers (Farber *et al.*, 1981). This indicates that cyclic AMP is evenly distributed between the photoreceptor and inner layers of the ground squirrel retina, whereas the low levels of cyclic GMP are localized only in the cone visual cells.

In summary, these studies provide a temporal sequence of morphological and biochemical observations through the early stages of cone cell damage and debris clearance in the cone-dominant retina of the ground squirrel. We have shown that the levels of cyclic AMP and cyclic GMP become elevated soon after iodoacetic acid injection and prior to the degeneration of the visual cells. However, it has not been established whether cyclic AMP or cyclic GMP independently or in a combined action may lead to the destruction of the cone photoreceptors. Future studies will have to answer this question.

ACKNOWLEDGEMENTS

We would like to thank Dennis Souza for his assistance in the laboratory and Louise V. Eaton and Inga L. Anderson for their help in the preparation of the manuscript. This work was supported by NIH grants EY 2651 and RCDA 5-K04-EY144 to Debora B. Farber and by the Medical Research Service of the Veterans Administration.

REFERENCES

Aguirre, G., Farber, D., Lolley, R., Fletcher, R.T. and Chader, G.J. (1978). Rod-cone dysplasia in Irish setters: a defect in cyclic GMP metabolism in visual cells. *Science* **201**, 1133-1134.

Farber, D.B. and Lolley, R.N. (1974). Cyclic guanosine monophosphate elevation in degenerating photoreceptor cells of the C_3H mouse retina. *Science* **186**, 449-451.

Farber, D.B. and Lolley, R.N. (1976). Enzymic basis for cyclic GMP accumulation in degenerative photoreceptor cells of mouse retina. *J. Cyclic Nucleotide Res*. **2**, 139-148.

Farber, D.B. and Souza, D.W. (1981). Phosphodiesterase of the cone-dominant ground squirrel retina. *Soc. Neurosci. Abstracts* **7**, 918.

Farber, D.B., Souza, D.W., Chase, D. and Lolley, R.N. (1981). Cyclic nucleotides of cone-dominant retinas. *Invest. Ophthalmol. Vis. Sci.* **20**, 24-31.

Lolley, R.N., Farber, D.B., Rayborn, M.E., and Holleyfield,
    J.G., (1977). Cyclic GMP accumulation causes degeneration
    of photoreceptor cells: simulation of an inherited disease.
    Science **196**, 664–666.
Lolley, R.N., Rayborn, M.E., Holleyfield, J.G. and Farber,
    D.B. (1980). Cyclic GMP and visual cell degeneration in
    the inherited disorder of *rd* mice: a progress report.
    Vision Research **20**, 1157–1161.
Noell, W.K., Delmelle, M.C. and Albrecht, R. (1971). Vitamin
    A deficiency effect on the retina: dependence on light.
    Science **172**, 72–76.

EFFECTS OF VITAMIN A DEPRIVATION ON RCS (DYSTROPHIC) AND RCS-rdy[+] (CONGENIC) RATS

[+]E.R. BERMAN, *M. KAITZ and [+]N. SEGAL

*[+]Eye Biochemistry Unit and *Vision Research Laboratory,
Department of Ophthalmology, Hadassah University Hospital,
Jerusalem, Israel*

INTRODUCTION

Accumulation of lamellar debris in the interphotoreceptor
matrix and impaired phagocytic capabilities of the pigment
epithelium are the morphological hallmarks of the inherited
dystrophy in the RCS rat (Dowling and Sidman, 1962; Herron
et al., 1969; Bok and Hall, 1971). The elegant studies of
Mullen and LaVail (1975) using chimeric rats leave little
doubt that the gene acts solely in the pigment epithelium.
Certain aspects of the dystrophy, such as loss of vision
and diminution of ERG amplitude, bear some resemblance
to a vitamin A deficiency state in albino rats (Dowling
and Wald, 1958; Dowling, 1960). However, despite these
superficial similarities, the inherited and induced degenerations are undoubtedly caused by unrelated mechanisms.
Nevertheless the possibility of a defect in retinoid metabolism in the RCS rat remains an open and compelling question.
For example, there are reports of a slight excess of retinol
in the pigment epithelium of RCS rats, with more accumulating in the light-adapted state (Reading, 1970) than in dim
cyclic illumination (Berman *et al.*, 1981). Curiously however, vitamin A deficiency accelerates the retinal degeneration as measured electrophysiologically in the RCS rat
(Delmelle *et al.*, 1975). In addition, it has been shown
that vitamin A-deficient RCS rats have less lipofuscin in
their pigment epithelium than dystrophic rats maintained
on normal vitamin A intake (Robison *et al.*, 1980). The
more recent finding of a defect in retinol esterifying
enzyme in the pigment epithelium of RCS rats also suggests
hitherto unsuspected complexities of vitamin A metabolism
in the RCS rat (Berman *et al.*, 1981).

These observations prompted us to undertake an integrated study of the effects of vitamin A deprivation on the physical characteristics, biochemistry and electroretinographic responses of both the RCS (dystrophic) and RCS-rdy^+* (congenic) strains of rats. We now report that retinoic acid does not maintain growth or epithelial differentiation to the same extent in vitamin A-deprived RCS strains as it does in albino rats. Moreover vitamin A deficient dystrophic RCS rats show a rapid and immediate loss of visual function (ERG) compared to their nondeprived counterparts (Kaitz, 1982). The RCS-rdy^+ and albino strains are similarly affected, but only after much more prolonged deprivation.

MATERIALS AND METHODS

The albino rats, descendants of the Wistar strain, were obtained from the Hebrew University breeding farm. The RCS and RCS-rdy^+ strains were descendants of breeding pairs kindly supplied by Drs M.O. Hall and M.M. LaVail. All animals were maintained in 12-hr cyclic light of 15 to 20 ft-candles. The diets for the control (A^+) animals consisted of standard laboratory pellets containing 10 mg/kg of vitamin A equivalent. For the deprived animals, vitamin A restriction was initiated in pregnant dams and continued throughout lactation and weaning of litters. This diet was prepared according to Muto *et al.* (1972) and contained 12 mg/kg of retinoic acid. Weights of both control and experimental animals were recorded 3 to 4 times a week. ERG studies (Kaitz and Auerbach, 1980) and biochemical analyses (Berman *et al.*, 1979, 1980) were performed at weaning, and at intervals of 10 days thereafter.

RESULTS

Growth Characteristics

As shown in Fig. 1, the RCS and RCS-rdy^+ strains have indistinguishable growth patterns on standard (A^+) diets, both being about 25% smaller than their albino counterparts. Whereas vitamin A deprivation had little detectable effect on the growth rates of the albino rats, the RCS strains on A^- diets were significantly smaller than A^+ controls. During

---

*Retinal dystrophy (rdy) is an autosomal recessive character occurring in the RCS rat. Its normal counterpart in the same (congenic) genetic background is referred to as rdy^+ (Eds)

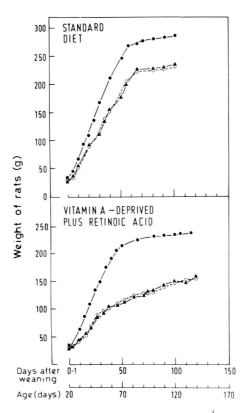

Fig. 1 *Growth rates of albino (●), RCS-rdy⁺ (○) and RCS (▲) rats on standard laboratory diets and on vitamin A-deficient diets supplemented with retinoic acid (12 mg/kg ration). Each point represents the average of 6 or more animals, with approximately equal numbers of males and females.*

the first 3 to 4 weeks of the dietary regime, the RCS rats weighed about 10 to 20% less than their A⁺ counterparts. Afterward their rate of growth was even slower, relative to RCS rats on A⁺ diets, and at maturity, the deprived RCS rats were about 50 to 60% of the size and weight of RCS animals on A⁺ diets. There was however great variability in body size among the A⁻ RCS animals, with individual weights varying from about 55 to 75% of those of A⁺ RCS rats. This variability could not be attributed to either the sex or the size of the litters. Correspondingly, the mortality rate of the deprived RCS strains was higher than that of either A⁺ RCS rats or A⁻ albino rats. We noted that a higher proportion of deprived RCS dystrophic rats died under this dietary regime than RCS congenic A⁻ animals,

and the deaths usually occurred between the 7th and 9th weeks
of life.

Physical Appearance

All of the animals on A^+ diets, regardless of strain, as well
as albino rats receiving A^- diets, were in good health and
normal in appearance. By contrast, the majority of RCS
animals on A^- diets showed abnormal fur from about 50 days
of age onward. Again, the variability in this characteristic
should be emphasized. Within a given litter, some rats showed
only small patches of thin or fallen hair while in more
extreme cases, the animals were completely denuded. Others
retained an essentially normal coat, which was however
usually lack-luster and pale in appearance. There was no
obvious correlation between the extent of hair loss, poor
weight gain, stunted growth or mortality.

Vitamin A in Liver and Blood

Hepatic vitamin A levels at weaning were nearly identical
in all animals fed A^+ diets regardless of strain. The absolute amount varied from 17 to 30 µg/g liver. Surprisingly,
by 20 days after weaning (40 to 42 days of age) the average
liver stores of vitamin A were about 20% higher in the albino
rats on A^+ diets than in the RCS strains fed the same rat
chow (Table 1). There was however again a broad range of
values among individual animals and the differences were
not statistically significant ($P > .05$).
     The decline of vitamin A stores in the liver of all de-
prived animals was similar. By 20 days of age, for instance, hepatic vitamin A levels had fallen to 7 to 14% of
those present in A^+ rats (Table 1). At the same age, blood
levels of vitamin A in the deprived animals were comparable
to those fed A^+ diets. These findings are in good accord
with previous ones (Dowling and Wald, 1958) and attest to
the fact that blood levels of vitamin A-deprived animals
do not decline until hepatic vitamin A is virtually depleted.

Electrophysiological Studies

Our results confirm earlier findings (Dowling and Wald, 1958;
Dowling, 1960) showing a reduction in ERG amplitude of vitamin
A-deprived albino rats after 6 to 8 weeks of dietary restric-
tion (Fig. 2). With continued deprivation the a-wave, b-
wave and log sensitivity progressively decline. Rats of the
RCS-rdy^+ strain show a similar time course in the decline of

TABLE 1

Analytical data on albino and RCS strains on vitamin A⁺
or vitamin A⁻ diets 20 days after weaning

Strains and diet	Weights of animals	Vitamin A		
		Protein	Liver	Serum
	g	mg/g liver	mg/g	μg/dl
Albino				
A⁺	107—118	233 (202—266)	91 (70—123)	61 (50—71)
A⁻	102—115	215 (198—245)	6.6 (5.7—7.3)	59 (47—63)
RCS-rdy⁺				
A⁺	85—98	218 (194—241)	70 (66—74)	62 (44—74)
A⁻	62—80	210 (186—215)	6.4 (4.7—7.7)	46 (37—56)
RCS				
A⁺	83—95	230 (216—259)	69 (41—109)	55 (41—66)
A⁻	55—75	235 (224—242)	9.7 (8.1—11.2)	50 (46—54)

The weights of animals are given as the range, and correspond to the averages shown in Fig. 1. Analyses of protein
and vitamin A are the means of 4 animals or more in each
group, with the range of values given in parentheses.

the ERG following vitamin A restriction. In line with the
findings of Delmelle and coworkers (1975), the electrophysiological response of the dystrophic RCS rats on A⁻
diets declined at an accelerated pace from about 5 days after
weaning compared to those on standard (A⁺) diets.

DISCUSSION

Albino rats reared on vitamin A-restricted diets show weight
loss, abnormal fur and diminished visual function commencing

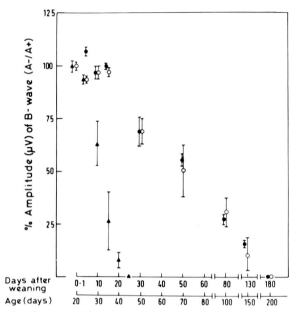

Fig. 2 *Relative amplitude of the b-wave responses of vitamin A-deprived albino (●), RCS-rdy⁺ (○) and RCS (▲) rats compared to animals on standard (A⁺) diets.*

at approximately 6 weeks of age (Dowling and Wald, 1958). Those supplemented with retinoic acid show only diminished ERGs, abnormal behavioural thresholds and decreased levels of visual pigment without the classical somatic symptoms of vitamin A deficiency (Dowling, 1960; Schneider *et al.*, 1977; Carter-Dawson *et al.*, 1979; Crouch and Katz, 1980). Morphological changes in the pigment epithelium (Yang *et al.*, 1978) as well as gross structural breakdown (Carter-Dawson *et al.*, 1979) or "thinning" (Herron and Riegel, 1974) of the photoreceptors have been reported in vitamin A-deprived albino rats supplemented with retinoic acid.

Our investigations have shown that, in contrast to the albino rat, retinoic acid does not completely fulfil the role of vitamin A for growth and epithelial differentiation in either the dystrophic or congenic strains of RCS rats. All animals showed fur abnormalities, albeit to varying degrees, commencing after about 3 to 4 weeks on the dietary regime. While for the first month, body weights in the deprived RCS rats were about 70 to 80% of those of RCS rats on A⁺ diets, the weight gains subsequently became relatively smaller and at maturity, the deprived RCS rats were about a half to two-thirds of the size of their A⁺ counterparts. There was great variability in responses to the diet, both within and between the various litters; moreover, there was no direct correlation between the extent of fur abnormality and the poor growth response. Our general observation was that, after about a month on the diet, all of the RCS animals showed abnormal fur and a small number of them (less than one per litter) died; the remainder continued to grow, but at a slower rate than in the preceding period. In addition to these somatic responses of both of the RCS strains, we have also noted, in agreement with previous observations (Delmelle *et al.*, 1975), that in vitamin A-deprived RCS rats, the decline in the b-wave amplitude is much more rapid than in dystrophic rats maintained on A$^+$ diets. This is not the case with either the RCS-rdy^+ or albino rats deprived of vitamin A. Taken together these findings suggest the possibility of specific inherited abnormalities in retinoid metabolism in the RCS rat strains.

The site of such a hypothetical defect in retinoid metabolism in the RCS strains can only be a matter of speculation. Figure 3 summarizes the metabolic fate of retinol and retinoic acid as we understand it today. Both retinoids support growth and epithelial differentiation in all animal species studied to date. One of the most important biological functions of retinoids involves their role as carriers of monosaccharides to cell surface membranes for the biosynthesis of essential glycoconjugates. The pathway for these glycosyl transfer reactions has been established for retinol and is known to involve mannosylretinyl phosphate (De Luca, 1977; De Luca *et al.*, 1979; Shidoji *et al.*, 1981). The intermediate in which retinoic acid acts as a carrier has not been characterized with certainty, nor have the resulting glycoconjugates, apart from a few isolated cell systems (Lotan *et al.*, 1980; Bhat and De Luca, 1981; King and Tabiowo, 1981). Despite the fragmentary information available, we could speculate that some stage in the synthesis of glycoconjugates mediated through retinoic acid is affected in the RCS strains of rats. Other possibilities such as abnormalities in retinoic acid-binding protein should not however be excluded in spite of normal levels found in the retina of adult RCS dystrophic rats (Wiggert *et al.*, 1978).

An additional defect in the metabolism, transport or storage of vitamin A or one of its metabolites in the pigment epithelium could underlie the accelerated rate of ERG deterioration in vitamin A-deprived RCS dystrophic rats. This would seem a reasonable hypothesis in view of the finding that this is the cellular site of the inherited defect (Mullen and LaVail, 1975). In further support of this notion, we have recently reported a marked deficiency in retinol esterifying activity in the pigment epithelium

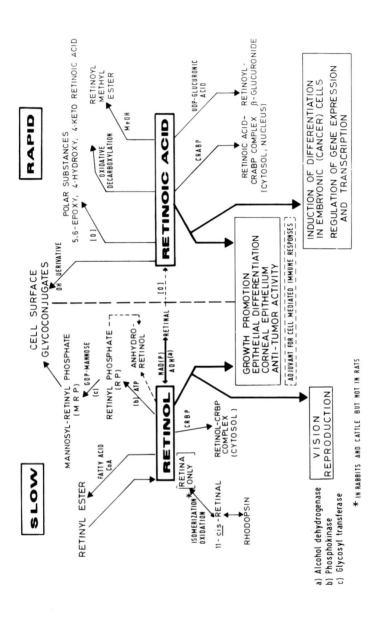

Fig. 3 *Summary of known metabolic pathways of retinol and retinoic acid*

of the RCS rat, and also found a concomitant small excess of
retinol in 10 to 12-day old dystrophic rats reared in dim
cyclic illumination (Berman *et al.*, 1981). It thus appears
that there may be a specific inherited enzymatic defect in
the RCS dystrophic rat confined to the pigment epithelium,
superimposed on a generalized abnormality in retinoid metabolism in both of the RCS strains.

Subsequent investigations on the effects of vitamin A deprivation in the RCS strains of rats have provided further insight
into the findings reported above. Factors such as the teratogenic and toxic effects of retinoic acid (even at the low
concentrations used) play an important role in the etiology
of the somatic abnormalities. Although these responses are
often erratic and highly variable, the effects of vitamin A
deficiency on the rapid deterioration of the ERG responses
in the RCS dystrophic rats are consistent. It is our general
impression that the RCS strains do not always thrive on basal
diets, regardless of their composition, to the same extent
as albino rats.

ACKNOWLEDGEMENTS

This work was supported in part by the U.S.-Israel Binational
Science Foundation and the Chief Scientists' Office, Ministry
of Health, Israel.

REFERENCES

Berman, E.R., Segal, N. and Feeney, L. (1979). Subcellar
    distribution of free and esterified forms of vitamin A
    in the pigment epithelium of the retina and in liver.
    Biochim. Biophys. Acta **572**, 167—177.
Berman, E.R., Horowitz, J., Segal, N., Fisher, S. and
    Feeney-Burns, L. (1980). Enzymatic esterification of
    vitamin A in the pigment epithelium of bovine retina.
    Biochim. Biophys. Acta **630**, 36—46.
Berman, E.R., Segal, N., Photiou, S., Rothman, H. and
    Feeney-Burns, L. (1981). Inherited retinal dystrophy
    in RCS rats: a deficiency in vitamin A esterification
    in pigment epithelium. *Nature* **293**, 217—220.
Bhat, P.V. and De Luca, L.M. (1981). The biosynthesis of a
    mannolipid containing a metabolite of retinoic acid by
    3T12 mouse fibroblasts. *In* "Annals of the New York
    Academy of Sciences", Vol. 359, Modulation of Cellular
    interactions by Vitamin A and Derivatives (Retinoids),
    (Eds L.M. De Luca and S.S. Shapiro) p. 135. The New York
    Academy of Sciences, New York.

Bok, D. and Hall, M.O. (1971). The role of the pigment epithelium in the etiology of inherited retinal dystrophy in the rat. *J. Cell Biol.* **49**, 664–682.

Carter-Dawson, L., Kuwabara, T., O'Brien, P.J. and Bieri, J.G. (1979). Structural and biochemical changes in vitamin A-deficient rat retinas. *Invest. Ophthalmol. Vis. Sci.* **18**, 437–446.

Crouch, R. and Katz, S. (1980). The effect of retinal isomers on the VER and ERG of vitamin A deprived rats. *Vision Res.* **20**, 109–115.

Delmelle, M., Noell, W.K. and Organisciak, D.T. (1975). Hereditary retinal dystrophy in the rat: rhodopsin, retinol, vitamin A deficiency. *Exp. Eye Res.* **21**, 369–380.

De Luca, L.M. (1977). The direct involvement of vitamin A in glycosyl transfer reactions of mammalian membranes. *Vitam. Horm.* **35**, 1–57.

De Luca, L.M., Bhat, P.V., Sasak, W. and Adamo, S. (1979). Biosynthesis of phosphoryl and glycosyl phosphoryl derivatives of vitamin A in biological membranes. *Fed. Proc.* **38**, 2535–2539.

Dowling, J.E. (1960). Night blindness, dark adaptation, and the electroretinogram. *Amer. J. Ophthal.* **50**, 875–887.

Dowling, J.E. and Wald, G. (1958). Vitamin A deficiency and night blindness. *Proc. Nat. Acad. Sci.* **44**, 648–661.

Dowling, J.E. and Sidman, R.L. (1962). Inherited retinal dystrophy in the rat. *J. Cell Biol.* **14**, 73–109.

Herron, W.L., Riegel, B.W., Myers, O.E. and Rubin, M.L. Retinal dystrophy in the rat — A pigment epithelial disease. *Invest. Ophthalmol.* **8**, 595–604.

Herron, W.L. and Riegel, B.W. (1974). Vitamin A deficiency-induced "rod thinning" to permanently decrease the production of rod outer segment material. *Invest. Ophthalmol.* **13**, 54–59.

Kaitz, M. (submitted for publication) Acceleration of retinal degeneration in RCS (dystrophic) rats by vitamin A deficiency.

Kaitz, M. and Auberbach, E. (1980). Light damage in dystrophic and normal rats. *In* "The Effects of Constant Light on Visual Processes" (Eds T.P. Williams and B.N. Baker) p. 179. Plenum Publishing Corporation, New York.

King, I.A. and Tabiowo, A. (1981). The effect of all-trans-retinoic acid on the synthesis of epidermal cell-surface-associated carbohydrates. *Biochem. J.* **194**, 341–350.

Lotan, R., Kramer, R.H., Neumann, G., Lotan, D. and Nicholson, G.L. (1980). Retinoic acid-induced modifications in the growth and cell surface components of a human carcinoma (HeLa) cell line. *Exp. Cell Res.* **130**, 404–414.

Mullen, R.J. and LaVail, M.M. (1975). Inherited retinal dys-
    trophy: primary defect in pigment epithelium determined
    with experimental rat chimeras. *Science* **192**, 799–801.
Muto, Y., Smith, J.E., Milch, P.O. and Goodman, D.S. (1972).
    Regulation of retinol-binding protein metabolism by
    vitamin A status in the rat. *J. Biol. Chem.* **247**, 2542–
    2550.
Reading, H.W. (1970). Biochemistry of retinal dystrophy.
    J. Med. Genet. **7**, 277–284.
Robison, W.G. Jr., Kuwabara, T. and Bieri, J.G. (1980). Phago-
    cytosis and vitamin A in retinal lipofuscin accumulation.
    Suppl. Invest. Ophthalmol. Vis. Sci., *abstr.* p. 189.
Schneider, B., Hood, D.C., Cohen, H. and Stampfer, M. (1977).
    Behavioral threshold and rhodopsin content as a function
    of vitamin A deprivation in the rat. *Vision Res.* **17**,
    799–806.
Shidoji, Y., Sasak, W., Silverman-Jones, C.S. and De Luca,
    L.M. (1981). Recent studies on the involvement of
    retinyl phosphate as a carrier of mannose in biological
    membranes. *In* "Annals of the New York Academy of Sciences"
    Vol. 359, Modulation of Cellular Interactions by vitamin
    A and Derivatives (Retinoids) (Eds L.M. De Luca and
    S.S. Shapiro) p. 345. The New York Academy of Sciences,
    New York.
Wiggert, B., Bergsma, D.R., Helmsen, R. and Chader, G.J. (1978).
    Vitamin A receptors. Retinoic acid binding in ocular
    tissues. *Biochem. J.* **169**, 87–94.
Yang, W.C., Hollenberg, M.J. and Wyse, J.P.H. (1978). Morpho-
    logy of the retinal pigment epithelium in the vitamin A
    deficient rat. *Virchows. Arch. B. Cell Path.* **27**, 7–21.

RETINAL-REDUCTASE ACTIVITY IN NORMAL AND DYSTROPHIC RATS

P.A.A. JANSEN, F.J.M. DAEMEN and W.J. de GRIP

Department of Biochemistry, University of Nijmegen, PO Box 9101, 6500 HB Nijmegen, The Netherlands

ABSTRACT

Among other abnormalities, dystrophic retinas show impaired retinol formation and transport. In order to investigate whether the retinal reductase (retinol dehydrogenase) present in the rod outer segment membrane might be responsible, normal (Wistar) and dystrophic (RCS) rats were raised either in continuous darkness or under cyclic (12/12) light. At various time-points after birth, retinas were excised in darkness and rhodopsin-concentration and maximal activity of retinal-reductase determined. Retinal-reductase activity followed the very same pattern as the rhodopsin-concentration in all experimental groups, indicating that the enzyme itself is not the primary target, but rather that the metabolic organization of the entire membrane is afflicted. Impaired accessibility of the extracellular cell debris, still containing the enzyme, for its (intracellular) coenzyme NADPH may be an important factor.

PART 1

Lolley was asked whether the search for changes in extraocular tissues proved that there was no substitute for eye
tissues. **LOLLEY** said that in the rd mouse and RCS rat the
vulnerability was photoreceptor-specific. He thought that
no extraocular markers would be found in the early differentiation type of lesion, but that they may be found in the
renewal types, because other cell systems must have similar
renewal processes. **HOLLEYFIELD** suggested that circulating
factors, to which the photoreceptor was particularly vulnerable, may be found. **LOLLEY** said that such a hormonal factor
fell under the definition of a maintenance defect.

Aguirre was asked how the changes in the dystrophic dog
retina differed from those in taurine deficiency. **AGUIRRE**
replied that they were morphologically different but that a
visual cell could only express degenerative changes by a
disarray of the rod outer segments. In the first 14.5 weeks,
the ERG recordings from normal and affected dogs were indistinguishable. He was asked whether the depression was of
total retinal protein metabolism rather than of rhodopsin.
AGUIRRE replied that this could be so, but he did not know
as they had not prepared rod outer segment extracts.

HOLLEYFIELD asked Chader if there was any calmodulin in
the retina when the phosphodiesterase (PDE) was calmodulin-
dependent. **CHADER** said that it was about 50% of normal
levels. However, they would have to examine other enzymes,
because the PDE assay might be simply a convenient assay of
calmodulin and PDE was only one of many calmodulin-dependent
enzymes. **LOLLEY** suggested a different interpretation. The
calmodulin-dependent PDE was not produced until differentiation was complete and the PDE of the inner nuclear layers
was a calmodulin-regulated enzyme, as Chader had found in
the young animal. In the normal retina, the high PDE
activity of the photoreceptors predominates, whereas in the
degenerate retina all that is found is the PDE of the inner

layers, since no photoreceptors exist to contain any PDE.
The "switch" is not a "switch" in the photoreceptors, but a
masking of the change by a change in cell population. **CHADER**
agreed that this was a possibility. He was testing his model
by injecting calmodulin into the vitreous of the young dog.
It was stated that antibodies to calmodulin and cyclic
nucleotide enzymes had been prepared and, significantly, no
binding of the calmodulin antibody had been found in outer
segments. **CHADER** said there was a lot of calmodulin present
in cow outer segments, but there was no calmodulin-dependent
PDE. **CLAYTON** suggested that if calmodulin (molecular weight
17,000) was very loosely bound to the tissue, the antibody
could leach it off.

   HAYWOOD asked Lolley if a calcium ionophore produced a
potentiation of the effect. **LOLLEY** replied that this had not
been done. He said that they had found that total calcium
in the developing rd mouse retina was lower than in normals
which suggested that intracellular calcium was lower. The
abnormal levels of cyclic GMP may interfere with the levels
of calcium. **READING** said that light exacerbates the lesion
in the RCS rat and that light increases intracellular calcium levels, so that it was paradoxical that Lolley had
found low levels of intracellular calcium in the affected
retina. **LOLLEY** said that this hypothesis may not hold,
since Hagin had found that light stimulates a release of
calcium from outer segments and it is not known what this
release does to the photoreceptor calcium concentration.
READING said that it may not be the calmodulin levels which
are important for PDE activation, but the free calcium levels.
CHADER said they were attempting to wash pigment epithelium
and interphotoreceptor layers in the light and dark to
measure calmodulin and calcium binding. This might help to
indicate whether calmodulin is acting as a calcium "sink".
LEE asked whether there was a disturbance in the cells of
the inner retina as well as the photoreceptors? **LOLLEY**
replied that if one looked at cAMP, one would see a different picture from cGMP and the dopamine-controlled cAMP
systems in the inner retina would be changed.

   Holleyfield was asked if he had looked at an all-cone
retina. He replied that he had only looked at the fovea.
HAYWOOD said that they had tried analogous experiments to
the dibutyrylcGMP and IBMX one, by using dibutyrylcAMP plus
IBMX on the cone-dominant chick retina. There was no damage
to the cones on 12h incubations, even though the cyclic AMP
levels were elevated. **FARBER** said that she would show some
experiments in her paper which showed that when the cyclic
AMP levels go up, then the cone photoreceptor cells degenerate.

PART 2

HAYWOOD asked Farber if the rods in the ground squirrel
retina might contain very high levels of cGMP, the fall
representing a rod as well as cone loss. FARBER replied
these were atypical, rod-like cells, but could have contained
cGMP. When asked if other varieties of squirrel had the same
type of retina, she said that they only looked at flying
squirrels which had a much higher rod content and had a cAMP
level comparable to the rat. The ground squirrel was chosen
to obtain as near as possible a pure cone retina. LAVAIL
pointed out that although Farber had suggested that cAMP in
the degenerating retina could be due to macrophage invasion,
as in other retinal degenerations, the level of cAMP would
rise four- to ten-fold dramatically. FARBER agreed that the
rise may not involve macrophages. VOADEN asked about the
relative sensitivities of ground squirrel and monkey cones.
FARBER replied that she had referred to Noell's original
experiments on monkeys before starting with squirrels and
used comparable doses based on body weight. Noell had
found rods degenerating faster than cones. There was some
discussion about the difficulty of producing retinal degeneration in the rat with iodoacetate and VOADEN quoted
Graymore's work in which he gave malate in conjunction with
the iodoacetate, which suggested that primate cones were
more damage-resistant than the squirrel-type. Farber did
not completely agree and said that toxicity and retinal
disease affect rods before cones. Discussion of the time
course of the toxic degeneration followed and it was established that the time course differed markedly in different
species, but whether this was due to different rod:cone
proportions was unclear. CHADER asked if anyone had found
lens abnormalities associated with the cone-type degeneration as seen with rod-type, but this had not been observed.
LAVAIL pointed out that Berman's data was a good example of
the advantages of using congenic strains. If non-congenic
controls had been used the lowered weight of the retinoic
acid RCS rats might have been interpreted as coupled to
retinal dystrophy. BERMAN agreed and said that the trait
may be present in other varieties of rat. LaVail said that
it was understandable that the RCS and RCS-rdy$^+$ strains
behaved similarly as they were 97 to 99% genetically
identical, whereas the albinos were genetically removed.
BERMAN said that she thought that there was a specific
deficit in the PE in esterification of retinol but superimposed upon this was the difference in the handling of
retinoic acid in its substitution for vitamin A for fur and

growth. **LAVAIL** added that if the abnormal handling of the
vitamin A in the RCS rat was important it would be possible
to develop an outbred stock by transferring the rdy gene to
a non-inbred strain. **BERMAN** thought that the abnormality in
vitamin A metabolism was related to the synthesis of the
receptors of the PE apical surface. This would explain the
phagocytic incapability of the PE. **LOLLEY** asked whether this
defect was because the RCS strain, dystrophic or not, did not
eat the diet, since both had the same kind of growth curve.
It transpired in discussion that the vitamin A-free diet was
powder, whereas the normal was pelleted and **BERMAN** confirmed
that experiments were in progress to administer retinoic acid
parenterally.

   READING suggested to de Grip that changes in retinal
reductase activity could have been due to inaccessibility of
the required coenzyme $NADP^+$. **DE GRIP** agreed that this could
have been so.

   LaVail was asked if it was possible to use chimaeras to
see if the IPM was necessary to ensure phagocytosis, and
LAVAIL replied that they had begun to do this. Staining of
plastic embedded material was difficult but with colloidal
iron their preliminary results showed that the normal IPM
band was missing between the mutant PE cells and the retina.
A question was raised concerning the general case of the
development of polymers of proteoglycans from monomers and
whether this could have been the case with the missing IPM.
LAVAIL said that this could have been so and could have
caused the defect in the differentiation of these cells resulting in the phagocytosis defect. It was clear that
proteoglycans and their changing sizes were quite important
in development. **ARDEN** said that one saw thick plates of
debris between the PE and the retina in the RCS rat. The
simple explanation of cell death could be the oily layer
under the PE. He suggested that LaVail's slides showed that
the water-soluble material was being squeezed out by the
thick oily material. **LAVAIL** answered that they were interested in the cause of the "plate" which clearly had an
abnormal composition. There was also a change in membrane
composition, When examined by electron microscopy the plates
were seen not to be solid and intercellular spaces existed so
that diffusion of metabolites could still occur. Their work
had shown that the proteoglycans which should be there were
missing and that this could be a stage in cell degeneration.
VOADEN asked if the IPM came from the PE rather than from
the inner limbs of the photoreceptors. **LAVAIL** said that
Berman's data had shown that the IPM came from the PE, whereas Young had shown that it could come from the inner segments

and be secreted into the intercellular space. Practically
every cell which bordered this zone could form material for
the IPM, probably by sloughing of the cell surface coat as
well as by secretion. He said that the defect in the PE
could have prevented mucopolysaccharide (MPS) synthesis.
VOADEN said that when the inner limbs were closer to the PE
the synthesis was inhibited, and it suggested that the
environment of the PE inhibited MPS synthesis, perhaps by PE
and by the photoreceptors. As they moved away from each
other the effect on the PE was to prevent proper phagocytosis.
LAVAIL did not agree and quoted Berman's finding that muco-
subtances are synthesized by the PE and said that in normal
animals, with long outer segments, the heaviest concentration of MPS was at the PE. Rather than being an interaction
of the photoreceptors and the PE, the primary lesion resided
in the PE. This was clear from the chimaeric model. Because
the apical band was not seen it did not mean that the PE was
not synthesizing material. The processes of the PE were
much longer in the mutant, and extended down into the outer
segment zone, and it was possible that the MPS being secreted
in that area accounted for the large accumulation there.
BERMAN asked if PAS staining would show up the "fuzzy coat"
of the photoreceptors which LAVAIL said might be done.
Excess retinol might feed back onto the synthesis of the
"fuzzy coat" and alter its formation. BERMAN replied that
they had not been able to show excess retinol diffusing out
of the PE. AGUIRRE asked if LaVail had found staining
differences in retinas from pigmented and non-pigmented rats.
LAVAIL said that there seemed to be more in the pigmented
rats. They wanted to look at the time course of this since
the pigmented retina degenerated more slowly than the albino.
LEE asked whether LaVail had seen evidence of lysosomal
activation by EM. LAVAIL noted that the lysosomal fragility
hypothesis had not been raised, yet this was one of the most
interesting ideas concerning the condition. Excess retinol
could account for lysosomal enzyme release. Chader's new
data on the collie supported this, and also some small
vesicular material was present in the pcd mouse. In the
debris zone there was material suggestive of lysosomal
activation. CHADER said that there was a lot of interchange
of material between the photoreceptors and the PE cells, and
that in the RCS rat the connections between the retina and
the PE cells were disrupted, pointing to transport problems.
A possible candidate for this defective transport was
retinol, which had to go back and forth for its esterification process to continue, Retinol did not do this by itself
and in all tissues it was bound to serum proteins or to

intracellular receptors which were soluble proteins like
steroid receptors. In rat retina there were two types of
protein, a small sepcies of an hormonal type and a much
larger type (8S) restricted to rod outer segments. This has
a probable transport function. They had examined dystrophic
rats to see what was in the washings of subretinal and subPE
fluid and in the matrix without rupturing the cells. There
were interesting light/dark differences in the amount of 8S
protein on the outer segments surface and the 8S protein was
greater than the 2S protein in the wash from dystrophic
tissues. They felt that this was a candidate as a marker
for the condition.

ANIMAL MODELS AND HUMAN DISEASE: SUMMING UP

J. HAYWOOD

*Department of Biochemistry, University of Edinburgh,
Edinburgh EH8 9XD, UK*

This third session of the symposium on animal models of human
retinal disease has taken us into quite different ground to
that of the first session with its focus on abnormal cyclic
GMP metabolism. Drs Arden and Barnett have given us two quite
distinct overviews. Dr Arden directed our attention to the
human side of the topic by comparing what we know about human
retinal degenerations with the models, while Dr Barnett described a wide range of potential animal models, many of
which are probably little known outside ophthalmic veterinarian
circles, and all of which are worthy of more investigation.
The existence of these further models emphasizes Dr LaVail's
comments at the end of the last session about our good for-
tune in this respect in comparison with researchers working
on other diseases of the human nervous system.

Dr Farber gave a new direction to our consideration of
cyclic nucleotides, by taking us away from the rods of the
rodent and canine retinas to the cones of the ground squirrel.
Her demonstration that cAMP in cones seems to fulfill a
similar function to that of cGMP in rods suggests that a comparative study of these two photoreceptor types is timely,
using the techniques developed for use in rod retinas. There
are rather few exceptions to the rule that photoreceptor biochemists are rod-orientated, in spite of the importance
of cones in many animals and especially in Man. A great deal
is known about colour vision at the psychophysical level but
rather little at the molecular level. In addition, although
cones seem to be less sensitive to damage than do rods (as
Dr Holleyfield's paper shows), many are lost from the human
retina in Retinitis Pigmentosa. The fact that we know so
little about this photoreceptor type in molecular terms probably stems from the less ready availability of cone-dominant
retinas. Birds have mixed (rod and cone) retinas which are
cone-enriched, and three of our contributions (Wolf; Pollock

et al; Wilson *et al*.) describe inherited defects in the chick
retina which could be explored further both morphologically
and biochemically.

The roles of Vitamin A and retinal were considered next
with particular reference to the RCS rat. Dr Berman's study
of the effects of a dietary lack of Vitamin A on RCS rats
and their congenic controls shows the importance of the use
of such control animals. Whatever the reasons for the differences between the RCS, the RCS-rdy$^+$ and the Wistar strains
of rats on Vitamin A-free diets, it is clearly not related
solely to the defect associated with retinal degeneration.
The production of animals congenic at most, if not all, loci
except those involved in the other retinal degenerations
which have been described in the symposium would be a great
help in specifying the relevant biochemical lesions. Both
Drs Berman and de Grip have shown defects and losses of
activity of the enzymes of retinol metabolism in RCS rats
which may have consequences for glycoconjugate metabolism
as well as rhodopsin function. The elegant studies on the
interphotoreceptor matrix (IPM) of the RCS rats, by Dr LaVail,
in which he has shown that there is an abnormal staining of
carbohydrate-containing material suggests that this may be
one morphological consequence of the biochemical defect in
the P.E.

In comparison to our knowledge of cyclic nucleotide involvement in visual transduction in rods, our knowledge of
the molecular interrelationships between the P.E. and the
photoreceptor outer segments in sparse. What are the bases
of adhesion between the two cell types and why does its
strength vary with species and strains? What is the trigger
and control for outer segment differentiation in which P.E.
plays some critical role, and how do P.E. cells recognize
shed outer segments? Dr Lolley has suggested a testable
hypothesis for animal models on the basis of which comparisons can be made. However, the diversity of models now
available, and the complexity of neural retina-pigment epithelium interactions make it very likely that a variety of
gene defects will be involved in some of these. To attempt
useful analyses we will need much greater information about
the workings of the normal retina.

RETINITIS PIGMENTOSA — A CLINICIAN'S VIEWPOINT:

A.C. BIRD

*Department of Clinical Ophthalmology,
Moorfields Eye Hospital, London, UK*

I plan to consider the subject of retinal degeneration from
the point of view of the clinician. It was interesting to
hear accounts of new information concerning retinal physiology during the last two sessions and to question how this
new information can be applied to clinical science. From
the clinician's standpoint it is clearly very important that
full advantage is taken of all new knowledge from wherever
it is derived, and the clinician must work towards this end.
What is the responsibility of the clinician in the assessment of Retinitis Pigmentosa in Man? It is fundamental that
all workers concerned with the retinal diseases and with an
interest in Retinitis Pigmentosa should appreciate that we
are considering a group of quite different conditions, that
have variable inheritance and variable severity, although
all produce a fairly typical fundus appearance. They are all
slowly progressive, though the rate of progression is variable from one condition to another.

The appreciation that many different disorders are included
within the term Retinitis Pigmentosa is important to all
workers in the field. If a collection of patients are subjected to investigative research, it is unrealistic to expect
any definite conclusions to be drawn from such patients concerning the pathogenesis of their diseases if each patient
within the group has a disease different from the others.
For this reason it is important to obtain purer samples of
the disease; this represents the initial responsibility of
the clinician. It is important to subdivide Retinitis Pigmentosa into groups in which there is a single disease or
at least a smaller number of nosological entities. This is
an essential prerequisite for further research, since if the
pathogenesis or a cure has been identified in an animal with
retinal degeneration, the question arises as to whether

there is any human disease that is homologous with the disease
in animals. The answer to such a question would probably be
yes. It is then the responsibility of the researcher to
identify which one. Similarly, if the therapist has identified
a cure for one patient with Retinitis Pigmentosa, this form
of treatment will be helpful only if they identify another
human with exactly the same disorder.

INHERITANCE

The first method of subdividing human disease is according
to its inheritance; this allows a subdivision into autosomal
dominant, autosomal recessive, and x-linked disease. Table
1 shows an initial analysis of the first 305 families seen
in the Genetic Clinic at Moorfields Eye Hospital, London.
Of these, 77 were identified as autosomal dominant, 52 were
x-linked and 19 autosomal recessive. In about 50% of the

TABLE 1

Genetic diagnosis in 305 families

Autosomal dominant	77
Autosomal recessive	19
x-linked	52
Simplex	106
Multiplex	29
Usher's syndrome	20
Adopted	2

families the inheritance had not been identified. These
comprised families in which there was only one member
affected (simplex) or where more than one affected member
is in the same sibship (multiplex).
    There are two surprising features of these results. The
first is the high prevalence of x-linked disease in our
clinical experience. This is in marked contrast to the very
low prevalance in other series. Whilst it is conceivable that
this is due to bias of ascertainment in our clinic, or that
the population of London differs significantly from populations elsewhere, neither seems likely. The second significant finding was the large proportion of the total in which
the inheritance could not be identified. From the researcher's
standpoint this implied that a large number of patients with
Retinitis Pigmentosa can not be subdivided according to the
inheritance of the disease. The second is that the clinician
wishing to give genetic advice can not do so. Both these

problems could be resolved if it were reasonable to assume
that all multiplex and simplex families had autosomal recessive disease, an assumption made universally in the ophthalmic literature.

Dr Marcell Jay has recently analysed patients seen at
Moorfields Eye Hospital in order to answer the various
questions brought to light by earlier studies. Within the
series she found that there was an excess of males amongst
the multiplex and simplex families and she found a large
excess of male multiplex over female multiplex families.
Both of these suggested that there was a significant number
of x-linked families within those labelled multiplex and
simplex. When she examined in some detail the clinical information available in families with possible x-linked
disease she found that in a large number of families with
males only affected, few or no additional males at risk of
having the abnormal gene were identified by family history, and
that females likely to be heterozygous for the abnormal gene
had not been examined or were not available for examination.
She then undertook a segregational analysis of the multiplex
and simplex families. This involved the examination of the
proportion of affected siblings to total number of siblings
of the propositus. If all multiplex and simplex families
have either autosomal recessive or x-linked disease, the
ratio should be 0.25. She found that the segregational
ratio was much lower than 0.25 in these families, implying
that many of these patients did not have autosomal recessive
or x-linked disease. She then subdivided the patients
according to the severity of the disease, using loss of
visual acuity to a lower level by the fourth decade of life
as the point of subdivision. In severely affected members
the segregational ratio was close to 0.25, implying that in
severe disease, female patients had probably inherited the
disease as an autosomal recessive characteristic, whereas
males had either autosomal recessive disease or x-linked
disease. The second conclusion was that of those with mild
disease, very few had inherited their disorder as an autosomal recessive characteristic.

These results imply that a severely affected male with
Retinitis Pigmentosa but without family history of disease
may have x-linked or autosomal recessive Retinitis Pigmentosa,
whereas a severely affected female is likely to have autosomal recessive disease. If the disorder is mild this may
represent autosomal dominant disease, either as a new mutation or as a disorder with variable expressivity, whereby
affected parents had not been identified by family history.
Alternatively, such a patient may have mild recessive disease
or the disorder may represent phenocopy, implying that the
eye disease is not genetically determined.

What conclusions can be drawn from the point of view of
the researcher? It is likely that Retinitis Pigmentosa
causing severe disease in a female or severe disease in a
mixed sibship is autosomal recessive. Severe disease in a
male or in a male sibship may be x-linked and this can only
be confirmed by examining heterozygotes. In mild disease
no firm conclusions can be drawn, and in particular the possibility of the disease being a phenocopy of Retinitis Pigmentosa serves as a warning against using such patients in
research into Retinitis Pigmentosa.

FUNDUS CHANGES

In what other ways can the clinician subdivide Retinitis
Pigmentosa? There are certain outer retinal dystrophies that
are easily recognizable. Choroideremia cannot be mistaken
for Retinitis Pigmentosa, particularly if female heterozygotes are examined. Similarly, Gyrate Atrophy has a very
specific appearance, but another well defined disorder,
Refsum's syndrome, can produce fundus changes indistinguishable from Retinitis Pigmentosa of unknown cause.
    Various subdivisions of Retinitis Pigmentosa have been
made on the basis of fundus appearance. Retinitis Pigmentosa, sine pigmento, has been considered by some as a separate disorder, although it is now clear this represents early
disease and such patients will develop typical pigmentation
with time. Retinitis albipunctatus has also been considered
as a separate disorder but this proposal has not been for-
mally tested. Most workers would not consider the presence
of white dots to be sufficient evidence for considering this
to be a disease entity different from the rest of Retinitis
Pigmentosa, although it is undeniable that Vitamin A deficient states cause distinctive white deposits at the level
of the pigment epithelium. Unilateral Retinitis Pigmentosa
is rarely genetically determined; such patients usually have
asymmetrical bilateral disease or the disorder represents a
phenocopy. Significantly, no patient with unilateral
Retinitis Pigmentosa has had an affected relative, although
in one instance it has been reported that such a patient
had consanguineous parents.
    In only one condition is there evidence that an entity
within Retinitis Pigmentosa can be identified on the basis
of fundus changes. There are several autosomal dominant
families in which the disorder is always sectorial. The
fact that the disorder breeds true implies that this is an
entity different from other disorders within Retinitis

Pigmentosa. However, the observation of one individual with
sectorial disease and with a dominant family history is insufficient evidence to subcategorize that particular patient
as having the nosological entity of sectorial Retinitis
Pigmentosa. Sectorial disease may be seen in a dominant
family in which other members do not have sectorial disease,
and females heterozygous for x-linked Retinitis Pigmentosa
may also appear to have sectorial disease. Classification of
sectorial Retinitis Pigmentosa can only be made if it is
found to breed true within the family.

The principle of identifying attributes of Retinitis Pigmentosa that are peculiar to one family is very important to
all analyses of Retinitis Pigmentosa. Comparison of inter-
and intra-familial variation of certain attributes is an
essential end point in all research which has the purpose
of subdividing Retinitis Pigmentosa into specific entities.

FUNCTIONAL ATTRIBUTES

As soon as it was identified that rods were responsible for
night vision it was assumed that Retinitis Pigmentosa was
due to a metabolic abnormality of some specific function of
rods. It was assumed that a disease of rods would produce
maximum changes in areas of the fundus where the rod population was highest, such that patients would become night-
blind and have fundus changes in the periphery of the fundus.
This conclusion stimulated intense research into rod function
and possible metabolic abnormalities in patients with
Retinitis Pigmentosa which would have a selected effect on
rods. However, if there were an abnormality of a specific
metabolic attribute of mid-peripheral receptors (both rods
and cones), it would also produce a disease with the attributes that we recognize as being typical of Retinitis Pigmentosa.

During the last few years psychophysicists have addressed
the problem concerning the relative extent to which rods and
cones are affected in Retinitis Pigmentosa. Although no
definite conclusions can yet be drawn from these observations,
there is some evidence that in some patients rods are affected
before cones and in others rods and cones are affected
equally in the mid-peripheral fundus. Further investigations imply that in some autosomal dominant families the
pattern of disease is constant in affected members and in
this respect differs from other autosomal dominant families.
It is clear that these hypotheses should be tested further.
The significance of these findings can not be underestimated.
If it is shown beyond doubt that a particular family has a

disorder affecting rods before cones it is likely that the
abnormality is one affecting a specific metabolic activity
of rods. This would contrast with another family where the
abnormality is one of a specific metabolic attribute of
peripheral receptors rather than central receptors. In the
first case there is a great deal of information about the
metabolic differences between rods and cones, but to date
there is little, if any, indication of metabolic differences
between peripheral and central receptors.

It is encouraging also that electro-physiological testing
appears to confirm the differential extent of effect on
functional characteristics identified by psycho-physics.

In future it is possible that psycho-physical and electrophysiological tests may provide additional subdivisions of
Retinitis Pigmentosa. Predictably, patchy disease over the
whole fundus will produce different properties to confluent
disease affecting only part of the fundus. Response to discontinuous stimuli, both spatial and temporal, may reveal
further functional deficits which may not be a reflection of
loss of sensitivity alone.

In conclusion, I believe that it is important to study
patients in whom the inheritance is well defined. Identification of attributes of disease which may be used to subdivide
Retinitis Pigmentosa can only be defined initially in autosomal dominant and x-linked disease where many affected members in a single family are recognized, before these attributes can then be used to study recessive disease. Such
studies will allow a purer sample of disease to be defined
within the population, and may also give some clues as to
the pathogenesis of the disorder or, at least, which cell
is the initial target of disease.

DIFFERENTIAL DIAGNOSIS — A BIOLOGICAL VIEWPOINT

R.M. CLAYTON

Department of Genetics, University of Edinburgh, West Mains Road, Edinburgh, UK

Different modes of familial transmission (Bird, this volume), the age of onset and the pattern of deterioration are all partial discriminants of the retinitis pigmentosa group of diseases. However a finer diagnosis is an essential pre-requisite for research which might lead to the identification of the specific lesions in the several forms, and thus to the positive identification of individuals or foetuses at risk. Differential diagnosis is equally required for the evaluation of possible methods of treatment, the efficacies of which might be (like the dietary treatment of some of the aminoacidurias) related to the specific biochemical lesions.

In general, a group of similar syndromes is brought about if a particular structure or function is the end result of a series of sequential stages. Failure to form a blood clot is associated with a number of genetically independent conditions, sex linked, autosomal, dominant, recessive, and partially dominant (reviewed Harris, 1975). There are more steps required than the number of modes of genetic trans-mission, which is therefore a necessary but insufficient dis-criminant.

An overlapping series of syndromes will also obtain where a series of steps, some sequential in development, some sequential in a biochemical sequence, some cooperative or interactive, are all required for the normal structure and function of a specific tissue or cell. Anaemia may be brought about by a range of different mechanisms (see for example, Russel, 1981), including various types of failure of maturation of the red cell: defects in the enzymes of glycolysis, certain changes in the structure of the haemo-globin chains, and by other mechanisms, some of them environ-mental rather than genetic.

Overlapping syndromes may be, in part, distinguished by

their pleiotropic effects on tissues other than the one of
immediate interest.   There are over thirty different genetic
conditions recorded which lead to a syndrome of head shaking
and circling in the mouse. The syndrome is due either to
dysplasia or to degeneration of the vestibular apparatus (and
in a few cases, both). Those with defects in developmental
processes, such as defective induction, are likely to manifest pleiotrophic defects in other systems, which can serve
to distinguish between them. Shaker short (st) also affects
some skeletal structures (Bonnevie, 1936), kreisler (kr) has
secondary effects on brain (Deol, 1964) and fidget (fi)
(Truslove, 1956) also affects the eye. The involvement of
eye and ear together may itself be due to different factors.
The competent areas for eye and ear inductive relationships
are similar; both are ciliated, the retina only during embryogenesis, and the vestibulae throughout life. A large group of
vestibular mutants develop normally, but the vestibular apparatus
deteriorates at various times after birth. Although the end results
of this group are indistinguishable histologically , they have
different sequences of degenerative events. For example, the sensory elements of the ampullae degenerate early in Va and je but late
in pi, deterioration in sacculus and utriculus is early in sh-2 and
deterioration in sacculus and utriculus is early in   -2 and
je but later in pi and Va (Deol, 1954, 1956).   The susceptibility of all the vestibular sensory structures together with
the different temporal sequences of their breakdown suggests
that there are a number of distinct factors required for the
maintenance which are widely, but differentially, distributed,
conferring quantitative differences in susceptibility for
each of these.   This might be due to different proportions
of receptors on sites on the cell surface of vestibular
structures, or of regionally specific isofactors which have
overlapping specificities, and therefore different efficiencies
of response to a hypothetical regulator.
     The patterns of deterioriation in different RPs similarly
suggests the interaction of a specific process with a gradient.
Gradients across the developing retina have been found for
relative adhesiveness of embryonic retina cells, (for example,
Gottlieb et al., 1976; Cefferata et al., 1979) and for specific
molecular species (Trisler et al., 1981 and this volume).
     The cause of a degenerative condition is unlikely to be
accessible to investigation from tissue in which the degeneration is far advanced, but rather from retina not yet deter-
iorated. Retina biopsies must be regarded as unacceptable,
but extra-retinal or extra-ocular patterns of pleiotropic
damage may serve not merely as a discriminant but may also,
in some cases, offer tissue more accessible to biopsy than
the retina, which may share the lesion. The more generally an

extra-ocular factor is shared with large numbers of families
with RP the less useful it will be for discriminant diagnosis
as distinct from a general indicator (which has a different
value). Thus, the structural anomalies of nasal cilia reported
by Arden and Fox (1979), the anomalies reported by Voaden (this
volume) and the protein profiles of RP cataracts (Cuthbert
and Clayton, this volume) are potentially useful for a dis-
criminant diagnosis, if they are not universally applicable.

In principle, RP may be due to a defect in the RPE, the
neural retina, a defect in a process shared by both tissues,
or be extrinsic to both. Cell culture studies may be of
value in assessing these possibilities, but in man, are
likely at present to be affected by serious problems over
and above the difficulties of obtaining material before
differentiation has occured, such as the variation in age,
and genotype. It is also likely that only small samples
may be obtained, yet growing cells for several generations to
obtain increased numbers may be vitiated by the known pro-
pensity of mammalian cells for spontaneous transformation
in culture and other changes in cell phenotype. Nevertheless, some culture procedures make it possible to retain
tissue specificity (reviewed Kaighn, 1976) so that it may be
worth developing miniaturized methods of analysis in order
to use material in primary culture.

Cell culture of three Bardet-Biedel foetal retinas (Gosden
and Clayton in prep.) have all shown a failure of the RPE
to plate on plastic dishes, and the presence of some unusually
spiky cells in primary cultures of neural retina. These two
tissues may therefore share a specific anomaly: a cell surface factor is one possible explanation.

Phenocopies of retinal degeneration produced by retinotoxic
agents may provide a model for RP, but certainly not for every
form: (even if the initial lesion produced is not sharply
defined). For this reason, it may be essential to determine
the response of all the retinal cell types to the agent, not
merely that of the cell type of greatest immediate interest
to the researcher. Chloroquine is retinotoxic (Rosenthal
et al., 1978) and its effect may be investigated in vitro,
where it affects photoreceptors (see Converse , this volume) and
pigment epithelium (Barishak et al., 1976). It produces
same specific effect on the protein profiles of embryo
neural retina and brain cells in vitro (Clayton and Zehir,
1982) and also affects other tissues in vitro such as
muscle (Bossen et al., 1973).

Pharmacogenetic variation occurs in all species so far
studied, including man, and heterozygotes for various defi-
ciencies may be more susceptible to specific agents than
normals. The interaction of a subliminally retinotoxic

agent with an appropriate pharmacogenetic susceptibility
may account for some at least of the so-called "simplex"
cases of RP, for which a familial basis cannot be ascertained.

It may be possible in the future to assess tissues of
such individuals, and their relatives, with various retinotoxic substances *in vitro*.

A genomic library may be constructed for the detection of
RP-like conditions due to deletions, as in the case of some
of the thalassaemias; or for linkage studies, which is, of
course, a less certain diagnostic: linkage studies may also
be made using the man-mouse cell hybrid technique. Recombinant cDNA probes, prepared to selected mRNAs, make it possible to investigate the genomic complement using Southern
transfers and any convenient tissue, and also the characteristics of the mRNA by Northern transfers or by cell-free translation following hybridization selection (reviewed Ruddle, 1981).
The problem is first to obtain a relevant mRNA. The most readily
available mRNAs for cloning will be those most abundant in retina
as judged by cell-free translation (Godchaux, 1978; Schechter
et al., 1979), but antigenic species shared between retina
and other tissues (see Clayton, this volume) may also be
relevant for some conditions, and minor mRNA species may be
selected by immune sequestration (for example Delovich *et al.*,
1972), provided only that an antiserum is available. It
may be hoped that the availability of increasingly powerful
techniques for molecular recognition will help to transform
RP studies in the near future.

REFERENCES

Arden, G.B. and Fox, B. (1979). Increased incidence of
    abnormal nasal cilia in patients with retinitis pigmentosa.
    Nature **279**, 545-536.
Barishak, Y.R., Barr-Nec, L. and Messer, Y. (1976). Effect
    of chloroquine upon the retinal pigmented epithelium in
    organ culture conditions. *Ophthal. Res.* **8**, 17-24.
Bird, A.C. (1981). Retinitis pigmentosa - A clinicians view-
    point. (this volume)
Bonnevie, K. (1936). Abortive differentiation of the ear
    vesicles. *Genetica* **18**, p. 105
Bossen, E.H., Lough, J.W. and Housen, S.L. (1973). The
    effects of chloroquine on chick skeletal muscle *in vitro*.
    Toxicol. appl. Pharmacol. **24**, 197-205.
Cafferata, R., Panosian, J. and Bordley, G.(1979). Develop-
    mental and biochemical studies of adhesive specificity
    among embryonic retina cells. *Dev. Biol.* **69**, 108-117.
Clayton, R.M. and Zehir, A. (1981). The use of cell culture

methods for exploring teratogenic susceptibility.
"Developmental Toxicology", (Ed. K. Snell), pp. 59-92,
Croom Helm Publ. London.

Converse, C.A. (1982). Chloriquine and Thioridazine-induced
retinopathies. (this volume)

Cuthbert, J. and Clayton, R.M. (1982). Cataract in association
with retinitis pigmentosa: analysis of the crystallin
subunit composition. (this volume)

Delovitch, T.L., Boyd, S.L., Tsay, H.M., Holme, G., Sehon,
A.H. (1972). Isolation of messenger like RNA from immuno-
chemically separated polysomes. *J. Mol. Biol.* **69**, 373-86.

Deol, M.S. (1954). The anomalies of the labyrinth of the
mutants variant-wadler, shaker-2 and jerker in the mouse.
J. Genet. **52**, 562-588.

Deol, M.S. (1956). The anatomy and development of the
mutants pirouette, shaker-1 and waltzer in the mouse.
Proc. Roy. Soc. B **145**, 206-213.

Deol, M.S. (1964). The abnormalities of the inner ear in
Kreisler mice. *J. Emb. exp. Morphol.* **12**, 475-490.

Godchaux, W. (1978). Protein biosynthesis in a cell-free
system from bovine retina. *Biochim. Biophys. Acta.* **520**,
428-440.

Gottlieb, D.I., Rock, K. and Glaser, L. (1976). A gradient
of adhesive specificity in developing avian retina.
Proc. Natl. Acad. Sci. U.S.A. **73** (2) 410-414.

Harris, H. (1975). "Principles of Human Biochemical Genetics",
N. Holland, Elsevier, Amsterdam.

Jacobson, A.G. (1966). Inductive processes in embryonic
development. *Science* **152**, 25.

Kaighn, M.E. (1976). In "Tests of Teratogenicity *In Vitro*"
(Eds J.D. Eberg and M. Marois), pp. 73-90, Elsevier/
N. Holland, Amsterdam.

Rosenthal, A.R., Kolb, H., Bergsma, D., Huxgoll, D. and
Hopkins, S.L. (1978). Chloroquine retinopathy in the
rhesus monkey. *Invest. Ophthal. Vis. Sci.* **17**, 1158-1175.

Russel, E.S. (1981). Hereditary Anaemias of the mouse. A
review for geneticists. *Adv. Genetics* **20**, 358-460.

Ruddle, F.H. (1981). A new ear in mammalian gene mapping;
somatic cell genetics and recombinant DNA methodologies.
Nature **294**, 115-120.

Schechter, I., Burstein, Y., Zemell, R., Ziv, E., Kantor, F.
and Papermaster, D.S. (1979). Messenger RNA of opsin from
bovine retina. Isolation and partial sequence of the
in vitro translation product. *Proc. Natl. Acad. Sci.
U.S.A.* **76**, 2654-2658.

Trisler, G.D., Schneider, M.D. and Nirenberg, M. (1981). A
topographic gradient of molecules in retina can be used
to identify neuron position. *Proc. Natl. Acad. Sci.
U.S.A.* **78**, (4) 2145-2149.

Truslove, G. (1956).   The anatomy and development of the
     fidget mouse. *J. Gen.* **54**, 64-86.
Voaden, M.J. (1982).   Taurine and retinitis pigmentosa.
     (this volume)

THE ULTRASTRUCTURAL CHARACTERISTICS OF CONGENITAL HYPERPLASIA OF THE RETINAL PIGMENT EPITHELIUM

KLAUS WIRZ[+] and WILLIAM LEE[*]

[+]*Abteilung Augenheilkunde der Medizinischen Fakultat, 5100 Aachen, Goethestrasse 27/29, West Germany*

[*]*The University Departments of Pathology and Ophthalmology, The University of Glasgow, Glasgow G11 6NT, UK*

INTRODUCTION

Flat, solitary, disc-shaped and heavily pigmented lesions, which are located toward the retinal periphery, are a rare but a well-recognized clinical entity and are known to have a very limited growth potential. Various terms have been applied to this entity, for example "benign melanoma" (Reese and Jones, 1956), "hypertrophy with hyperpigmentation of the RPE" (Purcell and Shields, 1975), "hamartoma of the retinal pigment epithelium" (McLean, 1976), but the name coined by Buettner (1975) — "congenital hypertrophy of the retinal pigment epithelium" (CHRPE) is now established in the literature (Morris and Henkind, 1979; Tso, 1979). CHRPE is characterized *in vivo* by a scalloped edge with a peripheral halo and lacunae of depigmentation within the dense black central part. This macroscopic variation in pigmentation does not correspond to the two histological and one ultrastructural descriptions (Kurz and Zimmerman, 1962; Buettner, 1975) which revealed a hyperpigmented and hypertrophic RPE monolayer. A detailed examination of an RPE malformation of the type described as CHRPE was carried out to further investigate the discrepancy between the macroscopic and microscopic descriptions. To exclude the possibility that CHRPE is a reactionary change or a neoplastic transformation, a typical example of a postinflammatory reactionary RPE hyperplasia (presumed toxoplasmosis) and an RPE adenoma were studied concurrently.

MATERIALS AND METHODS

The example of CHRPE was present at the superior mid-periphery in the globe of a 60 year old male. This eye was removed for treatment of a small temporal peripapillary choroidal melanoma and was fixed in glutaraldehyde (3%). The CHRPE was 5 mm in diameter and showed the characteristic sharply defined scalloped edge (lined by an inner zone of pallor) and two irregular foci of depigmentation. Samples from the abnormality were prepared for routine paraffin histologic, fluorescence microscopy and for conventional electron microscopy.

RESULTS

Morphological Appearances

The retina and choroid in the vicinity of the CHRPE were of normal appearance.

At the hyperpigmented periphery, the RPE cells were hypertrophic and engorged with melanin, lipofuscin and melano-lipofuscin complexes (Fig. 1). Internal to this the RPE

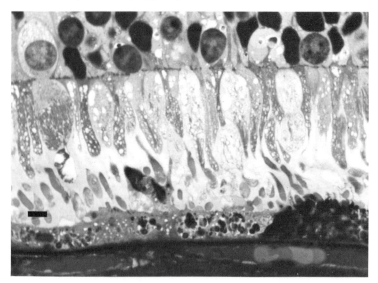

Fig. 1. *Light microscopy (toluidine blue/araldite section) to show the periphery of the malformation which is to the left. The extreme peripheral cells are enlarged by an excess of melanin and lipofuscin while internal to this the cells are atrophic (Bar marker 5μm).*

cells were flattened and atrophic and almost devoid of melanosomes (Fig. 1). Toward the central part there was a transition
from a hyperpigmented monolayer of RPE cells to multilayering
(3 to 4 layers) of the hyper-pigmented RPE cells and this was
paralleled by a progressive atropy of the photoreceptor layer
(Fig. 2). The inner retina, the choroid and the chorio-
capillaries showed no significant abnormality.

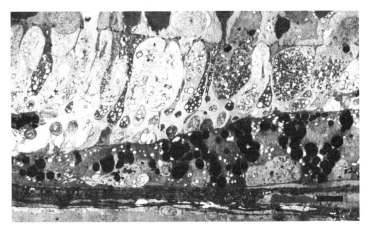

Fig. 2. *Electron micrograph to show the transition from an*
RPE monolayer to a multilayer which contains giant melano-
somes. Note the progressive atrophy of the photoreceptor
outer segments (Bar marker 5μm).

The cells in the macroscopically hyperpigmented area were
either of columnar shape (Fig. 3) or cuboidal and multilayered
(Fig. 4). In the latter situation the outermost layer of
cells showed a marked electron-lucency in the cytoplasm.
Junctional attachments (maculae adhaerentes and occludentes)
were maintained between the cells, but were atypical in
location. In the multilayered region, the cell processes
formed focal dense clusters and between these, the membrane
attachments were profuse. Extracellular material (ground
substance, basement membrane material, collagen of 60 and 100
nm banding) was located in foci between the cell layers.
Microcysts containing spike-like processes were present
in the outer layer of cells (Fig. 4).
The most significant abnormality was observed in the
nature and distribution of the melanosomes. In the outermost layer of RPE cells, round premelanosomes and partially
pigmented melanosomes (1 to 2 μm dia.) were prominent,
while in the inner layers the melanosomes were round and of
the order of 5 μm diameter (Fig. 4). The intermediate cells

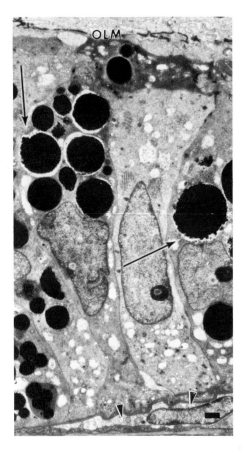

Fig. 3. *Electron micrograph to show cuboidal cells filling the space between the outer limiting membrane (OLM) and Bruch's membrane which contains a spindle cell (arrow heads). Note the giant melansome (arrow heads) (Bar marker 1 μm).*

contained smaller compound melanosomes which appeared to be a transition between the extremes. In the region of hyper-pigmentation, spindle cells were found within Bruch's membrane (Fig. 4); the cells contained melanosomes and were attached by maculae adhaerentes and maculae occludentes.

Blocks from the areas of pallor showed a total photo-receptor and RPE atrophy and here the residual Müller cells were in contact with Bruch's membrane.

DISCUSSION

Although the lesion most commonly described as "congenital

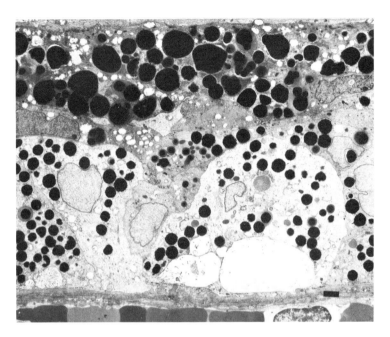

Fig. 4. *Electron micrograph to show the variation in architecture of the cells and the melanin granules between the
inner layer and the outer layer of the malformation (see
text) (Bar marker 2μm).*

hypertrophy of the retinal pigment epithelium" is now accepted
as a hamartomatous malformation (Purcell and Shields, 1975;
Norris and Cleasby, 1976; Cleary, *et al.*, 1976; Laqua and
Wessing, 1979), there is as yet no evidence that this abnormality of the RPE is present at birth. The assumption
that the abnormality is a malformation is based on the static
nature and absence of growth during many years of observation.
However, in one well-documented report, the enlargement of
a homogeneous black disc to the characteristic scalloped
and variegated lesion has been demonstrated (Norris and
Cleasby, 1976).

    Whatever the true nature of this entity, the histological
and ultrastructural features differ from processes which
might be considered as alternative aetiologies. The ultrastructural features of reactionary hyperplasia and neoplasia
have been documented (Wallow and Tso, 1972; Font *et al.*, 1972)
and are similar to those described in Table 1 which shows
that there are clear differences in the organization and
architecture of these three disorders of the RPE. Thus
there is additional morphological support for the clinical

TABLE 1

The ultrastructural features which distinguish CHRPE from post inflammatory reactionary hyperplasia (presumed toxoplasmosis chorioretinitis in a 69 year old man) and an adenoma of the RPE (60 year old man).

	Reactionary Hyperplasia	Congenital Hyperplasia	Adenoma
Cell Shape	Spindle	Columnar/cuboidal	Polygonal
Cell Orientation	Parallel to Bruch's Membrane	Perpendicular to Bruch's Membrane	Random
Maturation	To amelanotic cells	To heavy pigmentation	To amelanotic cells
Cytoplasmic Density	Uniform	Varies with maturation	Mainly uniform (low)
Organelles (Features of synthesis)	Prominent	Moderate	Sparse
Vacuoles	Occasional	Prominent	Absent
Processes	Focally profuse	Focally profuse and junctioned	Stunted and less common
Premelanosomes	Present	Present	Present
Malanosomes	Round and granular 1μm. diameter	Homogeneous and solid 2 to 6μm. dia. Complex malanosomes Giant melanosomes	Fragmentation ++ 1μm. dia.

Membrane attachments	m.a., m.o., gap. desmosomes	m.a., m.o., gap. desmosomes	m.a., m.o., gap. desmosomes
Basement membrane	Prominent	basal and focal	sparse
Extracellular material	60 nm and 100 nm collagen	60 nm and 100 nm collagen	50 nm and 100 nm collagen

---

Abbreviations: m.a., maculae adherentes, m.o., maculae occludentes, gap, gap junction.

opinion that "CHRPE" is a well-defined entity. The morphology
in the specimen under discussion differs from previous descriptions in that, in addition to hypertrophy and hyperpigmentation, as described by Buettner (1975), there is a hyperplasia. The morphological study of Buettner (1975) was performed on a small uniformly pigmented disc and it seems
reasonable to suggest that the present specimen is a more
advanced form of the same disease process.

The nature of this unique disturbance is speculative, but
the morphology suggests that a progressive disturbance in
melanogenesis is an important component. Whether or not the
basic abnormality is a disturbance in photoreceptor-RPE
interaction (see Morris and Henkind, 1979; for review) remains
open. This morphological study (which is considered in detail
elsewhere: Wirz and Lee, 1981) suggests that the outer retinal
atrophy is secondary to pressure and nutritional disturbance
and less to a specific disorganization of the process of
photoreceptor phagocytosis.

ACKNOWLEDGEMENTS

K. W. was supported by the Deutsche Forschungsgemeinschaft
Grant, W. 637/1-1. The authors wish to thank Mrs D.M.
Aitken for her technical assistance and Mrs P. Bonnar for
her secretarial assistance.

REFERENCES

Buettner, H. (1975). Congenital hypertrophy of the retinal
    pigment epithelium. *Amer. J. Ophthal.* **79**, 177—189.
Cleary, P.E., Gregor, Z. and Bird, A.C. (1976). Retinal
    vascular changes in congenital hypertrophy of the retinal
    pigment epithelium. *Brit. J. Ophthal.* **60**, 499—503.
Font, R.L., Zimmerman, L.E. and Fine, B.S. (1972). Adenoma
    of the retinal pigment epithelium. *Amer. J. Ophthal.*
    73, 544—554.
Kurz, G.H. and Zimmerman, L.E. (1962). Vagaries of the
    retinal pigment epithelium. *Int. Ophthalmol. Clin.* **2**,
    441—464.
Laqua, H. and Wessing, A. (1979). Congenital retino-pigment
    epithelial malformation previously described as a hamar-
    toma. *Amer. J. Ophthal.* **87**, 34—42.
McClean, E.B. (1976). Hamartoma of the retinal pigment
    epithelium. *Amer. J. Ophthal.* **82**, 227—231.
Morris, D.A. and Henkind, P. (1979). In "The Retinal Pig-
    ment Epithelium" (Eds K.M. Zinn and M.F. Marmor) pp.

247–266. Harvard University Press, Cambridge, Mass. and London, U.K.

Norris, J.L. and Cleasby, G.W. (1976). An unusual case of congenital hypertrophy of the retinal pigment epithelium. *Arch. Ophthal.* **94**, 1910–1911.

Purcell, J.J. and Shields, J.A. (1975). Hypertrophy with hyperpigmentation of the retinal pigment epithelium. *Arch Ophthal.* **93**, 1122–1126.

Reese, A.B. and Jones, I.S. (1956). Benign melanomas of the retinal pigment epithelium. *Amer. J. Ophthal.* **42**, 207–212.

Tso, M.O.M. (1979). In "The Retinal Pigment Epithelium" (Eds K.M. Zinn and M.F. Marmor) pp. 267–276. Harvard University Press, Cambridge, Mass. and London, U.K.

Wallow, I.H.L. and Tso, M.O.M. (1972). Proliferation of the retinal pigment epithelium over malignant choroidal tumours: a light and electron microscopic study. *Amer. J. Ophthal.* **73**, 914–926.

Wirz, K. and Lee, W.R. (1982). Congenital hyperplasia of the retinal pigment epithelium — an electron microscopic study. (Submitted for publication).

THE ELECTRORETINOGRAM IN DOMINANTLY INHERITED RETINITIS PIGMENTOSA

G.B. ARDEN

Department of Visual Science, Institute of Ophthalmology, Judd Street, London, UK

We have attempted to subdivide patients with Retinitis Pigmentosa (R.P.) into categories which might more nearly represent single disease entities, and wish to report on the preliminary results of electroretinogram (ERG) testing. These studies were in collaboration with Professor A. Bird, Mr B. Quinlon, Miss R. Lyness and Miss G. Clover (Retinal Unit, Moorfields Eye Hospital, London) and Dr W.J. Ernst (Institute of Ophthalmology, London).

The ERG is a postsynaptic phenomenon, and probably represents the current developed by glial (Müller) cells. Hence it is a most indirect way of analysing defects in photoreceptors. However, it is non-invasive and by altering the intensity and wavelength of the stimulating flashes, one can attempt to assess the sensitivity and supra-threshold function of the rods and cones.

In 55 subjects, all of whom suffered from autosomal, dominantly inherited R.P., we have measured the ERG, the extent of the visual field, and also the psychophysical threshold for rods and cones at numerous points within the visual field. In 36 patients we were unable to record any rod ERG at all. The remaining patients all had ERGs produced by weak blue light, of the characteristic slow rounded waveform associated with scotopic responses. The two groups were very sharply distinguished, by the amplitude of the ERG (10 µV for the cases with no rod waveform and 172 µV for the remainder) and also by its sensitivity. In patients without rod components, the sensitivity was raised more than 3 log units, while in the remainder the median increase was less than 1 log unit. In addition, the relationship between response amplitude and field size is quite different in those patients with rod ERGs. Thus, with a very superficial examination, human dominantly inherited disease can be divided

into two categories. Massof *et al.* (1981) have previously
subdivided patients with dominant R.P. on the basis that
in some (class I) there is no psychophysical evidence of rod
activity, and it appears that early in life the rods have
undergone a catastrophe. During the development of the R.P.
in adult life, the cones slowly deteriorate. In class II,
the degeneration affects rods and cones more or less equally,
and careful measurement of rod and cone thresholds indicates
that rods are active under certain circumstances. It seemed
possible that in our patients with no rod ERGs, the psychophysical characteristics would indicate similarity with
Massof's class I. This expectation was not however fulfilled;
16 of the 36 patients appeared to have preserved rod function,
even though this was undetectable on the ERG. Thus these
patients can again be subdivided, and by analysing other
aspects of the response, for example the amplitude, in
relation to age and field size, it appears that these subdivisions may be real, and the natural history of the condition is different in the two cases. One fairly trivial
possibility can easily be eliminated: in those patients with
no rod ERG but with psychophysical evidence of rod activity,
there is often a fairly large visual field, and a loss of
rod sensitivity to light intensity of no more than 2 log
units: it ought to be possible to record rod ERG responses.
We must, therefore, conclude that although the scotopic
system is functioning, the glial system responsible for the
production of the b- wave is secondarily affected. This is
not a new conclusion — for many years the "extinguished"
ERG in Retinitis Pigmentosa has been a puzzle. Our new
techniques enable us to see very small responses, and also
to pick up cone responses, but rod b- waves are not detected
in these patients, although in other R.P. patients the system
still functions. Thus it seems likely that in some of our
patients, there is a defect which is not limited to the
photoreceptors, since b- wave mechanism is more severely
affected than the rods themselves. Such findings, of course,
have bearing on the nature of the appropriate animal model
with which to compare our patients.

    Even further subdivision is possible. In the 19 patients
who have recognizable rod ERGs it was possible to determine
the sensitivity of the ERG b- wave. (This is done by determining the amount of light required to evoke a response which
is 50% of the size of a maximal response.) We found, much
to our surprise, that in many patients the result was within
0.5 log units of the normal average value. Thus, it is possible that the distribution of degeneration in the retina
is patchy, and in some areas the retina gives a response,
while in others the response is absent. However, when the

psychophysical threshold is measured, most patients with
dominant R.P. have obvious measurable losses of sensitivity
of the scotopic mechanism. We asked the question as to the
nature of the ERGs we would expect, given the losses of
visual sensitivity shown psychophysically. We assumed that
each small element of retina was capable of producing the sam
same ERG current, but the quantity of light required to
evoke the current varied, as was shown by the threshold determinations. We assumed that the voltage to light intensity
relationship of any particular small area of the retina
obeyed the same general relationship as is found in the normal.
In some cases the model results, which were calculated on a
computer, agreed well with the observed ERG results, both
when visual loss was mild and when it was severe. However,
in about half the cases there was a discrepancy which was
too great to account for by experimental error. In all these
cases the discrepancy was of the same kind, namely, that
although the patient reported night-blindness, when the
thresholds were determined the ERG sensitivity was near
normal. Thus it appears that the patients may be further
subdivided, and we may have four separate ERG categories of
autosomal dominant disease. Again, if the ERG (which is
developed in the outer plexiform and inner nuclear layers)
shows no loss of sensitivity, the simplest explanation is
that in R.P. of this type there is an additional post-photo-
receptor level in the retina where visual sensitivity is
lost. Therefore, this type of disease must also affect
more than the photoreceptors. Finally, in several instances,
it has been found that the retinas of patients with R.P.
contain considerable quantities of rhodopsin (Ripps *et al.*,
1978), and our ERG studies, which show so little loss of
sensitivity, would imply that this must be the case.

REFERENCES

Massoff, R.W., Johnson, M.A. and Finklestein, D. (1981).
    Peripheral absolute threshold spectral sensitivity
    curves. *Brit. J. Ophthalmol.* **65**, 112—121.
Ripps, H., Brin, K.P. and Weale, R.A. (1978). Rhodopsin
    and visual threshold in retinitis pigmentosa. *Invest.
    Ophthalmol. Vis. Sci.* **17**, 735—745.

TAURINE AND RETINITIS PIGMENTOSA

MARY J. VOADEN

Department of Visual Science, Institute of Ophthalmology, University of London, London, UK

INTRODUCTION

Taurine is distributed widely throughout the body, high concentrations having been reported in, for example, muscle,
lung, blood cells (platelets and leukocytes), spleen, bone
marrow, thymus, brain (in particular the neurohypophysis,
pituitary gland and olfactory bulb) and, of significance to
the present discussion on taurine and Retinitis Pigmentosa
(R.P.), the retina (Jacobsen and Smith, 1968; Mandel and
Pasantes-Morales, 1978; Sturman *et al.*, 1978 ; Voaden *et al.*,
1981). In the latter it is enriched in photoreceptor cells
and here may reach concentrations of 30 to 80mM (cf. Voaden
et al., 1981).

Apart from the well-established role for taurine as a con-
jugate in bile pigments our understanding of its functions
in the body remains tentative, being complicated by too many
rather than too few possibilities. It has, for example, been
implicated in mechanisms maintaining homeostasis of Na^+, K^+,
Ca^{2+} and Zn^{2+} in tissues (for reviews see Jacobsen and Smith,
1968; Barbeau and Donaldson, 1974; Huxtable and Barbeau,
1976; Barbeau and Huxtable, 1978) and, perhaps connected
with one or all of these, has anti-seizure activity in the
brain and inotropic action on the heart. It is neuro-active
and a putative neurotransmitter. Radiation-induced hyper-
taurinuria is well-documented and taurine administration will
increase the LD50 of radiation exposed mice (Abe *et al.*,
1968). It will also protect against, for example, the induction of diabetes by streptozotocin (Kuriyama *et al.*, 1981)
and has frequently been suggested as a membrane stabilizer.
It may participate in the regulation of osmotic pressure.
(Jacobson and Smith, 1968; Hoffman and Hendil, 1976; Thurston *et al.*, 1980).

In the retina taurine may serve with species variation, as

a neurotransmitter in some higher order retinal neurones but is not thought to have this role in photoreceptors (Voaden, *et al.*, 1981; Pourcho, 1981). In the latter, it may interact with and/or modulate Na^+, K^+ and Ca^{2+} movements perhaps playing a role in phototransduction (Pasantes-Morales *et al.*, 1979; Kuo and Miki, 1980) or possibly serving as an osmotic "buffer", protecting the cells against the ionic perturbations that occur in this process (Pasantes-Morales *et al.*, 1978; Miller and Steinberg, 1979). Light-stimulated release of taurine from both whole retinas and isolated outer limbs has been observed, (Salceda *et al.*, 1977; Pasantes-Morales *et al.*, 1978) occurring in the former at both the "on" and "off" of the light stimulus (Schmidt, 1978).

TAURINE DEFICIENCY AND THE RETINA

Kittens and cats maintained on a taurine-free diet develop and/or continue apparently normally, apart from a slight reduction in body weight. However, they go blind (Schmidt and Berson, 1978; Sturman *et al.*, 1978a; Anderson *et al.*, 1979). Vision is lost because of the selective degeneration of photoreceptor cells, cones being more susceptible in the earlier stages than rods. Although it has not, as yet, proved possible to duplicate this observation in other species, it is nevertheless suspected that a high endogenous level of taurine is essential for the maintenance of all photoreceptor cells, and it is this possibility that has led to the suggestion that a localized deficiency in taurine might be involved in the aetiology of some form(s) of R.P. It would appear that the cat is dependent on an adequate dietary supply of taurine because of the unfortunate combination of a low capacity for taurine synthesis from cysteine in its liver and the fact that it only conjugates bile acids with taurine (Jacobsen and Smith, 1978). The production of bile is one of the last body functions to be affected in the deficient animal, other body stores being depleted to maintain it. It is of interest, and perhaps a measure of the importance of taurine to the tissues, that the retina and olfactory bulb appear particularly resistant to depletion (Sturman *et al.*, 1978a; Anderson *et al.*, 1979).

Man also has a very low activity of cysteine sulphinate and cysteic acid decarboxylases in the liver (Jacobsen and Smith, 1968; Mandel and Pasantes-Morales, 1978) and the 1 to 2 week human neonate conjugates bile acids chiefly with taurine (Sturman and Hayes, 1980). However, with development, glycine is also introduced as a bile component until it constitutes 75% of the total amino acid pool. This may save man from

retinal problems associated with a dietary deficiency of
taurine. Nevertheless, it has been recognized that the neonate may be vulnerable and concern has been expressed about
the low levels of taurine in formulas based on cow's milk
(Sturman *et al.*, 1978a; Sturman and Hayes, 1980).

SOURCES OF RETINAL TAURINE

Taurine levels in the retina are normally maintained by two
mechanisms, endogenous synthesis and uptake from the blood
stream. We know that the former is insufficient to ensure
the structural integrity of the cat retina but the situation
in other species is unclear.

Retinas from several species, including the cat, contain
the anabolic enzymes cysteine oxidase and cysteine sulphinate
decarboxylase some being associated with photoreceptors
(Pasantes-Morales *et al.*, 1978), and evidence has been obtained for the synthesis of taurine from cysteine in guinea
pig and baboon retinas (Voaden *et al.*, 1981). Cysteine also
appears to readily enter most cells of the retina, including
photoreceptors; a particularly heavy uptake being observed in
cones of guinea pig and cat (Voaden *et al.*, 1981). Endogenous
synthesis of taurine in photoreceptors may well occur therefore. It is equally apparent, however, that the blood stream
is potentially a major source of this amino acid.

In the species so far examined, including primates (Table
1) the pigment epithelium (R.P.E.) has been found to possess
an active, high-affinity uptake mechanism for taurine (Voaden
et al., 1981) and it is known that the radio-labelled compound, when administered extra-ocularly, is taken up by the
R.P.E. before being transferred over a period of days, into
the neural retina. This may represent an adaptational mechanism developed to supply the specific needs of the tissue,
since, as with other neuroactive amino acids, taurine is
essentially excluded from free entry into the subretinal space
by the action of the blood-retinal barrier (i.e. membrane
carriers in the R.P.E. effecting a net transport of taurine
from retina to choroid: Miller and Steinberg, 1976). The
mechanism underlying the slow passage of taurine from the
R.P.E. to the neural retina is not understood. It may inter-
relate with the fluctuations in potassium and sodium transport occurring between photoreptors and the R.P.E. during
light and dark adaptation (Miller and Steinberg, 1979) but
no difference in the rate of taurine turnover was observed
in retinas from mice maintained in the dark or in a 12 h
light- 12 h dark cycle for a period of 8 weeks (Voaden
et al., 1981). It is known that in nutritionally-balanced

TABLE 1

3H Taurine uptake by Pigment Epithelium (R.P.E.)

A	Time Postmortem (h)	Km (μM)	V max pmol/min/3mm dia. disc R.P.E.
	1.0	30	7.5
	4.0	23	9.7
	96.0	45	5.1
	(at 4°C)		

B	Species studied	Km (μM)	V max nmol/h/μl cells
	Rat (cultured R.P.E.)	16	2.3
	Frog	23	0.8
	Baboon	30	5.8

To obtain the results shown in Section A, isolated baboon R.P.E. + choroid was incubated for 10 min, at 37°C, in glucose supplemented, Krebs' bicarbonate medium, containing from 1 to 60 μM ^{3}H-taurine. The tissue was then floated on to filter paper, drained, and 3mm dia. discs of the R.P.E. /filter paper preparation trephined out. Tissue was then solubilized in Triton X-100 and the radio-activity counted on a Packard 3375 liquid scintillation spectrometer. Values are based on 10 (1 and 4 h pm) and 24 (96 h pm) estimations (Hussain and Voaden unpub. obsv.). Section B shows data for 1 h pm baboon R.P.E., recalculated on a volume basis (taking the radial diameter of a R.P.E. cell as 10μ) and compared with values obtained by Edwards (1977) for rat, and Lake *et al.* (1977) for frog.

animals entry into the neural retina occurs by exchange with
the endogenous stores, the half-life being 9 to 11 days in
the cat (Sturman *et al.*, 1978*a*) and in the mouse (Voaden *et
al.*, 1981). In contrast net uptake is observed in deficient
cats (Sturman *et al.*, 1978*a*).

Catabolism of taurine in the retina, if existing, is slight
(Voaden *et al.*, 1981; cf. Fellman *et al.*, 1980).

The relative contributions of systemic supply and endogenous
synthesis to taurine levels in the retina are not known, nor
is the extent that one can substitute for the other if a
defect exists. However, it is apparent that the R.P.E. is
in part regulating the retinal supply of the amino acid and
it is clear that photoreceptors might be placed in jeopardy
if a defect should exist at this level.

TAURINE AND RETINITIS PIGMENTOSA

A breakdown of taurine homeostasis in the retina, leading to
or exacerbating photoreceptor degeneration could arise from
one or a combination of three general situations: a defect
in endogenous synthesis; an inability of the cells to retain
the amino acid once it is there; and a deficiency in the
systemic supply. We are only at the beginning of investigat-
ing these possibilities in the various forms of R.P., and
study is inevitably hindered by inaccessibility of the tissue
and lack of suitable postmortem material. In addition, should
affected retinas become available, allowance would have to be
made for photoreceptor loss, as this by itself would lead to
a change in the concentration and total tissue level of taurine,
and taurine uptake sites. It is essential, therefore, to
monitor morphology and if possible, to quantify, for example,
DNA protein and rhodopsin levels per unit area of tissue:
regional differences must also be considered. Observation
of a lowered endogenous level of taurine within the remaining
tissue would not necessarily mean that this was a causative
factor in the lesion, since it is possible that a reduction
might represent, for example, a secondary change occurring in
response to an osmotic imbalance.

A deficiency in the systemic supply of taurine or its precursors to the retina might arise from lowered levels in the
blood or from defects in the membrane carriers in the R.P.E.
and/or the photoreceptors. Defect in the carrier(s) could
be molecular or might result from secondary inhibition by,
for example, plasma factors. Some measurements relating to
these possibilities have been made, although, at present,
studies are limited by the low numbers of patients included
in the groups, or by inadequate patient classification. With

these reservations it would appear that normal plasma taurine
levels are present in "autosomal dominant", "X-hemizygote",
"autosomal recessive", "junior macular dystrophy", "choroidae-
mia" and "gyrate atrophy" patients (Berson *et al.*, 1976); in
"simplex" patients (Airaksinen *et al.*, 1981) and in patients
with macular dystrophy (Table 2). ("Simplex" cases may be
autosomal recessives.) A deficiency in cysteine found earlier,
by Fujiwara (1968) in serum from patients with "hereditary"
R.P. was not seen/investigated in these studies.

Several tissues of the body, including blood platelets,
possess "high-affinity" uptake mechanisms for taurine resembling that present in the R.P.E. Platelets are readily
accessible and can be used to see if there is a generalized
defect in taurine uptake in R.P. patients. Preliminary
observations by Airaksinen *et al.* (1981) have provided
evidence for a reduction in the uptake of taurine by platelets
(incubated in autologous plasma) from a predominantly simplex
group of R.P. patients (i.e. with no known relatives). Engo-
genous taurine was also lowered. In contrast, uptake by
platelets from patients with Usher's syndrome was normal.
The former is an interesting observation meriting further
study. However, normal taurine uptake has been found by
Voaden *et al.*, 1982 in platelets from "simplex" and "autosomal
dominant" patients. There was a reduction in the tissue to
medium ratio established by platelets, from "X-hemizygote" RP
patients, incubated in autologous plasma and a trend towards
an increase when the platelets were incubated in Ca^{2+}-free
Krebs bicarbonate medium — suggesting that there may be a plasma
factor affecting taurine handling. It is, therefore, of
interest that in a study of amino acid levels in whole blood
haemolysates from R.P. patients Arshinoff *et al.* (1981) have
found normal taurine levels in all but "X-hemizygote" patients,
where there was an 11% reduction. Although this might suggest
a decrease in endogenous taurine uptake in these patients and
would correlate well with the taurine uptake data, it should
be noted that we have also observed a high incidence (62%) of
thrombocytopaenia in the "X-hemizygote" patients studied.
Since platelets contain a high concentration of endogenous
taurine, lowered numbers in the blood could well account
for the decrease observed in the study of Arshinoff and
coworkers.

Normal taurine handling by platelets from R.P. patients
does not exclude the possibility of a localized defect in
taurine uptake in the R.P.E. or photoreceptors. Taurine uptake in the neural retina decreases rapidly postmortem
(Schmidt and Berson, 1980) and this must also be considered
in any future studies. However, the same may not be true
for the pigment epithelium (Table 1), where it may be possible

TABLE 2

Taurine levels in blood from patients with Macular Dystrophy

| | Normal (n = 7) | | Macular Dystrophy (n = 8) | |
	range	mean (μm $\pm$ SEM)	range	mean (μm $\pm$ SEM)
Whole blood haemolysate	160-285	206 $\pm$ 17	167-246	197 $\pm$ 11
Plasma	49-73	59 $\pm$ 3	40-68	51 $\pm$ 3

The "Macular Dystrophy" patients selected for this study were a heterogenous group representing various manifestations of the disease (including recessive and dominant inheritance). Freshly-drawn, heparinized, "fasting" blood was used, norleucine being added as internal standard. One ml of whole blood or plasma was mixed with 4 mls methanol, stood on ice 1 h and centrifuged. Supernatants were recovered and processed on a Technicion Amino Acid Analyser. The mean concentrations of all amino acids did not significantly differ from normal. Cystine was not recovered. (Bird, Huggins and Voaden, unpubl. observ.).

to obtain meaningful data from tissue several hours and, possibly, even days post—mortem. More studies are needed to
confirm these observations.

REFERENCES

Abe, M., Takahashi, M., Takeuchi, K. and Fukuda, M. (1968).
    Studies on the significance of taurine in radiation injury.
    Radiation Res. **33**, 563—573.
Airaksinen, E.M., Airaksinen, M.M., Sihvola, P. and Marnela,
    K.-M. (1981). Decrease in the uptake and concentration of
    taurine in blood platelets of Retinitis Pigmentosa patients.
    Met. and Ped. Ophthalmol. **5**, 45—48.
Anderson, P.A., Baker, D.H., Corbin, J.E. and Helper, L.C.
    (1979). Biochemical lesions associated with taurine
    deficiency in the cat. *J. Animal Science* **49**, 1227—1234.
Arshinoff, S.A., McCulloch, J.C., Macrae, W., Stein, A.N.
    and Marliss, E.B. (1981). Amino acids in Retinitis Pig-
    mentosa. *Brit. J. Ophthalmol.* **65**, 626—630.
Barbeau, A. and Donaldson, J. (1974). Zinc, taurine and
    epilepsy. *Arch. Neurol (Chicago)* **30**, 52—58.
Barbeau, A. and Huxtable, R.J. (Eds) (1978). "Taurine and
    Neurological Disorders" Raven Press, New York.
Berson, E.L., Schmidt, S.Y. and Rabin, A.R. (1976). Plasma
    amino acids in hereditary retinal disease: ornithine,
    lysine and taurine. *Brit. J. Ophthalmol.* **60**, 142—147.
Edwards, R.B. (1977). Accumulation of taurine by cultured
    retinal pigment epithelium of the rat. *Invest. Ophthal-
    mol.* **16**, 201—208.
Fellman, J.H., Roth, E.S., Avedovech, N.A. and McCarthy, K.D.
    (1980). The metabolism of taurine to isethionate.
    Arch. Biochem. Biophys. **204**, 560—567.
Fujiwara, H. (1968). Biochemical studies on Retinitis Pig-
    mentosa. 3. Study on amino acids metabolism of the
    patients with Retinitis Pigmentosa. *Folia Ophthal. Jap.*
    19, 741—753.
Hoffman, E.K. and Hendil, K.B. (1976). The role of amino
    acids and taurine in isosmotic intracellular regulation
    in Ehrlich ascites mouse tumour cells. *J. Comp. Physiol.*
    108, 279—286.
Huxtable, R. and Barbeau, A. (Eds) (1976). "Taurine". Raven
    Press, New York.
Jacobsen, J.G. and Smith, L.H. Jr. (1968). Biochemistry and
    physiology of taurine and taurine derivatives. *Physiol.
    Rev.* **48**, 424—511.
Kuo, C.-H., and Miki, N. (1980). Stimulatory effect of
    taurine on Ca^{2+}-uptake by disc membranes from photo-

receptor cell outer segments. *Biochem. Biophys Res. Commun.* **94**, 646–651.

Kuriyama, K., Yoneda, Y. and Maramatsu, M. (1981). Taurine: a sulphur containing amino acid possibly important for maintaining cellular integrity. In "The Effects of Taurine on Excitable Tissues". (Eds S.I. Baskin, J.J. Kocsis and S.W. Schaffer.) Spectrum Publications, New York.

Lake, N., Marshall, J. and Voaden, M.J. (1977). The entry of taurine into the neural retina and pigment epithelium of the frog. *Brain Research* **128**, 497–503.

Mandel, P. and Pasantes-Morales, H. (1978). Taurine in the nervous system. *Reviews of Neuroscience* **3**, 157–193.

Miller, S. and Steinberg, R.H. (1976). Transport of taurine, L-methionine and 3-o-methyl-D-glucose across frog retinal pigment epithelium. *Exp. Eye Res.* **23**, 177–190.

Miller, S.S. and Steinberg, R.H. (1979). Potassium modulation of taurine transport across the frog retinal pigment epithelium. *J. Gen. Physiol.* **74**, 237–259.

Pasantes-Morales, H., Ademe, R.M. and Lopez-Colomé, A.M. (1979). Taurine effects on $^{45}Ca^{2+}$ transport in retinal subcellular fractions. *Brain Research* **172**, 131–138.

Pasantes-Morales, H., Salceda, R. and Lopez-Colome, A.M. (1978). Taurine in Normal Retina. In "Taurine and Neurological Disorders" (Eds A. Barbeau and R.J. Huxtable.) pp. 265–279. Raven Press, New York.

Pourcho, R.G. (1981). ^{3}H Taurine — accumulating neurons in the cat retina. *Exp. Eye Res.* **32**, 11–20.

Salceda, R., Lopez-Colomé, A.M. and Pasantes-Morales, H. (1977). Light stimulated release of [^{35}S] taurine from frog retinal rod outer segments. *Brain Research* **135**, 186–191.

Schmidt, S.Y. (1978). Taurine fluxes in isolated cat and rat retinas: effects of illumination. *Exp. Eye Res.* **26**, 529–535.

Schmidt, S.Y. and Berson, E.L. (1978). Taurine in retinal degenerations. In "Taurine and Neurological Disorders" (Eds A. Barbeau and R.J. Huxtable). pp. 281-287. Raven Press, New York.

Schmidt, S.Y. and Berson, E.L. (1980). Postmortem metabolic capacity of photoreceptor cells in human and rat retinas. *Invest. Ophthalmol. and Vis. Sci.* **19**, 1274–1280.

Sturman, J.A. and Hayes, K.C. (1980). The biology of taurine in nutrition and development. *Adv. Nutr. Res.* **3**, 231–299.

Sturman, J.A., Rassin, D.K., Hayes, K.C. and Gaull, G.E. (1978a). Taurine deficiency in the kitten: exchange and turnover of [^{35}S] taurine in brain, retina and other tissues. *J. Nutrition*, **108**, 1462–1476.

Sturman, J.A., Rassin, D.K. and Gaull, G.E. (1978a). Taurine

in the development of the central nervous system.   In
"Taurine and Neurological Disorders" (Eds A. Barbeau and
R.J. Huxtable).   pp. 48-71.   Raven Press, New York.

Thurston, J.H., Hauhart, R.E. and Dirgo, J.A. (1980).   Taurine:
a role in osmotic regulation in mammalian brain and possible clinical significance.   *Life Sciences*, **26**, 1561—
1568.

Voaden, M.J., Oraedu, A.C.I., Marshall, J. and Lake, N. (1981).
Taurine in the retina.   In "The Action of Taurine on
Excitable Tissues".   (Eds S.I. Baskin, J.J. Kocsis and
S.W. Schaffer).   pp. 145—160.   Spectrum Publications,
New York.

Voaden, M.J., Chan, I.P.R. and Hussain, A.A. (1982).   Taurine
uptake by platelets from patients with retinitis pigmentosa.
(this volume).

TAURINE UPTAKE BY PLATELETS FROM PATIENTS WITH RETINITIS PIGMENTOSA

M.J. VOADEN, I.P.R. CHAN and A.A. HUSSAIN

*Department of Visual Science, Institute of Ophthalmology
University of London, London, UK.*

INTRODUCTION

In order to investigate whether a generalized defect in the mechanism(s) accumulating taurine into tissues exists in patients with Retinitis Pigmentosa (RP) we have undertaken a study of taurine uptake by blood platelets. Measurements have been made in autologous plasma, or in Ca^{2+}-free Krebs' bicarbonate medium containing 1.0 or 60.0μM ^{3}H-taurine. With the former the rate of entry will reflect activity of the "high affinity" carrier (Ahtee *et al.*, 1974). Whereas the latter may more closely simulate the levels found in plasma, as it is normally prepared (i.e., 30 to 150 μM: Berson *et al.*, 1976; Perry and Hansen, 1969).

MATERIALS AND METHODS

Patients who participated attended the Genetic and Electro-diagnostic Clinics of Moorfields Eye Hospital, London, where the category and extent of retinal dystrophy was defined genetically, clinically and, where possible, by psycho-physical and electro-physiological tests. The age range of patients was 15 to 67 years and that of randomly selected normal volunteers 22 to 64 years.

Blood (20ml) was obtained by venipuncture and was added to tubes containing potassium EDTA (final concentration 0.25%) to prevent coagulation. Approximately 1 h later it was centrifuged in 2 × 10 ml aliquots at 300g for 15 min at room temperature. The supernatants, composed of platelet rich plasma (PRP) were then drawn off and pooled. Aliquots were then either used immediately for assessment of taurine uptake, following the addition of trace amounts of ^{3}H-taurine

or were recentrifuged at 900g for 10 min. No haemolysis was
evident.

Resultant pellets of platelets were resuspended to a
volume equivalent to that of the original PRP, in $Ca^{2\pm}$ free
Krebs' bicarbonate medium containing 3.0mM EDTA (Ahtee *et al.*,
1974). One ml portions were then incubated for 20 min with
1.0 or 60.0µM ^{3}H-taurine (0.25µCi/ml, added in a volume of
20µl) at 37°C or 0°C, in an atmosphere of 95% O_2: 5% CO_2:
^{3}H-taurine (18Ci/m mol; 1mCi/ml) was obtained from The
Radiochemical Centre, Amersham. Packard "mini" counting
vials were used as incubation vessels. Ten minute incubations were also included in many of the tests, to establish
linearity of uptake of the radioactivity in all the groups
studied. The incubations were stopped by placing the tubes
in ice and the platelets then recovered by centrifuging
at 1,800g for 10 min at 4°C.

Ten µl of medium were removed at the beginning and end
of the incubation, the radioactivity counted, and a mean of
the two used to assess tissue/medium (T/M) ratios. The
remaining medium was poured from the tube, which was then
drained on filter paper and the sides of the tubes were
swabbed with small portions of filter paper to remove ad-
hering droplets of medium. In some estimations the platelets
were then washed once with fresh taurine-free medium. Although this lowered the background level of ^{3}H-taurine, it
made no difference to the final results. Triton X-100
(0.5 ml 10% V:V, aqueous solution) was then added to solu-
bilize the tissue, followed 30 min later by 4.5 ml scintillation fluid. Radioactivity was counted on a Packard 3375
liquid scintillation spectrophotometer.

Platelet counts were done on whole blood and also on
aliquots of PRP, and protein was estimated in known aliquots
of the platelet/Krebs' medium mixture. The protein standard
was bovine serum albumin.

Platelet wet weights were estimated from the protein
values by assuming a 10% protein content, and, for cal-
culation of T/M ratios, 1.0 mg wet weight then taken as
equivalent to 1.0µl incubation medium.

RESULTS AND DISCUSSION

A preliminary study, with platelets obtained from apparently
healthy volunteers, established that accumulation of the
^{3}H-taurine (exogenous concentration 1.0µM) was linear for
at least 60 min. The T/M ratios established after 20 min
by platelets from patients with photoreceptor dystrophy are
shown in Table 1. Uptake was normal in "autosomal dominant"

TABLE 1

^3H-Taurine uptake by platelets from patients with Retinitis Pigmentosa

Patient Classification	Taurine Uptake (T/M Ratio)			Whole blood platelet count × 10⁹/litre [1]	platelet size (μg protein/10⁶)
	1.0 μM	60.0 μm	Plasma		
Control	6.3 ± 0.4 (27)	3.0 ± 0.3 (15)	5.2 ± 0.3 (25) (range 2.7–7.6)	207 ± 12 (17)	2.9 ± 0.2 (30)
Autosomal Dominant	6.2 ± 0.3 (25)	3.3 ± 0.2 (17)	5.1 ± 0.2 (30) (range 3.0–8.6)	198 ± 10 (35)	3.4 ± 0.2 (27)
X-linked Hemizygote	7.7 ± 0.8 (12)	3.2 ± 0.3 (9)	4.2 ± 0.3 (10)* (range 2.5–6.2)	151 ± 13 (13)**	3.0 ± 0.3 (11)
Simplex [2]	6.9 ± 0.5 (16)	3.3 ± 0.2 (14)	4.8 ± 0.3 (15) (range 2.7–6.8)	185 ± 14 (17)	3.4 ± 0.4 (10)

*p < 0.5   **p < .01

Results are expressed as the mean ± SEM: the number of estimations is shown in brackets.

1) Refers only to platelets remaining in plasma after the initial centrifugation

2) No known relatives with the disease

and "simplex" patients but was slightly reduced when platelets
from "X-hemizygotes" were incubated in their own plasma. The
normal uptakes observed in the Krebs' bicarbonate medium
suggest that the plasma from these patients contains factor(s)
which are affecting uptake, or else the plasma contains more
taurine than normal. Normal plasma taurine levels were observed by Berson *et al*. (1976) in 3, "X-hemizygote" patients,
and a slightly lower than normal taurine concentration was
found by Arshinoff *et al*. (1981) in whole blood haemolysates
from this group (n = 8). More studies are needed to ascertain
if the latter result reflects a lowered endogenous level of
taurine within the blood cells, or is caused by a lowered
number of taurine-rich platelets in the blood. In the present
study we have observed a significantly lower number of platelets in the blood of "X-hemizygotes", 7 of the 13 patients
studied having counts of 140 or below. None were seen in our
normal group, although 8 presented amongst the "autosomal
dominants" and 4 amongst the "simplex" patients. Our observation of normal taurine uptake by platelets from "simplex"
patients contrasts with the results of Airaksinen *et al*. (1981).

ACKNOWLEDGEMENTS

Many people have provided essential background help in this
study ranging from the classification of patients to the
volunteering and taking of blood. We thank them all. In
particular, we are grateful for the encouragement and time
given by Miss G. Clover, Mr M. Quinlan, Dr L. Lyness, Prof.
G. Arden and Prof. A. Bird. We thank Prof. A. Garner,
Department of Pathology, Institute of Ophthalmology for
allowing us to use the facilities of his department, and
his staff for their help, in the initial phase of this study,
with platelet counting and general blood surveys.
    The study is being supported by grants from the National
Retinitis Pigmentosa Foundation and the M.R.C.

REFERENCES

Ahtee, L., Boullin, D.J. and Paasonen, M.K. (1974). Trans-
    port of taurine by normal human blood platelets. *Brit.
    J. Pharmacol.* **52**, 245-51.
Airaksinen, E.M., Airaksinen, M.M., Sihvola, P. and Marnela,
    K,-M. (1981). Decrease in the uptake and concentration
    of taurine in blood platelets of Retinitis Pigmentosa
    patients. *Med. and Ped. Ophthalmol.* **5**, 45-48.
Arshinoff, S.A., McCulloch, J.C., Macrae, W., Stein, A.N.

and Marliss, E.B. (1981). Amino acids in Retinitis Pigmentosa. *Brit. J. Ophthalmol*. **65**, 626–630.

Berson, E.L., Schmidt, S.Y. and Rabin, A.R. (1976). Plasma
amino acids in hereditary retinal disease: ornithine
lysine and taurine. *Brit. J. Ophthalmol*. **60**, 142–147.

Perry, T.L. and Hansen, S. (1969). Technical pitfalls leading
to errors in the quantitation of plasma amino acids.
Clin. Chim. Acta. **25**, 53–58.

CATARACT IN ASSOCIATION WITH RETINITIS PIGMENTOSA: ANALYSIS OF THE CRYSTALLIN SUBUNIT COMPOSITION

J. CUTHBERT and R.M. CLAYTON

Institute of Animal Genetics, University of Edinburgh, West Mains Road, Edinburgh EH9 3JN, UK

INTRODUCTION

Retinitis Pigmentosa (RP) includes a heterogeneous group of diseases differing in their genetic transmission (Sorsby, 1951; Duke-Elder, 1969) and in the secondary characteristics associated with each of them. Posterior subcapsular cataract (PSC) has been regularly observed in association with retinitis pigmentosa but the literature is contradictory as to whether the association is with the dominant or recessive form of the disease. Both Sorsby (1951) and Duke-Elder (1969) considered that PSC occurred more commonly in association with dominant RP, and to occur later and more occasionally in recessive forms of RP. However, an editorial article in the British Medical Journal (1981) suggested that cataracts occur especially in the x-linked form of the disease and Fishman (1980) suggests that earlier onset and more rapid development of PSC occurs with the autosomal recessive form and perhaps the x-linked form of the disease; lens changes in the dominant RP patient occurring late and with a less well defined association. In another study (Berson and Siminoff, 1979), of 18 patients with dominant RP only one had cataract, but 2 were aphakic due to surgical extraction. A recessive condition in the rat resembling RP was also associated with PSC (Bourne *et al.*, 1938*a*, *b*).

Dilley, *et al.*, (1976) and Eshagian *et al.* (1980) have shown that the ultrastructural changes observed in the posterior subcapsular cataracts associated with RP are very similar to those seen in "senile" PSC's and Dilley *et al.* (1976) suggest that the same mechanism of cataractogenesis may be invoked by different stimuli.

In this study, investigations have been carried out to determine the protein profile of a number of individual

cataractous lenses from patients with Retinitis Pigmentosa
so that comparisons could be made (a) between lenses of
similar cataract morphology from individuals with and without
the disease and (b) between individual lenses from RP patients
which differ in their cataract morphology. Table 1 lists the
information regarding the genetics of the disease and the
cataract morphology for each lens where this information is
available. Of the 14 lenses there are 3 pairs of bilateral
cataracts, numbers 3 and 10, numbers 7 and 9 and numbers 13
and 14.   Thus we have 14 lenses from 11 patients.   There is
no genetic or cataract information for lenses numbers 6 and
12, but of the remaining 12 lenses, 5 are from patients with
dominant RP and 7 are from patients with recessive RP; it is
not known for any of the latter group whether the reces-
sivity is autosomal or x-linked.   This table is based on
the information given by the respective surgeons.

    The cataract morphology is known for eight of the fourteen
lenses.   Posterior subcapsular cataract (PSC) occur in seven
patients, with some anterior polar opacities in three cases.
Of these seven PSC's two were from patients with dominant
RP and were from patients with recessive RP.   The other
cataract of known morphopathology had a brown nuclear
opacity with additional cuneiform involvement and was from
a patient with dominant RP.

MATERIALS AND METHODS

Most of the lenses were examined *in vitro* before extraction,
frozen on removal and transported in solid CO_2. On arrival,
they were transferred into storage in liquid N_2 until analysed.
Preparation of the water soluble (WS) and urea soluble (US)
fractions from the lens homogenates was carried out as
described previously (Cuthbert *et al.*, 1978). Isoelectric
focussing (IEF) and scanning of the IEF gels was also carried
out as described previously (Cuthbert *et al.*, 1978).

RESULTS

The densitometric traces of the IEF gels of the WS and US
fractions of the individual RP lenses did not form a homogeneous group but, instead, formed one major class of 12
lenses which gave similar traces, the remaining 2 giving
traces which were rather different both from one another and
from the group of 12 lenses. It is noteworthy, too, that
the 3 pairs of bilateral cataracts fall into the group of 12
lenses and similarity between the lenses of each pair is

TABLE 1

Lens No.	Type of RP	Type of Cataract
1	Dominant	Posterior Subcapsular
2	Recessive	Posterior Subcapsular
*3	Recessive	Posterior Subcapsular and Slight Anterior Capacities
4	Recessive	Posterior Subcapsular
5	Recessive	Posterior Subcapsular and Some Anterior Opacities
6	—	—
+7	Recessive	—
8	Dominant	Brown Nuclear and Cuneiform
+9	Recessive	—
*10	Recessive	Posterior Subcapsular and Slight Anterior Opacities
11	Dominant	Posterior Subcapsular
12	—	—
+*13	Dominant	—
+*14	Dominant	—

Information of the genetics of the RP disease and the morphology of the cataract for 14 individual cataractous lenses from RP patients. Three pairs of bilateral cataract are indicated
by the marks *, + and +*.

closer than between lenses from different individuals.

The group of 12 lenses includes 7 lenses (numbers, 2, 3, 4, 5, 7, 9 and 10) 5 of which are known to have PSC, from patients with recessive RP, and 4 lenses, 2 of which are known to have PSC (numbers 1, 11, 13, and 14) from patients with dominant RP. There is no information for the 12th lens. The lenses which give different traces are numbers 6 for which there is no information, and 8 which is from a patient with dominant RP who did not have PSC.

Comparisons of Cataractous Lenses from RP and Non-RP Patients

Using the integration values for the area under each peak, expressed as percentage values of the area under the trace, means values and standard deviations can be obtained for individual peaks, and statistical tests carried out to determine whether any peak is significantly raised or lowered in value in the RP compared to the non-RP lenses.

Traces from 12 lenses with PSC from individuals known not to have RP were compared with groups of cataracts of various morphopathologies (Cuthbert *et al.*, 1978). The PSC group were found to show a degree of similarity to each other and the groups as a whole showed significant differences from all other groups of cataract.

Traces from the 12 lenses from individuals with RP known to include 7 with PSC were more homogeneous as a group and a comparison of PSC lenses from RP and from non-RP patients show significant differences between them (Fig. 1, Table 2.)

These RP cataracts also differed significantly from those from patients with inflammatory changes in the retina and iris, such as a group of leprosy patients (Clayton *et al.*, 1980), and patients with uveitis (unpub. obsv.).

DISCUSSION

From the information and results given in this paper, little can be concluded about the association of any particular cataract morphology with any particular genetic form of RP, although PSC does seem to be particularly associated with the disease. Fifty percent of the lenses studied here are known to have PSC and 5 others show similar protein distribution and possibly have the same morphopathology.

In the population of approximately 500 non-RP cataract lenses, about 20% had PSC, but only 12 of these lenses had PSC with no other involvement. These are the 12 pure PSC's compared with the PSC's in this RP population.

The results arrived at in this study show that lenses

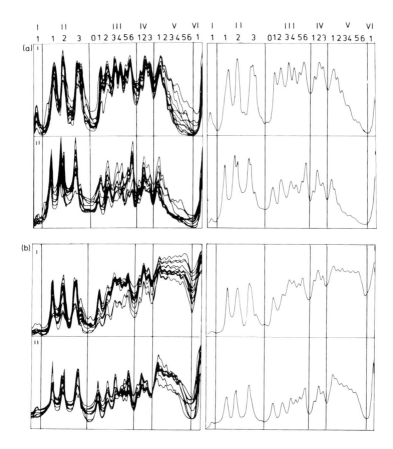

Fig. 1 *Superimposed densitometric traces of IEF gels for (a) the WS and (b) the VS functions of (i) PSC's from RP patients and (ii) PSC's from non-RP patients. On the right are the average traces obtained from them.*

from RP patients do form a distinct population of cataracts compared with those from non-RP patients, even though there is some degree of heterogeneity in the protein profiles obtained from the former. The RP lenses show some specific biochemical changes, in that a discrete group of lens proteins are either raised or lowered in amounts in the WS and US fractions. This particular change in profile has not been observed for any other group of lenses (Cuthbert *et al.*, 1978; Clayton *et al.*, 1980). However, it is not possible to determine from these data whether the RP specific lens changes are due to the expression of the genetic lesion in both retina and lens (which would require that the majority

TABLE 2

List of protein subunits which are significantly raised or lowered in value in PSC's from RP patients compared to PSC's from non-RP patients.

	Raised		Lowered	
Statistical significance	Water Soluble	Urea Soluble	Water Soluble	Urea Soluble
P 0.05	III_3 V_4	III_4	–	III_5 V_2
P 0.01	III_5	–	–	V_3 VI
P 0.005	–	III_3 V_6	II_2 VI	–
P 0.0005	III_0	III_0 III_6	–	–

of the RP patients in this small survey had a similar form of the disease), or to the response of the lens to biochemical changes in the RP retina.

ACKNOWLEDGEMENTS

We would like to thank the following surgeons for their kind cooperation in providing the RP lenses for analysis: P.L. Blaxter (Manchester Royal Eye Hospital), S.J. Crews (Birmingham and Midland Eye Hospital), D.V. Ingram (Sussex Eye Hospital), C.I. Phillips (Princess Alexandra Eye Pavilion, Edinburgh), N.S.C. Rice (Moorfields Eye Hospital), M.D. Saunders (St. Thomas's Hospital, London), S.K. Sharma (Pinderfields Hospital, Wakefield), N.L. Stokoe (Victoria Hospital, Kirkcaldy), J.P. Travers Noble's Isle of Man Hospital) and T. Wilson (Falkirk and District Royal Infirmary). We are also grateful to the British Retinitis Pigmentosa Society for liaising between some of these surgeons and ourselves.

We are most grateful to L.G. Hendrey for excellent technical assistance and to L. Dobbie for typing the manuscript.

J. Cuthbert is in receipt of a grant from the Iris Fund for the Prevention of Blindness.

REFERENCES

Berson, E.L. and Siminoff, E.A. (1979). Dominant retinitis pigmentosa with reduced penetrance. Further Studies of the Electroretinogram. *Arch. Ophthal.* **97**, 1286—1291.

Bourne, M.C., Campbell, D.A. and Pyke, M. (1938). Cataract associated with an hereditary retinal lesion in rats. *Br. J. Ophthal.* **22**, 608-612.

Bourne, M.C., Campbell, D.A. and Tansley, K. (1938). Hereditary degeneration of the rat retina. *Br. J. Ophthal.* **22**, 613-623.

Clayton, R.M., Cuthbert, J., Phillips, C.I., Bartholomew, R.S., Stokoe, N.L., Ffytche, T., Reid, J.McK., Duffy, J., Seth, J. and Alexander, M. (1980). Analysis of Individual Cataract Patients and their Lenses: a Progress Report. *Exp. Eye Res.* **31**, 553-566.

Cuthbert, J. (1981). Differential Diagnosis of Cataracts by Crystallin Subunit Quantitation Correlated with Clinical and Morphological Observations. Ph.D. Thesis, University of Edinburgh.

Cuthbert, J., Clayton, R. M., Truman, D.E.S., Phillips, C.I. and Bartholomew, R.S. (1978). Analysis of the Crystallin composition of individual human lenses: Characteristic modifications associated with different cataracts. *Interdiscipl. Topics. Gertont.* **13**, 183-192.

Dilley, K.J., Bron, A.J. and Habgood, J.O. (1976). Anterior polar and posterior subcapsular cataract in a patient with retinitis pigmentosa: a light-microscopic and ultra-structural study. *Exp. Eye Res.* **22**, 155-167.

Duke-Elder, S. (1969). System of ophthalmology. Vol. XI, p. 225. Kimpton, London.

Eshagian, J., Rafferty, N.S. and Goossens, W. (1980). Ultra-structure of human cataract in retinitis pigmentosa. *Arch. Ophthal.* **98**, 2227-2230.

Fishman, G. (1980). Hereditary retinal and choroidal disease: Electroretinogram and electrooculogram findings. In "Principles and Practice of Ophthalmology" Vol. II. (Ed. G.A. Peyman, D.R. Saunders, M.E. Goldberg) pp. 857-904. W.B. Saunders Company, Philadelphia, London, Toronto.

Sorsby, A. (1951). Genetics in Ophthalmology. pp. 136-138. Butterworths, London.

CONVERSE asked if, in the autosomal dominant type with incomplete penetrance, there were more males than females
affected. BIRD said that he was not aware of males being
more affected than females in dominant pedigrees. The main
alternative was x-linkage, but if there was male-to-male
inheritance this could be excluded. The interpretation of
pedigrees was very subject to ascertainment bias which could
give rise to a spurious excess of one or other sex. PHILLIPS
said that the simplex or sporadic cases had a high probabi-
lity of being autosomal recessive, since, in these days of
relatively small families, the chance of having only one
affected sib was quite high. BIRD replied that they correct-
ed for sibship size and the disparity between what was
expected and what was found remained. Sixty or 70% are
probably autosomal recessive, but the remainder are uncertain.
BERMAN asked about the degree of consanguinity in parents.
BIRD said that it was low in his series and could not be
used to calculate the frequency of autosomal recessives.
LOLLEY asked what Bird told his patients about what could be
done to help them. BIRD replied that he put them in touch
with the British R.P. Society and suggested that they do not
actively seek therapy at this stage. He advised dark glasses
since they all have poor function in bright illumination and
difficulty in dark adaptation. WRIGHT asked whether the
variable expression in female carriers in the x-linked
disorder could be explained by X-chromosome inactivation or
by different types of disease. BIRD said that severely
affected heterozygotes could be found in every big family
and several authors had suggested that there were x-linked
intermediate and x-linked recessive types. There was much
variability within families however, with mildly and
severely affected females. X-inactivation was clearly a
possible explanation, but there was no evidence either way.
Equally, there was no evidence that it was due to environmental factors such as climate. AGUIRRE asked if there
could be different diseases within the recessive group.
BIRD thought that it was probably a large number of diseases.

Four subdivisions of Leber's amaurosis had been recognized,
even though this was a minor subgroup, so it was likely there
were several disorders within the recessive group as a whole.
AGUIRRE asked if a subclassification within the recessive
groups was possible on the basis of clinical or other
features. BIRD said that in dominant disease this might be
possible, but in the recessive type there are too few affected members in any sibship to form the basis for subclassification. MCDEVITT asked if histocompatibility antigens (HLA)
had been ascertained in Retintis Pigmentosa (RP) patients.
BERMAN said that there were two HLA studies in RP, both
negative.

LOLLEY asked if there was any correlation in the rate of
change in the affected retina with sexual maturity or
pregnancy. BIRD replied that it was not specifically
documented but an adverse effect of pregnancy was observed
by many people. LOLLEY asked about the effect of oral
contraceptives. BIRD commented that their use was too
widespread, which made analysis difficult. LAVAIL commented
that Stein had published data showing the effect of sex
hormones on constant-light damage to the retina.

READING commented on Clayton's suggestion that different
types of disease could be distinguished by making probes to
look for abnormal gene products in an accessible tissue.
Would these probes have to be prepared from an altered
messenger RNA in a diseased patient's retina? CLAYTON said
that it could be done the other way round, by looking for a
normally-translated product that was missing in the patient,
although it would still be a minority product. Several
laboratories had isolated mRNA for a minority product such
as an enzyme by immune sequestration of polysomes, bearing
nascent chains. The process was laborious but feasible.
The search for a product not normally translated might require
small samples of patient material. READING asked whether,
assuming that the lesion was either in the neural retina or
in the pigmented epithelium, it would not be necessary to
obtain the material from a RP eye before deterioration,
otherwise the messenger RNA and DNA was likely to be damaged
or lost because of cell death. CLAYTON agreed, but added
that one could look for expression of the gene at low levels
in other tissues, or raise a probe in an animal model,
hoping that it would cross-hydridize with the human.
Hybridization to DNA did not require retina. WRIGHT said
that, as an alternative strategy, it was possible instead
to make DNA probes specific for randomly spaced regions
along a particular chromosome, starting from normal human
chromosome fractions. These could be used to detect

polymorphisms in restriction sites which are specifically
disposed throughout the genome, and act as markers to detect
linkage between a probe and the RP gene. One that was close
enough to the RP gene would be useful in counselling or
prenatal diagnosis without having any knowledge of abnormal
proteins or gene products at all. **CLAYTON** said that the
drawback was the enormous task of analysing all the chromosomes, so you would have to fix on a particular one. **WRIGHT**
agreed, but said that it was already possible to have probes
for the X chromosome. Several labs were separating chromosomes into different sized groups and isolating clones from
particular ones to act as probes. It might be 5 years before
there were probes for all the chromosomes. **CLAYTON** felt that
it would certainly take as long as that because if a library
was made from chromosomes of a particular size class, there
would still be a lot of screening for suitable probes. She
thought that these techniques, whether via DNA or gene
products, were not immediately round the corner but were not
impossible.

   READING asked Voaden if there might be value in doing
taurine release studies, after preloading the platelet with
the radio-labelled compound. It was possible that the uptake
mechanism was normal but retention was abnormal. **VOADEN**
replied that there was insufficient patient material at present. **BERMAN** said that, as a general rule the melanin content decreased with age and lipofuscin was evident by 69
years, yet in Lee's 69 year old patient the reverse was seen.
She asked if there were few lipofuscin granules and whether
some of the particles were melanin. She suggested that some
of the cells had been extruded to Bruch's membrane. **LEE**
replied that his control retina was as expected. He had no
explanation for the absence of lipofuscin and of breakdown
in the malformation which was presumably congenital. The
cell type was uncertain, but they resembled PE cells rather
than exogenous macrophages. **HOLLEYFIELD** commented that in
this eye the condition of the retina over an abnormal PE was
very similar to what LaVail had found in some of his
chimaeras in the RCS rat. **LOLLEY** said that the stacked-up
layers of PE looked like repeating layers of Bruch's membrane. **LEE** replied that it was clumps of extra-cellular
material and the basement membrane was not folded.
HOLLEYFIELD remarked that there was extracellular, collagenous-
like material and **LEE** agreed.

FINAL DISCUSSION

HOLLEYFIELD posed the highly important question of what investigations would anyone receiving an eye carry out in the light of our knowledge to date.

LAVAIL suggested that the eye should be subdivided but that the morphological identity was of extreme importance, since abrupt changes in appearance were not uncommon in the degenerating retina. One of the problems was that biochemists generally require more tissue than other researchers. What was most important was the need to correlate the morphology with the biochemistry and to examine as wide a range of characteristics of the degenerating retina as possible in any study of human material. For morphologists this should include looking at the interphotoreceptor matrix, rod and cone photoreceptors, melanosomes and in fact every organelle and cell type. He felt that there was still scope for this in the existing animal models. He and his colleagues were ready to go back and look for changes in the interphotoreceptor matrix in previously embedded human eyes. **CLAYTON** also stressed the need to correlate morphology with whatever other study was being undertaken. Since static and dynamic information are both important she suggested taking a series of punch cores rather than segments of the retina. Adjacent cores could be used for morphology and biochemistry. She questioned whether electron microscope morphology or immunohistology required a lot of tissue and thought that most sorts of biochemistry could be miniaturized.

CLAYTON made two further practical suggestions for any eye which became available. First, to freeze portions of the eye in liquid nitrogen to use when monoclonal antibody probes became available. Second, to do cell culture studies which are possible using very small numbers of cells. She stressed the importance of recognizing that continued culture of retinal cells can lead to divergence of the primary characteristics and the expression of properties that have nothing to do with Retinitis Pigmentosa (RP). She raised the question of enlisting the support of people who have

developed specialized techniques but have not been involved
in RP research. **HOLLEYFIELD** replied directly that "button"
type procedures with a 3mm trephine had been used in his lab
quite extensively. He mentioned the difficulties of separating the retina and pigment epithelium and again emphasized
the need to share human retinal material as it becomes
available. **BERMAN** questioned the usefulness of retina in an
advanced state of degeneration as a source of research material and this view was supported by **FARBER,** who said that
information from autolysed tissue was often minimal. She
stressed the importance not only of animal models but of
building up a baseline of information on normal human retinas
and suggested splitting up the material between different
labs proficient in different techniques. **AGUIRRE** pointed out
that to divide an eye into a large number of small portions
could be a disadvantage, in that correlation of morphology
and biochemistry becomes more difficult the smaller the
portions. He stressed the need to obtain good clinical,
genetic and electrophysiological documentation for any eye
samples, since if this was lacking, some of the analyses
could be meaningless. **ARDEN** asked about the possibility of
looking at protein uptake and synthesis. He pointed out that
eyes from patients in the end-stage of the condition were
most likely to become available and asked if this technique
could be used to see if there is potential for making rod
outer limb material. **LOLLEY** argued the case for there being
some sort of central control through which RP eye material
would be distributed. He felt it was essential that anyone
wanting to work on this priceless material should first have
shown beyond doubt that they were able to do the necessary
assays and that they had normal data for comparison. **CLAYTON**
said that the improper use of such material would be tragic,
but **LOLLEY** re-emphasized that who got the eye was often
largely a matter of chance. **CLAYTON** suggested there was also
a need to obtain biopsy samples from other RP tissues.
BERMAN described her work on retinol-esterifying enzyme in
skin fibroblasts of RP patients, which produced equivocal
results and said that they were moving to granulocytes and
lymphocytes to look for biochemical changes in extraocular
tissues. Both **FARBER** and **AGUIRRE** said that they had looked
in many extraocular tissues in both mouse and dog and yet
had found no anomalous biochemical process like that occurring
in the retina. **WRIGHT** pointed out that even in RP tissue at
a late stage of degeneration it should still be possible to
look for a change reflecting a difference in the primary
structure of an enzyme, such as the heat stability.
HOLLEYFIELD said that the main problem was that, after a

period , degenerate cells disappear completely. **LOLLEY** sounded a practical note of caution when he stressed that eye material is most likely to end up in fixative prior to pathological examination and that much educative ground work remained to be done to obtain such eye material. **CLAYTON** asked about possible protocol arrangements in the United States for obtaining human eye material. **FARBER** explained that the Central American RP Foundation had collected protocols from all the researchers and laboratories interested in receiving material and that the country was divided geographically with respect to patient/laboratory allocation. In the general discussion that followed, it appeared that in the United States there were reasonable facilities for interested scientists to obtain freshly enucleated normal eyes but that RP eyes were just as scarce as in the U.K. It was also the general opinion that even if many RP eyes become available, most would be of limited use for research owing to their advanced state of degeneration. As **LOLLEY** succinctly pointed out, "You're gonna have to do a lot of bad ones before you get a good one."